Hunsaker

EMERGENCY MEDICINE

AF815009

PEARLS OF WISDOM

WRITTEN BOARD REVIEW

Fifth Edition

Dwight Collman, M.D.

Scott H. Plantz, M.D.

Jonathan Adler, M.D.

NOTE

The intent of Emergency Medicine *Pearls of Wisdom*, Fifth Edition is to serve as a study aid to improve performance on a standardized exam. It is not intended to be a source text of the knowledge base of emergency medicine, nor to serve as a reference in any way for the practice of clinical emergency medicine. The authors do not warrant that the information in this text is complete or accurate. The reader is encouraged to verify each answer in several references. All drug use indications and dosages must be verified by the reader before administration of any compound.

Copyright © 2000 by Boston Medical Publishing Corporation, Boston, MA.

Printed in USA

All rights reserved, including the right of reproduction, in whole or in part, in any form.

The editors would like to extend thanks to Terri Lair for her excellent managing and editorial support.

This book was produced using Times and Symbols fonts and computer based graphics with Macintosh® computers

ISBN: 1-58409-022-7

DEDICATION

To Kris, Katie, and Ryan, there are no words for the joy you bring me.
To C.J. and Tara our loyal friends, we love you. To Barbara Herman and Barbara Schwartz,
thank you for pressing on through a constant flood of work. You are truly loyal.

I would also like to thank the followings physicians for contributing their radiographs, photographs and ECG's:
Thomas P. Habif, M.D., Nora Klinker, M.D., Lawrence Heiskell, M.D.,
Thomas Guillot, M.D., Jose Pollack, M.D., F.A.A.P., and A. Molson, M.D.

Thank you Natalia for the love and nurturing you continue to give my children.

Dwight

For my father, Alan Huntly Plantz, whose love, support and brilliance has always been my guiding light.

Scott

For my brothers, David and Peter, for your fellowship, love, and your wonderful extended families!

Jonathan

AUTHORS AND EDITORS

Dwight Collman, M.D.
President, The Collman Institute
Boca Raton, FL

Scott H. Plantz, M.D., FAAEM
Asst. Prof. of Emergency Medicine
Chicago Medical School
Mt. Sinai Medical Center
Chicago, IL

Jonathan Adler, M.D., FAAEM
Assistant in Emergency Medicine, Massachusetts General Hospital
Instructor in Medicine,
Harvard Medical School
Boston, MA

CONTRIBUTING AUTHORS AND EDITORS

Bobby Abrams, M.D., FAAEM
Attending Physician
Macomb Hospital

Felix Ankel, M.D.
Assistant Professor, Emergency Medicine
University of Wisconsin Medical Center
Madison, WI

Steven M. Anneken, M.D., FACEP
Staff Physician, Department of Emergency Medicine
EHS Christ Hospital and Medical Center
Oak Lawn, IL

David F.M. Brown, M.D.
Assistant Chief
Department of Emergency Medicine,
Massachusetts General Hospital
Instructor in Medicine,
Harvard Medical School
Boston, MA

Edward Castro, M.D.
Assistant in Emergency Medicine, Massachusetts General Hospital
Instructor in Medicine,
Harvard Medical School
Boston, MA

C. James Corrall, M.D., MPH
Clinical Associate Professor of Pediatrics
Clinical Associate Professor of Emergency Medicine
Indiana University School of Medicine
Indianapolis, IN

Leslie S. Carroll, M.D.
Asst. Prof. of Emergency Medicine
Chicago Medical School
Mt. Sinai Medical Center
Chicago, IL

Clive Stuart, M.D.
Practicing Physician
Immanuel St-Joseph-Mayo Health System
Mankato, MN

Jesse A. Cole, M.D.
Charlotte, NC

Alasdair K. Conn, M.D.
Chief of Emergency Services, Massachusetts General Hospital
Assistant Professor of Surgery,
Harvard Medical School
Boston, MA

Michael Cruz, M.D.
Clinical Instructor of Emergency Medicine
University of Illinois College of Medicine
St. Francis Medical Center
Peoria, IL

Stephen Emond, M.D.
Research Director,
Department of Emergency Medicine
New York Hospital
N.Y., NY

Craig Feied, M.D.
Clinical Associate Professor
George Washington University
Washington Hospital Center
Washington, D.C.

Bill Gossman, M.D., FAAEM
Assistant Professor of Emergency Medicine
Chicago Medical School
Mt. Sinai Medical Center
Chicago, IL

David Hendricksen, M.D., Ph.D.
Staff Physician, University of Illinois College of Medicine
St. Francis Medical Center
Peoria, IL

George Z. Hevesy, M.D.
Project Medical Director,
Peoria Area EMS;
Clinical Associate Professor of Emergency Medicine
University of Illinois
College of Medicine;
Vice Chairman,
Department of Emergency Medicine
St. Francis Medical Center
Peoria, IL

James Holmes, M.D.
Division of Emergency Medicine
U of C, Davis School of Medicine
Sacramento, California

Eddie Hooker, M.D., FAAEM
Assistant Professor,
Department of Emergency Medicine
University of Louisville
Louisville, KY

Lance W. Kreplick, M.D., FAAEM
Associate Chair, University of Illinois
Research Director, Department
of Emergency Medicine
EHS Christ Hospital and Medical Center
Oak Lawn, IL

Michael J. Lambert, M.D.
Staff Physician, Department of Emergency Medicine
EHS Christ Hospital and Medical Center
Oak Lawn, IL

Gordon Larsen, M.D.
University of Illinois
St. Francis Medical Center
Peoria, IL

Bernard Lopez, M.D., FAAEM

Nicholas Y. Lorenzo, M.D.
Department of Neurology
Cellular Neurobiology Laboratory
Mayo Clinic
Rochester, MN

Grant Mansell, M.D.
University of Illinois
St. Francis Medical Center
Peoria, IL

Mary Nan Mallory, M.D., FAAEM

Chuck McCart, M.D.
University of Illinois
St. Francis Medical Center
Peoria, IL

Rick Miller, M.D.
Director of Emergency Medical Services
St. Francis Medical Center;
Clinical Associate Professor of Emergency Medicine
University of Illinois College of Medicine
Peoria, IL

David Morgan, M.D., FAAEM
Assistant in Emergency Medicine
Southwest Medical Center

Edward Panacek, M.D., FAAEM
Associate Prof. of Medicine
Division of Emergency Medicine
U of California, Davis School of Medicine
Sacramento, California

Stewart Reingold, M.D.
Staff Physician, Department of Emergency Medicine
EHS Christ Hospital and Medical Center
Oak Lawn, IL

Karen Rhodes, M.D.
Dept. of Emergency Medicine
University of Chicago Medical Center
Chicago, IL

Carlo Rosen, M.D.
Beth Israel Medical Center
Instructor in Medicine,
Harvard Medical School
Boston, MA

Tony Russo, M.D.
University of Illinois
St. Francis Medical Center
Peoria, IL

Timothy J. Schaefer, M.D.
Clinical Assistant Professor
University of Illinois College of Medicine
Assistant Program Director,
Emergency Medicine Residency
St. Francis Medical Center
Peoria, IL

Marc D. Squillante, D.O.
Program Director,
Emergency Medicine Residency
University of Illinois College of Medicine
St. Francis Medical Center
Peoria, IL

Dana Stearns, M.D.
Assistant in Emergency Medicine, Massachusetts
General Hospital
Instructor in Medicine,
Harvard Medical School
Boston, MA

Jack "Lester" Stump, M.D., FAAEM
Attending Physician
Rogue Valley Medical Center
Medford, OR

Joan Surdukowski, M.D.
Assistant Professor of Emergency Medicine
Chicago Medical School
Mt. Sinai Medical Center
Chicago, IL

Loice Swischer, M.D., FAAEM
Toxicology Staff Physician
Medical College of Pennsylvania/
Misericordia Hospital
Pennsylvania, PA

Greg Tudor, M.D.
University of Illinois
St. Francis Medical Center
Peoria, IL

José M. Vega, M.D.
Assistant in Emergency Medicine, Massachusetts
General Hospital
Instructor in Medicine,
Harvard Medical School
Boston, MA

Therese M. Whitt, M.D.
Asst. Prof. of Emergency Medicine
University of Illinois College of Medicine
St. Francis Medical Center
Peoria, IL

Joseph P. Wood, M.D., J.D.
Associate Professor of Emergency Medicine
University of Illinois
Chairman, Department of Emergency Medicine
EHS Christ Hospital and Medical Center
Oak Lawn, IL

WE APPRECIATE YOUR COMMENTS!

We appreciate your opinion and encourage you to send us any suggestions or recommendations. Please let us know if you discover any errors, or if there is any way we can make our *Pearls of Wisdom* Text more helpful to you. We are also interested in recruiting new authors and editors. Please call, write, fax, or e-mail. We look forward to hearing from you.

D.C., S.H.P. & J.N.A.

Return to:

Boston Medical Publishing Corporation
237 S. 70th Street, Suite 206, Lincoln, NE 68510

888-MBOARDS
402-484-6118
FAX: 402-484-6552
E-MAIL: bmp@emedicine.com

Visit our on-line Bookstore at
www.emedicine.com

INTRODUCTION

Congratulations! Emergency Medicine *Pearls of Wisdom*, Fifth Edition, Revised will help you learn some emergency medicine. Originally designed as a study aid to improve performance on the EM Written Boards/Recertification or EM Inservice exam, "Pearls" is full of useful information. First intended for EM specialists, we have learned that "Pearls" unique format has also been found to be useful by house officers and medical students rotating in the ED.

The primary intent of "Pearls" is to serve as a study aid to improve performance on the EM Written Boards/Recertification or EM Inservice Exam. To achieve this goal the text is written in rapid-fire question/answer format. Misleading or confusing "foils" are not provided. This eliminates the risk of erroneously assimilating an incorrect piece of information that made a big impression. Questions themselves often contain a pearl intended to be reinforced in association with the question/answer. Additional hooks are often attached to the answer in various forms including mnemonics, evoked visual imagery, repetition and humor. Additional information not requested in the question may be included in the answer. The same information is often sought in several different questions. Emphasis has been placed on distilling true trivia and key facts that are easily overlooked, are quickly forgotten and that somehow seem to be needed on Board exams.

Many questions have answers without explanations. This is done to enhance ease of reading and rate of learning. Explanations often occur in a later question/answer. It may happen that upon reading an answer the reader may think - "Hmm, why is that?!" or, "Are you sure...?!" If this happens to you, GO CHECK! Truly assimilating these disparate facts into a framework of knowledge absolutely requires further reading of the surrounding concepts. Information learned in response to seeking an answer to a particular question is retained much better than that passively observed. Take advantage of this! Use "Pearls" with your preferred source texts handy and open!

The short question/answer format of the First Edition has been retained. The structure and content of "Pearls" has been enhanced significantly in the Second, Third, Fourth and Fifth Editions. The first half of the text is presented in descending order of relative importance on the EM board exam. Information presented in the Pearls Topics sections is mostly limited to straightforward and more basic facts. The second section of the book consists of random pearls - questions grouped into small clusters by topic presented in no particular order. The random pearls section repeats much of the factual information contained in the Pearls Topics and builds on this foundation with greater emphasis on linking information and filling in gaps from the Pearls Topics.

"Pearls" has limitations (directly proportional to those of the senior editor/authors!). We have found *many* conflicts between sources of information. Variation between the definition of "apneustic" breathing provided in Tintinalli vs. Stedman's causes little consternation. Variations between half-life of paralyzing agents and of naloxone, or between rankings of stability of cervical spine fractures, provided in Tintinalli vs. Rosen are more concerning. We have tried to verify in other references the most accurate information. Some texts have internal discrepancies further confounding clarification of information.

"Pearls" risks accuracy by aggressively pruning complex concepts down to the simplest kernel - the dynamic knowledge base and clinical practice of emergency medicine is not like that! For the most part, the information taken as "correct" is that indicated in the texts, Emergency Medicine A Comprehensive Study Guide, edited by Tintinalli, Krome and Ruiz and The Clinical Practice of Emergency Medicine, edited by Harwood-Nuss, Linden, Luten, Shepherd, and Wolfson.

Further, new research and practice occasionally deviates from that which likely represents the "right" answer for test purposes. In such cases we have selected the information that we believe is most likely "correct" for test purposes. This text is designed to maximize your score on a test. Refer to your most current sources of information and mentors for direction for practice. "Pearls" is designed to be used, not just read. It is an *interactive* text. Use a 3x5 card and cover the answers; attempt all questions.

A study method we strongly recommend is oral, group study, preferably over an extended meal or pitchers. The mechanics of this method are simple and no one ever appears stupid.

One person holds "Pearls", with answers covered, and reads the question. Each person, including the reader, says "Check!" when he or she has an answer in mind. After everyone has "checked" in, someone states their answer. If this answer is correct, on to the next one, if not, another person says their answer or the answer can be read. Usually the person who "checks" in first gets the first shot at stating the answer. If this person is being a smarty-pants answer-hog, then others can take turns. Try it, it is almost fun!

"Pearls" is also designed to be re-used several times to allow, dare we use the word, memorization. One co-author (Plantz), a pessimist, suggests putting a check mark in each box provided every time a question is missed. Thus, two boxes have been arbitrarily provided. If you fill all the boxes on two re-uses of "Pearls", forget this question! You will get it wrong on the exam!

Another suggestion is to place a check mark when the question is answered correctly once; skip all questions with check marks thereafter. Utilize whatever scheme of using the check boxes you prefer.

For additional instruction, we recommend the Collman Institute board review prep programs either for preparing for board certification examinations, or a review for your current medical practice. Please call 800-54-BOARD.

We welcome your comments, suggestions and criticism. Great effort has been made to verify these questions and answers. There will be answers we have provided that are at variance with the answer you would prefer. Most often this is attributable to the variance between original sources (previously discussed). Please make us aware of any errata you find. We hope to make continuous improvements in a next edition and would greatly appreciate any input with regard to format, organization, content, presentation, or about specific questions. Leave a message with Terri Lair at 1-888-MBOARDS (626-2737) or email: bmp@emedicine.com. We look forward to hearing from you.

Study hard and good luck!

D.C., S.H.P. & J.N.A.

TABLE OF CONTENTS

AIRWAY, RESUSCITATION AND VENTILATOR PEARLS

"The king shall drink to HamLet's better breath"
HamLet, Shakespeare

❐❐ Speaking of rapid sequence induction, discuss some agents that may be used to induce unconsciousness.

Thiopental, etomidate, fentanyl and midazolam. Thiopental and etomidate are preferred in most situations of rapid sequence induction.

❐❐ What is the benefit to rapid sequence induction in the emergency setting?

The use of a paralytic agent, as succinylcholine, enhances the ease of intubation and prevents aspiration by paralyzing the muscles. Paralytic agents should not be used without agents that induce unconsciousness.

❐❐ In a trauma patient with multiple fractures, internal injuries and an unstable airway, emergent endotracheal intubation in the emergency department is considered prior to definitive surgical therapy. What are the most likely hemodynamic consequences of intubation and initiation of mechanical ventilation in this subject?

Hypotension may occur during or following endotracheal intubation and the institution of positive pressure ventilation. This cardiovascular decompensation is due to a decrease in venous return associated with both the use of sympatholytic agents for induction and the positive pressure-induced increase in intrathoracic pressure.

❐❐ What is the average distance from the external nares to the carina in males and females?

32 cm and 27 cm, respectively.

❐❐ What is the only abductor muscle of the vocal cords?

The posterior cricoarytenoid muscle.

❐❐ At what thoracic vertebral level is the carina situated during full inspiration and full expiration?

At the sixth and fourth thoracic vertebral level, respectively.

❐❐ How long should a patient be preoxygenated to achieve a denitrogenation level such that apnea for 3 to 5 minutes maintains the oxygen saturation above 90%?

5 minutes in the normal individual.

❐❐ What is the mean average rise of carbon dioxide in apneic oxygenation?

3 mmHg/min.

❒❒ **What are the optimal angles of flexion of the neck and extension of the atlanto-occipital joint to achieve axial alignment before intubation ("sniffing" position)?**

30° and 15°, respectively.

❒❒ **How difficult is conventional endotracheal intubation in a patient with rheumatoid arthritis who presents with a stiff neck and limited mouth opening?**

Impossible.

❒❒ **What is the failure rate at first attempt and the final failure rate with blind nasal intubation?**

70% and 20%, respectively.

❒❒ **In which clinical situation is retrograde and lightwand intubation considered better choices than fiberoptic assisted intubation?**

Bleeding in the oral cavity.

❒❒ **What is the maximum safe dose of lidocaine for topical anesthesia of the airway?**

3 mg/kg.

❒❒ **T/F: Too much lidocaine may cause seizures.**

True.

❒❒ **Which are the only "fail safe" ways to verify correct placement of an endotracheal tube?**

Fiberoptic confirmation and adequate visualization with direct laryngoscopy. Calorimetric CO_2 monitoring is most commonly used.

❒❒ **What is the safest technique to intubate a child with epiglottitis?**

Intubation in the operating room after induction of anesthesia with an inhaled anesthetic (halothane or sevoflurane) in the semi-sitting position.

❒❒ **Are there any differences between endotracheal and Combitube intubation with regard to oxygenation and ventilation?**

Yes. The $PaCO_2$ is higher with the Combitube. The PaO_2 is also higher due to the physiologic PEEP maintained by the vocal cords.

❒❒ **What is the incidence of impossible mask ventilation?**

1 in 5000 to patients.

❒❒ **What should be done immediately after a failed intubation and impossible mask ventilation?**

A laryngeal mask airway should be inserted.

❒❒ **At what peak inspiratory pressure should an air leak be detected in pediatric patients intubated with an appropriate sized endotracheal tube?**

25 to 30 cm H_2O.

❒❒ **What are the initial ATLS steps of a trauma resuscitation?**

A - Airway maintenance with cervical spine control
B - Breathing – oxygenation and ventilation
C - Circulation with hemorrhage control
D - Disability - neurologic assessment
E - Exposure/Environmental control - completely undress the patient and prevent hypothermia

❑❑ **In what circumstances should the above order be modified?**

When a patient in a monitored setting arrests with sudden pulseless ventricular fibrillation. This requires immediate defibrillation.

❑❑ **What is the most common cause of upper airway obstruction?**

The tongue occluding the posterior oropharynx.

❑❑ **Name some important adjuncts often needed to help establish basic airway control.**

Suction equipment to remove secretions from mouth and throat, chin lift-jaw thrust maneuver, oral/nasal airway and bag-valve-mask device.

❑❑ **What are some advanced techniques for airway management?**

Orotracheal intubation, nasotracheal intubation, esophageal obturator airway (EOA), esophageal gastric tube airway (EGTA), pharyngotracheal airway, combination esophageal-tracheal tube, cricothyroidotomy and tracheostomy.

❑❑ **What are some indications for intubation?**

Apnea, burns, acute airway obstruction, expanding neck hematomas, hemodynamic instability, severe head injuries, poor oxygenation, poor ventilation, prevention of aspiration, inability to maintain a patent airway and impending or potential compromise of the airway.

❑❑ **What must be kept in mind when performing endotracheal intubation in a trauma patient?**

The potential for cervical spine injury.

❑❑ **What is a potential problem with bag-valve-mask ventilation?**

Air can enter the stomach via the esophagus causing gastric distention and aspiration.

❑❑ **How many people does it take to effectively ventilate a patient via the bag-valve-mask technique?**

Two. One to hold the mask securely to the face and a second to squeeze the bag with two hands.

❑❑ **Does tracheal intubation prevent aspiration?**

No. Microaspiration can still occur.

❑❑ **What characteristic of gastric contents causes the greatest harm following aspiration?**

Although particulate matter can clog the airways leading to atelectasis, it is the acidity of the gastric contents that leads to the greatest injury.

❑❑ **Name some factors that place a patient at risk for aspiration.**

Full stomach, trauma, intra-abdominal pathology (obstruction, inflammation, gastric paresis), esophageal disease (symptomatic reflux, motility disorders), pregnancy and obesity.

❑❑ Are esophageal obturator, combination esophageal-tracheal tube or pharyngotracheal airways better than orotracheal intubation?

No. These are substitutes when no trained personnel are available for orotracheal intubation.

❑❑ What properties of succinylcholine make it particularly useful as an aid for intubation?

Succinylcholine, a depolarizing paralytic agent, has a brief duration of action (3 to 5 minutes) and a rapid onset of action (within 60 seconds).

❑❑ T/F: Succinylcholine has sedative and amnestic effects as well as muscle relaxant properties.

False.

❑❑ What maneuver should be performed during any tracheal intubation?

The Sellick maneuver (occlusion of the esophagus by pressure on the cricoid cartilage). It can help prevent aspiration during tracheal intubation.

❑❑ What equipment is needed to assist with endotracheal intubation?

Suction for the mouth and pharynx, bag-valve-mask system for oxygenation, functioning laryngoscope, stylet and endotracheal tubes.

❑❑ What type of endotracheal tube is used in children?

Uncuffed.

❑❑ Why are uncuffed tubes used in children?

Uncuffed tubes help avoid subglottic edema and ulceration. Young children have a narrow subglottic area.

❑❑ What is the correct tube size for the typical adult male and female?

Male 8.0 mm ± 1.0 and female 7.0 mm ± 1.0.

❑❑ T/F: Female patients have larger airways compared to males but actually need smaller sized tubes.

False. Female patients have smaller airways necessitating smaller tubes.

❑❑ What three axes should be aligned when attempting to perform endotracheal intubation when motion of the patient's cervical spine is not contraindicated?

Pharyngeal, oral and laryngeal.

❑❑ Where is the tip of the curved blade placed during orotracheal intubation?

Into the vallecula just anterior to the epiglottis.

❑❑ Where is the tip of the straight blade placed during orotracheal intubation?

Beneath the epiglottis to directly lift the epiglottis anteriorly.

❑❑ T/F: To use the laryngoscope correctly, the back of the blade is placed against the upper front teeth and the handle is rotated posteriorly, thus lifting the epiglottis anteriorly.

False. Once positioned correctly, the handle and blade are lifted anteriorly and inferiorly (relative to the patient) without rotation to lift the epiglottis and expose the cords.

❒❒ In the typical male patient, what length of ET tube should lay distal to the lips?

23 cm.

❒❒ In the typical female patient, what length of ET tube should lay distal to the lips?

21 cm.

❒❒ What is the consequence of an ET tube placed too far distally?

Respiratory insufficiency secondary to right mainstem bronchus intubation.

❒❒ How is right mainstem intubation diagnosed?

Decreased breath sounds on the left that corrects with repositioning of the ET tube.

❒❒ What type of endotracheal tube cuff is presently used?

High-volume, low pressure cuffs. (Pressure = 20 to 25 mmHg.)

❒❒ When does tracheal ischemia occur?

When the pressure in the endotracheal tube cuff exceeds capillary perfusion pressure (typically 25 to 35 mmHg).

❒❒ Immediately after inserting an ET tube, what is the next most appropriate step?

Confirm tube placement.

❒❒ How is proper endotracheal tube placement confirmed?

Symmetric chest expansion, breath sounds in axillae but not over the epigastrium, tube fogs with respirations, end-tidal CO_2, monitoring of oxygen saturation and visualizing the tube passing through the vocal cords.

❒❒ Does a chest x-ray guarantee correct endotracheal tube placement?

No. Clinical signs (see last question) are needed for confirmation of endotracheal tube placement.

❒❒ What is the correct position of the tip of the endotracheal tube?

Approximately 4 cm above the carina.

❒❒ What is the most common complication of nasotracheal intubation?

Epistaxis.

❒❒ When is an emergent cricothyroidotomy indicated?

When a patient cannot be adequately oxygenated or ventilated, orotracheal intubation and bag ventilation cannot be performed and alternate airway devices have failed (or there is insufficient time to attempt these).

❒❒ T/F: Cricothyroidotomy is generally contraindicated in children.

True. Needle jet insufflation is considered a better choice to avoid injuring the cricoid cartilage

❒❒ Why is emergent tracheostomy usually not recommended?

The trachea lies deeper in the neck than the cricothyroid membrane. The trachea is surrounded by a number of veins and the isthmus of the thyroid gland. Complications such as recurrent laryngeal nerve injury, pneumothorax and esophageal perforation can occur.

❒❒ When may emergent tracheostomy be performed instead of emergent cricothyroidotomy?

In pediatric patients. Cricothyroidotomy is generally contraindicated in the pediatric population. Because of the smaller size and greater soft tissue compliance of the pediatric airway, the cricoid cartilage plays a major role in maintaining patency of the tracheal lumen. An injury to this structure could be disastrous.

❒❒ What are the three divisions of the airway?

1. Extrathoracic - nose to the trachea before it enters the thoracic inlet
2. Intrathoracic, extrapulmonary - trachea at the thoracic inlet to the right and left mainstem bronchi before they enter the lungs
3. Intrapulmonary - bronchi within the lungs

❒❒ According to Poiseuille's law, if the airway radius of the conducting airway is reduced from 4 mm to 2 mm, how much will resistance to airflow increase?

Sixteen-fold.

❒❒ What is the narrowest part of the adult airway?

The glottic opening.

❒❒ What is the most common offender in foreign body aspiration?

Organic substances such as nuts and corn.

❒❒ Which site is used to evacuate a tension pneumothorax by using needle thoracentesis?

The second intercostal space at the midclavicular line or the fifth intercostal space at the midaxillary line.

❒❒ What are the signs of tension pneumothorax on physical exam?

Tachypnea, unilateral absent breath sounds, tachycardia, pallor, diaphoresis, cyanosis, tracheal deviation, hypotension and neck vein distention.

❒❒ What is the directional change in intrathoracic pressure in a ventilated patient versus a spontaneously breathing patient?

It decreases during spontaneous inspiration and increases during positive-pressure inspiration.

❒❒ Under normal conditions at rest, what percentage of the cardiac output goes to the respiratory muscles?

Less than 3%.

❒❒ In patients with COPD, what percentage of the total cardiac output may be directed to the muscles of respiration?

25 to 30%.

❐❐ Positive end-expiratory pressure (PEEP) primarily impairs cardiac output by what mechanism?

Decrease in LV preload.

❐❐ To the extent that LV preload is maintained, positive pressure ventilation has what effect on cardiac output in patients with normal cardiovascular function?

No measurable effect as compared to spontaneous ventilation.

❐❐ When two different modes of ventilation, such as pressure support and inverse ratio ventilation, have similar changes in intrathoracic pressure and ventilatory effort, how do their hemodynamic effects compare?

They are similar.

❐❐ An intubated patient with ischemic heart disease develops mild inspiratory stridor upon extubation associated with severe chest pain and marked ST segment elevations across the precordium. The immediate treatment of this condition should include what ventilatory therapy?

Eliminate the markedly negative swings in intrathoracic pressure by re-intubation.

❐❐ In a patient with impaired right ventricular dysfunction following anterior chest trauma, excessive positive end-expiratory pressure (PEEP) therapy may induce cardiovascular decompensation by any of three mechanisms, name one.

1) Hyperinflation will increase pulmonary vascular resistance impeding right ventricular ejection.
2) Hyperinflation will increase intrathoracic pressure reducing venous return and limiting right ventricular filling.
3) Hyperinflation that compresses the heart is similar to tamponade restricting right ventricular filling.

❐❐ A mechanically ventilated patient with chronic obstructive lung disease is breathing spontaneously on assist-control mode with a measured intrinsic PEEP of 12 cm H_2O. What will the application of 8 cm H_2O extrinsic PEEP (from the ventilatory circuit) do to the patient's work of breathing?

In general it will decrease the work of breathing by reducing the amount of airway have a deleterious pressure drop needed to trigger the positive pressure breath. Some patients with intrinsic PEEP may have deleterious effect when adding PEEP to the ventilator circuit. Careful monitoring of the patient is mandatory. The level of added PEEP should be less than the amount of intrinsic PEEP.

❐❐ What causes peripheral cyanosis?

Peripheral cyanosis is due to shunting or increased O_2 extraction.

❐❐ Name the two primary causes (groups) of peripheral cyanosis.

Cyanosis with a normal SaO_2 can be due to:
- Decreased cardiac output.
- Redistribution - may be 2° to shock, DIC, hypothermia, vascular obstruction.

❐❐ Is succinylcholine a depolarizing or a non-depolarizing neuromuscular blocking agent?

It is the only commonly used depolarizing agent. It binds to post-synaptic acetylcholine receptors causing depolarization. It is enzymatically degraded by pseudocholinesterase. Onset is within 1 minute with duration of paralysis of 7 to 10 min.

❑❑ **What is the rationale for pre-treating a patient with a sub-paralytic ("defasciculating") dose of a non-depolarizing agent prior to administration of succinylcholine?**

The pre-treatment agent attenuates fasciculations from succinylcholine induced depolarization. This may decrease subsequent muscle pain. This also blunts increased intragastric and intraocular pressure associated with succinylcholine.

❑❑ **Which patients are at risk for developing aspiration pneumonia?**

Patients undergoing emergency surgery, pregnant patients, obese patients, those with gastrointestinal obstruction, depressed level of consciousness and laryngeal incompetence.

❑❑ **What is the appropriate treatment following aspiration?**

Secure the airway, administer oxygen, suction any aspirate, consider bronchoscopy if large particulates are present, ventilatory support and bronchodilators as needed for bronchospasm.

❑❑ **T/F: Acute lung injury of the entire lung causes lung compliance to decrease similarly in each region of the lung.**

False. Marked regional differences in the degree of lung consolidation and compliance characterize all forms of acute lung injury.

❑❑ **Which lobes of the lung can develop atelectasis from intubation of the right mainstem bronchus?**

Right upper lobe, left upper lobe and left lower lobe.

❑❑ **What are the determinants of $PaCO_2$?**

Carbon dioxide production and alveolar ventilation.

❑❑ **What are the components of tidal volume?**

Alveolar volume and dead space volume.

❑❑ **What is the maximum acceptable endotracheal tube cuff pressure?**

Approximately 25 cm H_2O at the end of expiration.

❑❑ **What is the potential harm of excess endotracheal tube cuff pressure?**

It can induce ischemia and necrosis of the underlying tissue.

❑❑ **Adequacy of alveolar ventilation is reflected by which component of arterial blood gas analysis?**

$PaCO_2$.

❑❑ **$PaCO_2$ is mathematically related to alveolar ventilation in what manner?**

There is an inverse relationship.

❑❑ **What factors interfere with the bellows function of the chest?**

Abdominal binding, massive obesity, trauma with flail chest, massive effusion and ascites, pneumothorax, thoracic burn with eschar, neuromuscular blockade and strapping of ribs.

❒❒ **What is the principal mechanism of increased $PaCO_2$ with increased FIO_2?**

Worsening V/Q mismatch and the Haldane effect.

❒❒ **How does malnutrition contribute to respiratory failure?**

Respiratory muscle weakness.

❒❒ **Respiratory failure is worsened in spinal injuries at or above which nerve root?**

C2.

❒❒ **What infectious syndromes can lead to ventilatory insufficiency?**

Botulism, tetanus, Campylobacter, polio, diphtheria and Guillain-Barré Syndrome.

❒❒ **Deficiency of phosphorous may affect oxygen transfer from erythrocytes as a result of its contribution to what compound?**

2,3-diphosphoglycerate (2,3-DPG).

❒❒ **What processes cause the work of breathing to increase markedly in patients with COPD?**

Increased dead space ventilation, decreased respiratory muscle efficiency and increased airway resistance.

❒❒ **What are the most common causes of increased dead space in critically ill patients?**

Decreased cardiac output, pulmonary embolism, pulmonary hypertension, ARDS and excessive PEEP.

❒❒ **The total work of breathing is divided into what two parts?**

Overcoming lung and chest wall compliance and overcoming airway resistance.

❒❒ **What are the ventilation and perfusion relationships between Zone 1, Zone 2 and Zone 3 of the lung?**

Zone 1 represents dead space (ventilation occurs without perfusion); zone 2 contains high V/Q mismatch (ventilation occurs in excess of perfusion); zone 3 represents areas of optimal V/Q matching.

❒❒ **What is the equation for determining a patient's oxygen extraction ratio?**

Oxygen extraction ratio = $(CaO_2 - CvO_2)/CaO_2$ where CaO_2 is arterial blood oxygen content and CvO_2 is the mixed venous blood oxygen content.

❒❒ **What is the normal whole lung V/Q ratio?**

4 liters of ventilation to 5 liters of blood flow or 0.8.

❒❒ **What is the hemodynamic response to an acute complete spinal cord injury at the C7 level?**

Initially there is hypertension and tachycardia secondary to increased circulating catecholamines at the time of the injury followed shortly by hypotension due to vasodilatation and bradycardia secondary to loss of cardiac accelerator input.

❒❒ **During the first minute of apnea, how much would you expect the $PaCO_2$ to rise?**

During apnea, the $PaCO_2$ will increase approximately 6 mmHg during the first minute and then 3 to 4 mmHg each minute thereafter.

❑❑ **What is the most important factor in control of ventilation under normal conditions?**

Arterial $PaCO_2$.

❑❑ **How does one assess oxygenation?**

Skin color, pulse oximetry and blood gas analysis.

❑❑ **How does one assess ventilation?**

End tidal CO_2 monitoring and blood gas analysis.

❑❑ **What is a tension pneumothorax?**

An injury to the lung allowing intrapleural air to collect without escaping via the chest wall or trachea. This accumulation of air compresses the lung and shifts the mediastinum, leading to impaired venous return and hypotension.

❑❑ **What are the physical findings in tension pneumothorax?**

Distended neck veins, hypotension, tracheal deviation and a hyperresonant hemithorax.

❑❑ **What is the treatment for tension pneumothorax?**

Immediate needle decompression of the hyperresonant hemithorax, based on clinical suspicion. Radiography should not be used to confirm tension pneumothorax.

❑❑ **What is adequate urinary output to gauge resuscitation in adults?**

0.5 cc/kg or about 50 cc/hr.

❑❑ **How does one assess for disability in ATLS?**

A rapid assessment to establish level of consciousness (alert, arouses to voice, arouses to pain or unresponsive) and pupillary appearance and reaction constitute the initial assessment. A more detailed examination is performed later.

❑❑ **How can the work of breathing with mechanical ventilation associated with intrinsic PEEP be reduced?**

Add a small amount of PEEP, reduce tidal volume, reduce inspiratory time and increase expiratory time.

❑❑ **What complications are associated with mask ventilation?**

Skin breakdown, aspiration pneumonia, aerophagia, pneumothorax and barotrauma.

❑❑ **Through what mechanism does PEEP decrease cardiac output?**

Reduced preload.

❑❑ **How can static compliance of the lung/chest wall be approximated from airway pressure measurements during mechanical ventilation?**

Tidal volume/(inspiratory plateau pressure - end expiratory (pause) pressure).

❑❑ **What evidence of barotrauma can be observed on chest x-ray?**

Pneumomediastinum, pneumothorax, pneumopericardium, subcutaneous emphysema and pulmonary interstitial emphysema.

❑❑ What are the primary determinants of the work of breathing?

Minute ventilation, lung/chest wall compliance, airway resistance and presence of intrinsic PEEP.

❑❑ What are some conditions under which CO_2 production is increased?

Lipogenesis, fever and hyperthyroidism.

❑❑ What is the preferred FIO_2 for patients with ARDS?

The lowest that will maintain a hemoglobin oxygen saturation of about 90%.

❑❑ How is oxygen delivery calculated?

Cardiac output x arterial blood oxygen content (x 10 to get units correct).

❑❑ What is the primary determinant of the oxygen content of arterial blood?

The product of hemoglobin concentration and the percent hemoglobin oxygen saturation of arterial blood. The amount of oxygen dissolved in the plasma (a function of the PaO_2) is negligible at one atmosphere of pressure.

❑❑ How can adequate tidal volume be delivered to a patient undergoing volume cycled mechanical ventilation whose endotracheal tube cuff is failing to maintain an adequate seal (without changing the tube)?

Increase the mandatory tidal volume.

❑❑ What combination of medications, often used in the treatment of status asthmaticus requiring mechanical ventilation, may result in prolonged weakness?

Steroids and neuromuscular blocking agents.

❑❑ T/F: Pulse oximetry is a reliable method for estimating oxyhemoglobin saturation in a patient suffering from CO poisoning.

False. COHb has light absorbance that can lead to a falsely elevated pulse oximeter saturation level. The calculated value from a standard ABG may also be falsely elevated. The oxygen saturation should be determined by using a co-oximeter that measures the amounts of unsaturated O_2Hb, COHb and metHb.

❑❑ When may end-tidal carbon dioxide detectors prove inaccurate?

In patients with very low blood flow to the lungs or in those with a large dead space (e.g., following a pulmonary embolism).

❑❑ What is the most common complication of endotracheal intubation?

Intubation of a bronchus. Other complications include esophageal intubation, lacerations of the lip, tongue and pharyngeal or tracheal mucosa, resulting in bleeding, hematoma or abscess. Tracheal rupture, avulsion of an arytenoid cartilage, vocal cord injury, pharyngeal-esophageal perforation, intubation of the pyriform sinus, gastric content aspiration, hypertension, tachycardia and arrhythmias may also occur.

❑❑ What oxygen flow rate is recommended for face mask ventilation?

At least 5 L/min. Recommended flow is 8 to 10 L/min., which will produce oxygen concentrations as high as 40% to 60%.

❑❑ What oxygen concentration can be supplied with a face mask and oxygen reservoir?

6 L/min. provides approximately 60% oxygen concentration and each liter increases the concentration by 10%. 10 L/min. is almost 100%.

❑❑ What are the four commonly used modes of ventilation?

Intermittent mandatory ventilation (IMV), pressure support (PS), assist control (AC) and pressure control (PC).

❑❑ What is the difference between pressure control ventilation and pressure support ventilation?

In pressure support ventilation, a breath is spontaneously initiated by the patient. The ventilator delivers a flow of gas to reach a target pressure. This flow is maintained until a flow threshold is reached during the decelerating phase of inspiration. At this time expiration begins.

In pressure control ventilation, a patient receives a mechanical breath at a predetermined rate. Once again the ventilator delivers a flow of gas to reach a certain pressure. Unlike pressure support, the ventilator assists the breath until a predetermined time is reached. This is called time-cycling.

In neither mode is the tidal volume controlled. Instead, the tidal volume is determined by pulmonary compliance, duration of inspiration and synchrony between the ventilator and the patient.

❑❑ Describe the events associated with auto-PEEP.

Also known as air trapping and intrinsic PEEP (positive end-expiratory pressure), auto-PEEP occurs mostly in patients with asthma, chronic obstructive pulmonary disease and acute respiratory distress syndrome. Auto-PEEP occurs when a patient with lung disease is unable to completely exhale each tidal volume. The accumulation of pressure results in a persistent difference between alveolar pressure and external airway pressure at end expiration. The persistent pressure difference results in continued airflow at end exhalation.

❑❑ What are the consequences of auto-PEEP?

Auto-PEEP results in tidal volumes that occur at the upper limit of total lung capacity where compliance is low. Thus higher pressures are required to achieve a given tidal volume and the patient is at increased risk for barotrauma. In a patient who is initiating breaths on the ventilator (e.g., spontaneously breathing with pressure support), auto-PEEP increases the work of breathing. Like extrinsic PEEP, auto-PEEP can compromise cardiac function by decreasing venous return and cardiac output.

❑❑ An intubated patient is left on 100% oxygen for 20 hours. Describe changes that can be attributed to oxygen toxicity.

Tracheobronchial irritation (coughing, substernal discomfort), decreased vital capacity, decreased lung compliance, decreased diffusing capacity, decreased tracheal mucus velocity, increased arteriovenous shunting, absorption atelectasis and increased dead space to tidal volume ratio.

❑❑ What ventilator steps can be taken to optimize an ARDS patient's respiratory function?

Using pressure control to minimize barotrauma, decreasing tidal volume to minimize volutrauma, using inverse ratio ventilation and permissive hypercapnia to maximize inspiration time. None of these strategies have been proven by clinical trials.

❑❑ What factors shift the oxygen-hemoglobin dissociation curve to the right?

Acidemia hypercarbia, increased 2,3 DPG and increased temperature.

❐❐ What is the equation that relates total pulmonary compliance to lung compliance and chest wall compliance?

1/total pulmonary compliance = 1/lung compliance + 1/chest wall compliance.

❐❐ During sleep what is the normal, expected change in $PaCO_2$ and PaO_2 from the baseline, awake state?

Normally, $PaCO_2$ increases 4 to 8 mmHg and PaO_2 decreases 3 to 10 mmHg.

❐❐ Define compliance.

The change in volume divided by the change in distending pressure. Elastic recoil is usually measured in terms of compliance. Compliance measurements can be obtained for the chest, the lung or both together.

❐❐ What is the predominant stimulus for activation of hypoxic pulmonary vasoconstriction?

Decreased alveolar oxygen tension.

❐❐ What components contribute to physiologic shunting (venous admixture)?

The bronchial, pleural and thebesian veins and abnormal arterial to venous communications in the lungs.

❐❐ What is the respiratory quotient?

The rate of carbon dioxide production divided by the rate of oxygen consumption.

❐❐ Which neuromuscular and spinal diseases can lead to ventilatory insufficiency?

Muscular dystrophy, polymyositis, myotonic dystrophy, polyneuritis, Eaton Lambert syndrome, myasthenia gravis, amyotrophic lateral sclerosis, trauma, Guillain-Barré syndrome, multiple sclerosis, Parkinson's Disease and stroke.

❐❐ Patients on mechanical ventilation can develop hypoventilation based on what pulmonary factors?

Increased dead space (including length of ventilator circuit proximal to the "Y" piece separating the inspiratory and expiratory limbs), decreased tidal volume, overdistention of lung, air leaks and massive pulmonary embolism.

❐❐ Patients with failure of which organs are at increased risk of developing prolonged paralysis following neuromuscular blocker administration?

Liver and kidney.

❐❐ What are the principal complications of nasal endotracheal intubation (as opposed to oral)?

Maxillary sinusitis, amputation of turbinates, septal perforation and increased airway resistance associated with a narrower tube.

❐❐ How is the work of breathing affected by patient-triggered positive pressure ventilation?

It can increase, decrease or remain the same.

❐❐ What should be done first when tension pneumothorax is suspected?

Needle thoracostomy followed by tube thoracostomy.

❑❑ **How can the presence of intrinsic PEEP be confirmed in patients undergoing mechanical ventilation?**

Just prior to the onset of inspiration, one of three may be seen:
1) Expiratory flow has not ceased
2) Positive pressure is measured with an esophageal balloon
3) Positive pressure is measured during an airway occlusion maneuver

❑❑ **Under what circumstances should dead space be added to the ventilator circuit?**

None. Never.

❑❑ **What is the FIO_2 at the top of Mount Everest?**

21%.

❑❑ **What position is preferred for patients suspected of having an air embolism?**

Left lateral decubitus/Trendelenburg position.

❑❑ **What are the clinical signs of hypercarbia?**

Flushed hot hands and feet, bounding pulses, confusion or drowsiness, muscular twitching and engorged retinal veins (all secondary to vasodilatation).

❑❑ **Under normal conditions (pH 7.4, PCO_2 40mmHg, T 37°C) what are the corresponding PO_2 values to oxygen saturations of 60%, 90% and 95%?**

PO_2 of 30, 60 and 85, respectively.

❑❑ **What is the primary cause of hypercapnia?**

Hypoventilation.

❑❑ **A 50 year-old woman presents with pneumonia in the right lower and middle lobes. On 50% oxygen by face mask, her PaO_2 is 75 mmHg. Should the patient be positioned right side down or up?**

From an oxygenation perspective, right side up. Blood flow is gravity dependent. If the patient is positioned right side down, blood flow will preferentially go to the right side. However, because of the pneumonia, this will increase the amount of shunt, lowering the PaO_2 further.

From a pulmonary hygiene perspective, right side down. The infected material may move with gravity from the infected lung to the uninfected lung.

❑❑ **A 65 year-old male presents with dyspnea and a dry cough. Chest x-ray reveals bilateral interstitial infiltrates and biopsy reveals idiopathic pulmonary fibrosis. Room air PaO_2 is 60 mmHg. What is the mechanism of hypoxemia?**

Ventilation-perfusion inequality. It is a common mistake to attribute the hypoxemia as secondary to diffusion impairment because of the pulmonary fibrosis. Diffusion impairment is a rare cause of hypoxemia. In general, diffusion capacity must be less than 25% of normal for it to cause hypoxemia.

❑❑ **T/F: If a patient presents with a $PaCO_2$ of 75, he/she should be emergently intubated.**

False. There is no $PaCO_2$ level at which a patient must be intubated. Intubation is based upon the total clinical condition of a patient, not just upon a blood gas result.

❒❒ What is the treatment for carbon monoxide poisoning?

100% oxygen, which increases carbon monoxide clearance by competing for binding to hemoglobin. Hyperbaric oxygen (oxygen provided at higher than atmospheric pressure) is recommended in more severe cases.

❒❒ T/F: A normal $PaCO_2$ in a patient with an asthma exacerbation is a good sign.

Maybe. A normal $PaCO_2$ in an asthmatic is good if the patient is feeling improved and less dyspneic. However, it can be a sign of impending respiratory failure if the patient continues to feel dyspneic and is working hard to breathe.

❒❒ T/F: Oxygen should never be given to a hypoxemic patient with COPD who has chronic CO_2 retention.

False. Oxygen should always be given to a patient who is hypoxemic.

❒❒ What considerations should be addressed while giving the above patient oxygen?

It has been shown that giving oxygen to a chronic CO_2 retainer usually does not result in a significant decrease in minute ventilation. The $PaCO_2$ will go up, but the rise is probably a result of changes in the ventilation-perfusion inequalities.

Oxygen should be given judiciously with repeat $PaCO_2$ determinations to ensure that the $PaCO_2$ does not rise precipitously.

❒❒ What are the indications for chronic oxygen therapy?

1. Resting $PaO_2 < 55$ mmHg or $SaO_2 < 88\%$.
2. Resting PaO_2 56-59 mmHg or SaO_2 89% in the presence of evidence of cor pulmonale or polycythemia.
3. During exercise if the PaO_2 falls below 55 mmHg or the SaO_2 below 88% with a low level of exertion.

❒❒ What are the major mechanisms of hypoventilation and what clinical conditions are associated with each?

1. Failure of the central nervous system ventilatory centers - drugs (narcotics, barbiturates) and stroke.
2. Failure of the chest bellows - chest wall diseases (kyphoscoliosis), neuromuscular diseases (amyotrophic lateral sclerosis) and diaphragm weakness.
3. Obstruction of the airways – asthma and chronic obstructive pulmonary disease.

❒❒ How can hypoxemia secondary to hypoventilation alone be distinguished from other causes of hypoxemia?

If the hypoxemia is from hypoventilation alone, the A-a O_2 gradient is normal. It is elevated in all other causes.

❒❒ What are the most common clinical conditions in which shunt is the primary mechanism for hypoxemia?

Alveolar filling with fluid (pulmonary edema) or pus (pneumonia). Any condition that fills or closes the alveoli preventing gas exchange can lead to a shunt.

❒❒ How can shunt be distinguished from the other causes of hypoxemia?

If given 100% oxygen, the hypoxemic patient with a shunt will not have a significant increase in their PaO_2. There will be a significant increase in PaO_2 when 100% oxygen is given to patients with hypoventilation or ventilation-perfusion inequality.

❐❐ T/F: A leftward shift in the oxyhemoglobin dissociation curve indicates an increased hemoglobin affinity for oxygen.

True.

❐❐ Changes in temperature, $PaCO_2$ or pH or the level of 2,3-diphosphoglycerate (2,3-DPG) cause a shift in the oxyhemoglobin dissociation curve. To cause a rightward shift, what are the changes that must occur?

Increased temperature, increased $PaCO_2$, decreased pH and increased 2,3-DPG level. An easy way to remember this is that these conditions are often associated with decreased tissue oxygen levels. By right-shifting the curve, more oxygen is released from hemoglobin to the tissues.

❐❐ Which types of hemoglobin are associated with a leftward shift of the oxyhemoglobin dissociation curve?

Hemoglobin F (fetal hemoglobin), carboxyhemoglobin and methemoglobin.

❐❐ What drugs cause methemoglobinemia?

Oxidant drugs, such as antimalarials, dapsone, nitrites/nitrates (nitroprusside) and local anesthetics (lidocaine). Methemoglobinemia occurs when the iron moiety of hemoglobin is oxidized from the ferrous to the ferric state.

❐❐ Which common enzyme deficiency predisposes to the development of methemoglobinemia in the presence of the above drugs?

G-6-PD deficiency.

❐❐ What is the treatment of methemoglobinemia?

Methylene blue.

❐❐ What are the determinants of the oxygen content of blood?

Hemoglobin concentration, PaO_2 and SaO_2. The equation to determine the oxygen content of blood is: $CaO_2 = (1.34 \times [Hgb] \times SaO_2) + (PaO_2 \times 0.003)$. The first term is the hemoglobin bound oxygen and the second is the dissolved oxygen. Dissolved oxygen content is a minor portion of total oxygen content unless PaO_2 is very high.

❐❐ How does the shape of the oxyhemoglobin dissociation curve effect the oxygen content of blood?

Since SaO_2 does not increase significantly if the $PaO_2 > 60$ mmHg, the oxygen content of blood will increase significantly above this level only by increasing the hemoglobin concentration.

❐❐ What are some common causes of respiratory alkalosis?

Respiratory alkalosis is defined as a pH above 7.45 and a pCO_2 less than 35. Common causes of respiratory alkalosis include any process that may induce hyperventilation: shock, sepsis, trauma, asthma, PE, anemia, hepatic failure, heat stroke, exhaustion, emotion, salicylate poisoning, hypoxemia, pregnancy and inadequate mechanical ventilation.

❐❐ Calculate the alveolar-arterial oxygen (A-a O_2) gradient given the following arterial blood gas obtained at sea level: pH 7.24, $PaCO_2$ 60 and PaO_2 45.

30 mmHg.

To calculate the alveolar-arterial oxygen gradient, you must first calculate the expected alveolar partial pressure of oxygen (PAO_2) using the alveolar gas equation. The alveolar gas equation is commonly written: $PAO_2 = PIO_2 - PaCO_2/R$, where PIO_2 is the partial pressure of oxygen in the inspired gas and R is the respiratory exchange ratio, commonly estimated at 0.8. PIO_2 is calculated as follows: $PIO_2 = FIO_2\ (P_B - P_{H2O})$ where FIO_2 is the inspired concentration of oxygen (0.21 at sea level), P_B is the atmospheric pressure (760 mmHg at sea level) and P_{H2O} is the partial pressure of water (47 mmHg). At sea level, PIO_2 is equal to 150 mmHg. For this example, PAO_2 = 150 - 60/0.8 or 75 mmHg.

The A-a O_2 gradient is $PAO_2 - PaO_2$. Therefore, in this example, the A-a O_2 gradient is 75 - 45 or 30 mmHg.

❑❑ What is the normal A-a O_2 gradient?

10 mmHg in a 20 year-old.

❑❑ What is the age related decline in PaO_2?

The PaO_2 declines by 2.5 mmHg per decade. Given that a PaO_2 of 95-100 mmHg is normal for a 20 year-old, a PaO_2 of 75 to 80 would be normal for an 80 year-old. This decline is secondary to an increase in the A-a O_2 gradient, which increases from about 10 mmHg in a 20 year-old to 20 to 25 mmHg in an 80 year-old.

❑❑ What are the principal mechanisms that lead to hypoxemia?

Hypoventilation, diffusion limitation, shunt, ventilation-perfusion inequality, low inspired oxygen concentration, and low mixed venous oxygen in the presence of V/Q mismatch.

❑❑ Which of the above mechanisms is the most common?

Ventilation-perfusion inequality.

❑❑ Why does hypoventilation lead to hypoxemia?

Hypoventilation results in an increase in $PaCO_2$, which in turn decreases the PAO_2 (see the alveolar gas equation above).

❑❑ Can a shunt be seen in patients without alveolar abnormalities?

Yes. A shunt can occur if venous blood enters the left atrium without being oxygenated. This can occur in pulmonary arteriovenous malformations and intracardiac shunts.

❑❑ T/F: Diffusion limitation is an important cause of hypoxemia clinically.

False. Diffusion limitation is rarely a cause of hypoxemia.

❑❑ Does oxygen or carbon monoxide bind to hemoglobin with more affinity?

Carbon monoxide has a 240-fold greater affinity for hemoglobin than oxygen.

❑❑ What are the effects of carbon monoxide on hemoglobin?

Carbon monoxide bound to hemoglobin, carboxyhemoglobin, impairs tissue oxygenation by two mechanisms:
1: It decreases oxygen carrying capacity by decreasing the amount of hemoglobin available for oxygen binding.
2: It shifts the oxyhemoglobin dissociation curve to the left.

❑❑ What are the common clinical signs and symptoms of acute hypoxia?

1. Respiratory: tachypnea, dyspnea and cyanosis.
2. Cardiovascular: tachycardia, palpitations, arrhythmias and angina.
3. Central nervous system: headache, impaired judgment, inappropriate behavior, confusion and seizures.

❑❑ What is the normal tidal volume and minute ventilation in an average 70 kg subject?

The normal tidal volume (V_T) is 500 to 600 mL and the normal minute ventilation (V_E) is 5 to 6 L/min.

❑❑ What is the difference between anatomic and physiologic dead space?

Dead space refers to areas of lung that are ventilated but not perfused. Anatomic dead space refers to the conducting airways (trachea, bronchi and bronchioles) where there is no gas exchange because there are no alveoli. Physiologic dead space includes the anatomic dead space and any diseased lung in which there is ventilation but no perfusion.

❑❑ What is the normal dead space in an average 70-kg subject?

150 mL.

❑❑ Why do most asthmatics present with a decreased PCO_2?

First, the increased $PaCO_2$ associated with the increased dead space stimulates the central nervous system chemoreceptors to increase minute ventilation, which in turn decreases $PaCO_2$. Also, the associated hypoxemia and sensation of dyspnea causes the patient to hyperventilate, which lowers the $PaCO_2$.

❑❑ Why do asthmatics eventually have an increased $PaCO_2$ if untreated?

As the asthma attack continues untreated, the work of breathing will continue to increase. Eventually, the diaphragm fatigues and the patient hypoventilates. The hypoventilation, in association with the increased dead space and increased CO_2 production, increases the $PaCO_2$.

❑❑ What is the normal $PaCO_2$ and does it vary with age?

The normal $PaCO_2$ is 35 to 45 mmHg and does not vary with age.

❑❑ What is the normal expected change in pH if there is an acute change in the $PaCO_2$?

The pH will increase or decrease 0.8 units for every 10 mmHg decrease or increase (respectively) in $PaCO_2$.

❑❑ In chronic respiratory acidosis or alkalosis, what is the expected change in pH?

The pH will increase or decrease 0.3 units for every 10 mmHg decrease or increase (respectively) in $PaCO_2$.

❑❑ What is the expected change in serum bicarbonate in chronic respiratory acidosis or alkalosis?

Bicarbonate increases by approximately 3 mEq/L for each 10 mmHg increase in $PaCO_2$ in chronic respiratory acidosis. Bicarbonate decreases by 4 to 5 mEq/L for each 10 mmHg decrease in $PaCO_2$ in chronic respiratory alkalosis.

❑❑ What are the consequences of hypercapnia?

Acute hypercapnia has physiologic consequences due to the increased $PaCO_2$ and to the decreased pH.

Physiologic effects of the $PaCO_2$ increase include:
1. Increase in cerebral blood flow.

2. Confusion, headache ($PaCO_2 > 60$mmHg), obtundation and seizure ($PaCO_2 > 70$mmHg).
3. Depression of diaphragmatic contractility.

The primary consequences of the decreased pH are on the cardiovascular system with in decreased cardiac contractility, decreased fibrillation threshold and vasodilatation.

❒❒ What are the consequences of hypocapnia?

Acute hypocapnia has physiologic consequences due to the decreased $PaCO_2$ and to the increased pH.

Physiologic effects of the $PaCO_2$ decrease include:

1. Decreases in cerebral blood flow (this reflex is used in the management of neurologic disorders with high intracranial pressures as a short-term measure to decrease the increased intracranial pressure).
2. Confusion, myoclonus, asterixis, loss of consciousness and seizures.

The primary consequences of the increased pH are again primarily on the cardiovascular system with increased cardiac contractility and vasodilatation.

❒❒ A 32 year-old male presents to the emergency room obtunded. Examination is significant for a respiratory rate of 8 and pinpoint pupils. An arterial blood gas reveals pH 7.28, $PaCO_2$ 55 and PaO_2 60. What is the cause of the hypercapnia?

Acute narcotic overdose leading to hypoventilation.

❒❒ T/F: A chest x-ray in the above patient would most likely show signs of aspiration pneumonia.

True. The A-a O_2 gradient is 21 (PAO_2 is 150 - 55/0.8 or 81), which is high, indicating that there are two reasons for the hypoxemia.

❒❒ A 30 year-old female presents with dyspnea and signs of right sided heart failure. The PaO_2 on room air is 55 mmHg and on 100% oxygen is 70 mmHg. What is the cause of the hypoxemia?

Shunt, as there is no significant increase in the PaO_2 on 100% oxygen.

❒❒ The chest x-ray on the above patient reveals no pulmonary parenchymal lesions but does show prominent hila and an enlarged right ventricle. What diagnostic test should be performed?

The patient has no pulmonary parenchymal lesions to cause a shunt. She most likely has an intracardiac right-to-left shunt (most likely a previously undiagnosed atrial septal defect). An echocardiogram should be performed.

❒❒ A 45 year-old obese male presents with dyspnea, peripheral edema, snoring and excessive daytime sleepiness. A room air arterial blood gas shows the pH is 7.34, $PaCO_2$ 60 mmHg, PaO_2 58 mmHg and the calculated HCO_3^- is 28 mEq/L. What is the acid-base disturbance?

Chronic compensated respiratory acidosis. If this were acute, the pH would be 7.28 with a normal HCO_3^-.

❒❒ What is the cause of the hypoxemia in the above patient?

Hypoventilation is one cause. However, since the A-a O_2 gradient is elevated, there is another cause in addition to the hypoventilation. In an obese patient, both ventilation-perfusion inequality and shunt (secondary to atelectasis) can contribute to the development of hypoxemia.

❒❒ What is the cause of the hypoventilation?

Obesity-hypoventilation syndrome.

❒❒ A 25 year-old woman with a history of mitral valve prolapse presents with anxiety, chest tightness, hand numbness and mild confusion. Arterial blood gas reveals: pH 7.52, $PaCO_2$ 25 mmHg and PaO_2 108 mmHg. What is the most likely diagnosis?

An acute anxiety attack.

❒❒ Why is the PaO_2 elevated in the above patient?

Because the lower $PaCO_2$ means a higher PAO_2 (see alveolar gas equation above).

❒❒ What is the treatment?

Having the patient breathe in and out of a bag can terminate the acute hyperventilation. Anxiolytics can also be provided.

❒❒ In which pulmonary disease has long term continuous oxygen therapy been proven to be of clinical benefit?

Studies in both the United States and Great Britain have shown that mortality is reduced in patients with chronic obstructive pulmonary disease and hypoxemia who use long-term oxygen.

❒❒ What are the maximal oxygen concentrations that can be achieved by nasal cannula and face mask?

6 L/min. of nasal cannula oxygen can achieve an FIO_2 of ~44%. A simple face mask can achieve an FIO_2 of ~60%.

❒❒ What is a nonrebreather mask?

A nonrebreather mask has a one-way valve between the mask and a reservoir bag, such that the patient can only inhale from the reservoir bag (which contains 100% oxygen) and exhale through separate valves on the side of the mask.

❒❒ What is a Venturi mask?

An oxygen delivery device in which room air and 100% oxygen are mixed in a fixed ratio allowing for the delivery of an accurate FIO_2 up to 50%.

❒❒ Why is a Venturi mask clinically useful?

The Venturi mask is mostly commonly used for patients with chronic CO_2 retention and acute hypoxemia, where precise titration of the FIO_2 is necessary to prevent a precipitous increase in the $PaCO_2$.

❒❒ What should treatment for malignant hyperthermia include?

A change in the anesthetic agent to remove possible triggers, administration of dantrolene and the procedure should be terminated.

❒❒ T/F: Severe auto-PEEP may cause pulseless electrical activity.

True.

SHOCK PEARLS

"For he was great of heart"
Othello, Shakespeare

❑❑ **What is a normal oxygen extraction ratio in a healthy adult?**

(20 vol% - 15 vol%)/20 vol% = 5/20 or 25%

❑❑ **What is Beck's triad for the diagnosis of cardiac tamponade?**

Hypotension, distended neck veins and muffled heart tones.

❑❑ **What is the equation for calculating arterial oxygen content (CaO_2)?**

$CaO_2 = (1.39 \times Hgb \times \text{arterial } O_2 \text{ Sat}) + (.003 \times PaO_2)$ where Hgb is hemoglobin, O_2 sat is oxygen saturation and PaO_2 is arterial partial pressure of oxygen.

❑❑ **What hemodynamic changes are associated with sepsis?**

Increased cardiac index, decreased systemic vascular resistance (early stage), increased systemic vascular resistance (late stage), normal to decreased cardiac filling pressures and normal or elevated mixed venous oxygen saturation (early stage).

❑❑ **What are the indicators of global oxygen transport insufficiency?**

Decrease in mixed venous oxygen saturation, increase in arterial-venous oxygen content difference and development of lactic acidosis.

❑❑ **What are the clinical manifestations of the systemic inflammatory response syndrome (SIRS)?**

Fever or hypothermia, tachypnea, tachycardia and increased WBCs with a left shift.

❑❑ **What are the mechanisms of obstructive shock?**

Impedance to filling (e.g., tamponade and restrictive cardiomyopathies) and impedance to outflow (e.g., valvular stenosis and pulmonary embolism).

❑❑ **What is the classic hemodynamic finding of cardiac tamponade?**

Equalization of the diastolic pressures of the heart chambers.

❑❑ **Why does removal of very little pericardial fluid in tamponade greatly improve the clinical picture?**

Tamponade occurs at the right side of the pericardial compliance curve where small increases in volume cause large increases in pressure.

❑❑ **What causes electrical alternans on the ECG of a patient with cardiac tamponade?**

Cyclic motion of the heart in the fluid-filled pericardial sac.

❑❑ **What is pulsus paradoxus?**

A greater than normal decrease in systolic arterial pressure with inspiration.

❒❒ What is the differential diagnosis for pulsus paradoxus?

Cardiac tamponade, status asthmaticus, severe chronic obstructive lung disease, pulmonary embolus, constrictive pericarditis and tension pneumothorax.

❒❒ What clinical finding distinguishes cardiac tamponade from constrictive pericarditis?

Kussmaul's sign (increase in venous pressure during inspiration) is not seen in tamponade.

❒❒ What is the most common clinical finding in cardiac tamponade?

Tachypnea followed by pulsus paradoxus and tachycardia.

❒❒ What are the underlying pathogenetic mechanisms of cardiogenic shock?

Loss of contractile muscle, valvular failure, dysrhythmias and myocardial rupture.

❒❒ What is the classic clinical sign of systolic ventricular dysfunction?

An S3 gallop.

❒❒ Can preload and PCWP be used as synonyms?

No. PCWP is determined by juxtaventricular pressures, ventricular compliance and left ventricular end diastolic volume (LVEDV). LVEDV and preload are synonyms.

❒❒ What major conditions are associated with distributive shock?

Sepsis, anaphylaxis, neurogenic shock and adrenal insufficiency.

❒❒ What are the key endogenous molecular mediators of septic shock?

Cytokines (mainly TNF-α, IL-1, IL-6 and IFN-γ), prostaglandins, complement factors, platelet-activating factor and nitric oxide.

❒❒ What is the pathogenesis of anaphylactic shock?

Anaphylactic shock is an extreme manifestation of an immediate hypersensitivity reaction. It occurs through the interaction of an inciting antigen with mast cells and basophil-bound IgE. These effector cells then release numerous mediators that produce the clinical findings.

❒❒ What are the effects of septic shock on cardiac function?

There is transient dilatation of one or both ventricles, reduced contractility and low ejection fraction. These changes typically last several days and normalize after 7 to 10 days.

❒❒ What are the typical clinical findings that distinguish distributive shock from other types of shock?

Warm, well-perfused skin, wide pulse pressure and reduced diastolic blood pressure.

❒❒ What degree of blood loss is required to induce hypotension?

20 to 25% of the blood volume.

❒❒ What are the typical values of mixed venous oxygen saturation in septic shock?

It is often elevated above normal secondary to inadequate oxygen extraction by tissues.

❒❒ T/F: The finding of a hyperdynamic hemodynamic profile can confirms or excludes a septic etiology of shock.

False.

❒❒ What are the initial priorities during shock resuscitation?

Hemodynamic stabilization and cause-specific correction of the systemic and regional circulatory failure.

❒❒ What are the metabolic goals of shock resuscitation?

Correction of oxygen debt, anaerobic metabolism and tissue acidosis.

❒❒ What is the importance of the splanchnic circulation during shock and the post-shock phase?

The splanchnic tissues are preferentially underperfused relative to their metabolic demands during shock. Left uncorrected, this underperfusion is associated with increased morbidity and mortality.

❒❒ What is the initial blood pressure goal in shock resuscitation?

Mean arterial pressure (MAP) of 70 mm Hg.

❒❒ What is the significance of blood lactate determination in shock patients?

Mortality is directly related to the degree of lactic acidosis.

❒❒ T/F: Normal cardiac output values exclude cardiac dysfunction.

False.

❒❒ What is the optimal hematocrit in shock patients?

Approximately 30%.

❒❒ What is the role of catecholamines in the resuscitation of shock?

Inotropic or vasopressor support once effective intravascular volume has been restored.

❒❒ What are the major drawbacks of catecholamine use in shock?

Catecholamines can increase myocardial and systemic oxygen demands, induce arrhythmias and cause excessive vasoconstriction, resulting in ischemia.

❒❒ T/F: Normalization of vital signs, such as blood pressure and heart rate indicate complete resuscitation of shock.

False. Systemic vital signs do not reliably reflect the physiologic end-points of shock resuscitation.

❒❒ What is the most common cause of death of shock patients?

Multiple organ failure (MOF).

❒❒ Which parameter obtained on routine vital signs usually indicates a hypodynamic state?

A narrowed pulse pressure.

❒❒ In which lung zone should a pulmonary artery catheter tip be located?

Zone III.

❒❒ How is oxygen consumption (VO_2) calculated?

$VO_2 = CO \times C(a\text{-}v)O_2 \times 10$.

❒❒ What is the normal mixed venous blood oxygen saturation?

Approximately 75%.

❒❒ How is arterial oxygen content (CaO_2) calculated?

$CaO_2 = (Hgb \times 1.39 \times SaO_2) + (PaO_2 \times 0.0031)$.

❒❒ What are the typical PA catheter measurements in early septic shock?

High cardiac output (CO), low systemic vascular resistance (SVR) and low or normal pulmonary capillary wedge pressure (PCWP). In later stages, CO will drop and SVR may rise.

❒❒ What is the treatment of septic shock?

Volume infusion. Once euvolemia is achieved, vasopressor agents for hypotension or inotropic agents for inadequate tissue delivery of oxygen should be considered.

❒❒ How is cardiogenic shock managed?

Euvolemia first, then inotropic or vasopressor support.

❒❒ What are typical PA catheter measurements in neurogenic shock?

High or low CO, low SVR and low PCWP.

❒❒ How is neurogenic shock managed?

Volume infusion followed by vasopressors, if needed.

❒❒ What are the characteristics of dopamine?

It is primarily a dopaminergic agonist at low doses, a β-1 agonist at moderate doses and an α-agonist at high doses.

❒❒ How is oxygen delivery (DO_2) calculated?

$DO_2 = CO \times CaO_2 \times 10$.

❒❒ What is the definition of preload?

End-diastolic sarcomere length.

❒❒ T/F: Colloid solutions are preferred for resuscitation.

False.

❒❒ T/F: Blood products should be given as the initial resuscitation fluid for patients with presumed large blood loss.

False.

❐❐ What parameters indicate successful resuscitation?

Return of normal vital signs and signs of end organ perfusion (as urine output and clear mentation).

❐❐ What are the indications for central venous cannulation?

As a conduit for PA catheters, lack of peripheral access, CVP monitoring and infusion of vasoactive medications or medications requiring high flow veins.

❐❐ What is the preferred site for central venous catheterization?

Controversial. All three major sites (femoral, internal jugular and subclavian) have advantages and disadvantages that must be weighed.

❐❐ T/F: Femoral vein catheters have the highest infection rates and should not be used routinely.

False.

❐❐ What are the most common immediate complications of central venous catheterization?

Pneumothorax, hemothorax, arrhythmias, arterial puncture, air embolus and malposition.

❐❐ What are the common delayed complications from central venous catheterization?

Infection, thrombus formation, erosion through the SVC or atrium and delayed pneumothorax.

❐❐ How is ejection fraction (EF) calculated?

EF = SV / EDV, where SV = stroke volume and EDV = end diastolic volume.

❐❐ What catheter tip culture result is suggestive of catheter sepsis?

Greater than 15 colonies of the same organism.

❐❐ A patient has the following pulmonary artery catheter readings: Cardiac index (CI) of 2.0 L/min., CVP of 2 mm Hg, pulmonary artery occlusion pressure (PAOP) of 7 mmHg and SVR of 1600 dyne/sec/cm^2. What is the most likely diagnosis and what is the appropriate therapy?

The patient is hypovolemic and would benefit from fluid resuscitation.

❐❐ A patient's pulmonary artery catheter readings reveal a CVP of 12 mm Hg, PAOP of 18 mm Hg, CI of 1.7 L/min. and SVR of 1650 dyne/sec/cm^2. What is the most appropriate treatment?

Inotropic support. However, this must be judiciously balanced against the side effect of increasing myocardial oxygen demand. Depending on the patient's condition, an intraaortic balloon pump may be preferred. Echocardiography is necessary to rule out a structural cause for the decrease in cardiac index.

❐❐ What is the average survival rate for patients with septic shock?

40 to 60%.

❐❐ T/F: The circulatory derangements of septic shock precede the metabolic abnormalities.

False.

❒❒ Why has bicarbonate use been de-emphasized?

Because of its harmful effects, which include hyperosmolarity, alkalemia, hypernatremia, paradoxical CSF acidosis and increased CO_2 production.

❒❒ T/F: Vasodilators should be employed early in the management of hemorrhagic shock.

False.

❒❒ Which class of hemorrhagic shock is consistent with a drop in systolic blood pressure?

Class III.

❒❒ What are the CNS symptoms of acute volume loss?

Lethargy and apathy, progressing to coma.

❒❒ What is the best initial fluid management for a patient with hemorrhagic shock?

Lactated Ringer's.

❒❒ What are the signs of volume overload?

Distended veins, bounding pulse, functional murmurs, peripheral edema and basilar rales.

❒❒ What are the characteristics of Class II hemorrhagic shock?

Loss of 15 to 30% of circulating blood volume, tachycardia and a decrease in the pulse pressure.

❒❒ What is the most common volume disorder encountered in surgery?

Volume deficit. (Loss of isotonic fluid is the most common cause.)

❒❒ Which fluids flow faster through IV lines?

Crystalloid and colloids are faster than red cells

❒❒ T/F: Colloid solution is the preferred solution for resuscitation.

False. In terms of volume required, resuscitation with a colloid solution requires less volume than with a crystalloid solution. However, crystalloid is less expensive and yields no difference in outcome.

❒❒ T/F: Blood products should be given as the initial resuscitation fluid for patients with presumed large blood loss.

False. Non-blood containing fluids can be infused faster and therefore will more quickly support perfusion. Blood, usually in the form of packed red blood cells, should be given early in those patients with presumed large volume blood loss.

❒❒ What are the indications for invasive arterial monitoring?

Need for constant pressure monitoring due to a hemodynamic instability, vasoactive medications and need for frequent arterial blood gas monitoring.

❒❒ What are the preferred and acceptable alternative sites for arterial lines?

The radial artery is preferred due to a very high percentage of collateral flow to hand. Femoral and dorsalis pedis arteries are acceptable.

❐❐ T/F: Non-invasive arterial pressure measurements are more accurate than direct arterial measurements.

False.

❐❐ Do these assumptions hold true in a typical critically ill patient?

No.

❐❐ What are sources of error in these assumptions?

PCWP can be different from LA pressure or LVEDP due to pulmonary venous resistance, valvular abnormalities, positive pressure ventilation, positive end expiratory pressure (PEEP) and catheter placement in lung zones 1 or 2.

❐❐ Compare nitroglycerin and sodium nitroprusside.

Both are vasodilators. Nitroglycerin is a greater venous vasodilator than an arterial vasodilator. In contrast, nitroprusside is primarily an arterial vasodilator. Unlike nitroprusside which is used primarily to manage hypertension and hypertensive crisis, nitroglycerin is also used to treat angina and congestive heart failure. Prolonged use of nitroprusside may cause thiocyanate toxicity.

❐❐ What is the survival benefit of patients with massive PE in shock given thrombolytic therapy compared to heparin alone?

Faster clot lysis and improvement of right ventricular pressures have clearly been shown with thrombolytic agents. No study has ever been designed to demonstrate a survival advantage with thrombolytic agents.

❐❐ What is the treatment for patients with massive PE and hypotension?

Vasopressors, heparin and thrombolytic agents. Embolectomy is a consideration as well.

❐❐ Under which circumstances should a surgical embolectomy be strongly considered?

In any hemodynamically unstable patient with documented massive PE and absolute contraindications to thrombolytic therapy.

❐❐ What are the four Killip classes and how do they relate to mortality?

Killip 1: no heart failure, mortality 8%; Killip 2: mild to moderate failure (bibasilar rales, S3 gallop), mortality 30%; Killip 3: pulmonary edema, mortality 44%; Killip 4: cardiogenic shock, mortality 80 to 100%.

❐❐ What is the classical hemodynamic picture seen in cardiogenic shock?

Low cardiac index, high systemic vascular resistance and high pulmonary capillary wedge pressure (PCWP). The PCWP may not be elevated in right ventricular infarction.

❐❐ How much left ventricular muscle needs to be involved in the setting of an acute myocardial infarction (MI) to cause cardiogenic shock?

40% or more.

❐❐ What are the causes of cardiogenic shock in the setting of an acute MI?

> 40% loss of left ventricular myocardium, ventricular wall rupture, septal rupture, left ventricular aneurysm and acute mitral regurgitation due to papillary muscle rupture/dysfunction.

❒❒ What is the suspected diagnosis if a patient's blood pressure drops significantly with administration of nitroglycerin in the setting of an acute MI?

Inferior wall MI with right ventricular involvement.

❒❒ What is the survival benefit of patients with an acute MI in Killip class 4 after receiving thrombolytic therapy?

Probably none. One study found no difference in 30 day mortality in those treated with thrombolytics compared to placebo (subgroup analysis).

❒❒ What is the treatment of choice for a patient in cardiogenic shock in the setting of an acute MI?

Primary angioplasty.

❒❒ What seems to be the main predictor of survival of patients with cardiogenic shock due to an acute MI?

Successful myocardial reperfusion.

❒❒ How often does a careful clinical examination fail to correctly predict a patient's cardiac output and left ventricular filling pressure?

In 30% of cases an experienced clinician incorrectly predicts those parameters.

❒❒ How often does septal rupture occur in the setting of an acute MI?

1 to 3% of cases. All occur within one week, with 20 to 30% occurring during the first 24 hours.

❒❒ T/F: Septal rupture occurs more commonly in anterior infarcts than in inferior infarcts.

False. The incidence is approximately the same.

❒❒ Why does the posteromedial papillary muscle of the mitral valve rupture most often?

It is perfused from only one of the coronary arteries, whereas the anterolateral is perfused from the left and right coronary circulation.

❒❒ What are predisposing factors for free ventricular wall rupture?

Age >60, peri-infarct hypertension, a large area of infarcted myocardium, a transmural MI and poor collateral circulation.

❒❒ What percentage of deaths in patients with acute MI are caused by ventricular wall rupture?

10 to 15%. Mortality approaches 100%. 84% of the ruptures occur within the first week and 33% within the first 24 hours.

❒❒ How often is right ventricular (RV) involvement seen in patients with inferior acute MI?

40% of cases.

❒❒ What is the incidence of pure right ventricular MI?

2%.

❒❒ What is a simple way of predicting RV dysfunction in the setting of an acute inferior MI?

Elevation of the ST segment in lead V3R is seen only in patients with RV dysfunction. One study found that no patient with normal RV ejection fraction had this finding whereas all patients with ST elevation had RV ejection fractions of < 40%.

❒❒ What is the first line treatment of a patient in cardiogenic shock due to RV infarction?

Aggressive volume replacement as the right ventricle is "volume sensitive." Treatment may need to be guided by pulmonary artery catheter measurements.

❒❒ What is the role of anti-mediator therapy in septic shock?

Anti-mediator therapy has been most extensively studied in septic shock. At this time, none of the studied agents appear to clearly improve patient outcome.

❒❒ How should cardiac output (CO) values be interpreted during shock resuscitation?

CO is the total systemic blood flow. Normal or high values do not exclude cardiac dysfunction and do not assure matching of systemic or regional metabolic demands. Thus, CO determinations should be interpreted in combination with other hemodynamic and metabolic indicators.

❒❒ What is a common electrolyte abnormality associated with transfusion of packed red blood cells?

Hypocalcemia secondary to citrate toxicity. Citrate, when rapidly infused, binds ionized calcium and therefore decreases the calcium level. Hyperkalemia may also develop with rapid packed red blood cell transfusion, especially if the patient is in renal failure or if the blood products are old.

❒❒ What are the determinants of stroke volume?

Preload, contractility and afterload.

❒❒ How would you calculate systemic vascular resistance (SVR)?

$$SVR = \frac{MAP - CVP}{C.O.} \times 80 \left[\frac{dyne - sec}{cm^5}\right]$$

❒❒ How would you calculate pulmonary vascular resistance (PVR)?

$$PVR = \frac{PAP - PAOP}{C.O.} \times 80 \left[\frac{dyne - sec}{cm^5}\right]$$

❒❒ What is afterload?

Afterload is either ventricular wall tension during systole or arterial impedance to ejection. Wall tension is usually described as the pressure the ventricle must overcome to reduce cavity size.

❒❒ What is the baroreceptor reflex?

Increase in blood pressure stimulates peripheral baroreceptors located at the bifurcation of the common carotid arteries and the aortic arch. These baroreceptors then send afferent signals to the brainstem circulatory centers via the glossopharyngeal and vagus nerves, allowing an increase in vagal tone and, consequently, vasodilatation and a decrease in heart rate.

CARDIOVASCULAR PEARLS

The life so short, the craft so long to learn.
Hippocrates, c. 460-357 B.C.

❑❑ What is the most common symptom of aortic dissection?

Interscapular back pain.

❑❑ What is the most common side effect of esmolol, labetalol, and bretylium?

Hypotension.

❑❑ What side effect is expected with too rapid an infusion of procainamide?

Hypotension. Other side effects include: myocardial depression, QRS/QT prolongation, V-fib, and torsade de pointes.

❑❑ Adverse drug effects of lidocaine?

Drowsiness, nausea, vertigo, confusion, ataxia, tinnitus, muscle twitching, respiratory depression, and psychosis.

❑❑ What are the three stages of CXR findings in CHF?

1st - PAWP 12-18 mmHg. Blood flow increases in upper lung fields (cephalization of pulmonary vessels).
2nd - PAWP 18 -25 mmHg. Interstitial edema with blurred edges of blood vessels and Kerley A and B lines.
3rd - PAWP > 25. Fluid exudes into alveoli with generation of the classic butterfly pattern of perihilar infiltrates.

❑❑ Do nitrates affect predominantly preload or afterload?

Mostly preload.

❑❑ Does hydralazine affect preload or afterload?

Afterload.

❑❑ Do prazosin, captopril, and nifedipine affect predominantly preload or afterload?

Afterload.

❑❑ When is dobutamine used in CHF?

Potent inotrope with some vasodilation activity, used when heart failure is not accompanied by severe hypotension.

❑❑ When is dopamine selected in CHF?

Vasoconstrictor and positive inotrope, used if shock is present.

❑❑ Causes of MAT?

COPD is a common cause. CHF, sepsis, and methylxanthine toxicity are other causes, particularly among the elderly. Treat the underlying disorder. Magnesium, verapamil, and ß-adrenergic agents are thought to be helpful.

❑❑ How is atrial flutter treated?

Initiate A-V nodal blockade with ß-adrenergic or calcium channel blockers or with digoxin. If necessary, in a stable patient, attempt chemical cardioversion with a class IA agent such as procainamide or quinidine after digitalization. If such treatment fails, or if patient is unstable and requires immediate electrocardioversion, do so with 25-50 J.

❑❑ What are the causes of atrial fibrillation?

Hypertension, rheumatic heart disease, pneumonia, thyrotoxicosis and ischemic heart disease are common causes. Pericarditis, EtOH intoxication, PE, CHF and COPD are other causes.

❑❑ How is atrial fibrillation treated?

Control rate with digitalis or verapamil then convert with procainamide, quinidine, or verapamil. Synchronized cardioversion at 100 to 200 J in an unstable patient requiring cardioversion. In a stable patient with a-fib of unclear duration anticoagulation for 2-3 wk should be considered prior to chemical or electrical cardioversion.

❑❑ Causes of SVT?

Ectopic SVT may be due to digitalis toxicity (25% of digitalis induced arrhythmias), pericarditis, MI, COPD, preexcitation syndromes, mitral valve prolapse, rheumatic heart disease, pneumonia, and EtOH.

❑❑ How is SVT caused by digitalis toxicity treated?

Stop digitalis, treat hypokalemia. Give Mg or phenytoin. Provide digoxin specific antibodies in the unstable patient. Avoid cardioversion.

❑❑ Treatment of stable SVT not caused by dig toxicity?

Adenosine, verapamil, ß-blockers, vagal maneuvers, Mg.

❑❑ Describe the key features of Mobitz I (Wenckebach) 2° AV block.

Progressive prolongation of the PR interval until atrial impulse is not conducted. If symptomatic, atropine and transcutaneous/transvenous pacing.

❑❑ Describe the features and treatment of Mobitz II 2° AV block.

Constant PR interval. One or more beats fail to conduct. Treat with atropine and transcutaneous/transvenous pacing.

❑❑ What artery is most commonly associated with embolism in mesenteric ischemia?

Superior mesenteric artery.

❑❑ Name 5 causes of mesenteric ischemia.

Arterial thrombosis at sites of atherosclerotic plaques, emboli from left atrium in patients with a-fib or rheumatic heart disease who are not anticoagulated, arterial embolism most commonly to the superior mesenteric artery, insufficient arterial flow, and venous thrombosis.

❑❑ **What is the most common source for acute mesenteric ischemia.**

Arterial embolism 40-50%. Source is usually the heart, most often from a mural thrombus. Most common point of obstruction is the superior mesenteric artery.

❑❑ **What lab abnormalities are expected in a patient with mesenteric ischemia?**

Leukocytosis >15,000, metabolic acidosis, hemoconcentration, and elevation of phosphate and amylase.

❑❑ **For how long do ST and T changes persist after an episode of pain in unstable angina?**

Up to several hours.

❑❑ **What is the cause of Prinzmetal's variant angina?**

Spasm of epicardial coronary arteries.

❑❑ **Contraindications to ß-blockers?**

CHF, variant angina, AV block, COPD, asthma (relative), bradycardia, hypotension and IDDM.

❑❑ **What percentage of LV myocardium must be damaged to cause cardiogenic shock?**

40%. 25% results in heart failure.

❑❑ **What percentage of MI's are clinically unrecognized?**

About 5 - 10%.

❑❑ **What may a new systolic murmur indicate in a patient with an AMI?**

Ventriculoseptal rupture or mitral regurgitation as a result of papillary muscle rupture or dysfunction.

❑❑ **A non-Q-wave infarction is associated with:**

Non-Q-wave infarctions are more commonly associated with subsequent angina or recurrent infarction. They also have a lower in-hospital mortality than Q-wave MI.

❑❑ **Why do T waves invert in an AMI?**

Infarction or ischemia causes a reversal of the sequence of repolarization (endocardial-to-epicardial as opposed to normal epicardial-to-endocardial).

❑❑ **What ECG changes are seen in a true posterior infarction?**

Large R-wave and ST depression in V1 and V2.

❑❑ **What conduction defects are commonly seen in an AWMI?**

The dangerous kind. Damage to the conducting system results in a Mobitz II 2° or in a 3° AVB.

❑❑ **What conduction defects are commonly seen in an IWMI?**

IWMI affects the autonomic fibers in the atrial septum which increases vagal tone and impairs AV nodal conduction; 1° AV block and Mobitz type I 2° (Wenckebach) AV block are common.

❑❑ **How should PSVT be treated during an AMI?**

Vagal maneuvers, adenosine, or cardioversion. Stable patients may be able to tolerate verapamil or even ß-adrenergic blockers which are negative inotropes.

❑❑ A patient presents 1 day after discharge for an AMI with a new harsh systolic murmur along the left sternal border and pulmonary edema. Diagnosis?

Ventricular septal rupture. Diagnosis is confirmed with Swan-Ganz catheterization or echo. Treatment includes nitroprusside for afterload reduction and possible intra-aortic balloon pump followed by surgical repair.

❑❑ In a patient who has suffered an AMI, when would cardiac rupture be expected?

50% in the 1st 5 d and 90% within the 1st 14 d post MI.

❑❑ What type of infarct commonly leads to papillary muscle dysfunction?

IWMI. Signs and symptoms include a mild transient systolic murmur and pulmonary edema.

❑❑ A patient presents 2 wk post AMI with chest pain, fever, and pleuropericarditis. A pleural effusion is seen on CXR. Diagnosis?

Dressler's (postmyocardial infarction) syndrome which is caused by an immunologic reaction to myocardial antigens.

❑❑ Can patients be retreated with streptokinase or APSAC?

Antibodies persist for 6 mo. Retreatment is not recommended.

❑❑ What type of thrombolytic agent is fibrin specific?

Tissue plasminogen activator. It is a human protein with no antigenic properties.

❑❑ What maneuvers will increase hypertrophic cardiomyopathy murmurs?

Valsalva, standing, and amyl nitrate.

❑❑ What maneuvers will decrease hypertrophic cardiomyopathic murmurs?

Handgrip, squatting and leg elevation in the supine patient.

❑❑ What is the most common symptom of acute pericarditis?

Sharp or stabbing retrosternal or precordial chest pain. Pain increases when supine and decreases when sitting-up and leaning forward. Pain may be increased with movement and deep breaths. Other symptoms include fever, dyspnea described as pain with inspiration, and dysphagia.

❑❑ What physical findings are associated with acute pericarditis?

Pericardial friction rub is the most common. Rub is best heard at the left sternal border or apex in a sitting leaning forward position. Other findings include fever and tachycardia.

❑❑ What ECG changes are seen in acute pericarditis?

ST segment elevation in the precordial leads, especially V5 and V6 and in lead I. PR depression is seen in leads II, aVF, V4-V6.

❑❑ **What percentage of patients with angiogram proven pulmonary embolism have an initial ventilation-perfusion scan reported as low probability.**

12%!

❑❑ **What are the most common symptoms and signs of PE?**

CP (88%).
Tachypnea (92%).
Dyspnea (84%).
Anxiety (59%).
Fever (43%).
Tachycardia (44%).
DVT (32%).
Hypotension (25%).
Syncope (13%).

❑❑ **Can a patient with a PE have a PaO_2 greater than 90 mmHg?**

About 5% have a PaO_2 > 90 mmHg.

❑❑ **What is the most common CXR finding in PE?**

Elevated dome of one hemidiaphragm as a result of decreased lung volume observed in 50% of PEs. Other common findings include pleural effusions, atelectasis, and pulmonary infiltrates.

❑❑ **What are two relatively specific findings in PE on CXR?**

Hampton's Hump - Area of lung consolidation with a rounded border facing the hilus.
Westermark's sign - Dilated pulmonary outflow tract ipsilateral to the emboli with decreased perfusion distal to the lesion.

❑❑ **What does a normal perfusion scan rule out?**

Rules out a PE. An abnormal scan can be caused by PE, asthma, emphysema, bronchitis, pneumonia, pleural effusion, carcinoma, CHF, and atelectasis.

❑❑ **What does normal ventilation with decreased perfusion suggest?**

PE.

❑❑ **What are some of the indications for pulmonary angiography in a patient thought to have a PE?**

1. Patients at high risk for bleeding complications with anticoagulation.
2. Negative test for DVT and low or medium probability lung scans.
3. Unstable patients for whom fibrinolytic therapy is being considered.

❑❑ **What is the most common cause of mitral stenosis?**

Rheumatic heart disease. The most common initial symptom is dyspnea.

❑❑ **What is the earliest chest x-ray finding seen with mitral stenosis?**

Straightening of the left heart border as a result of left atrial enlargement.

❑❑ **What physical findings may be found with mitral stenosis?**

Prominent a-wave, early-systolic left parasternal lift, 1st heart sound is loud and snapping, and early-diastolic opening snap with a low-pitched, mid-diastolic rumble that crescendos into S1.

❑❑ **What are the most common causes of acute mitral regurgitation?**

Rupture of the chordae tendineae, rupture of the papillary muscles, or perforation of the valve leaflets. Common causes include AMI and infectious endocarditis.

❑❑ **What are the two most common causes of valvular aortic stenosis?**

Rheumatic heart disease or congenital bicuspid valve.

❑❑ **What triad of symptoms is characteristic of aortic stenosis?**

Syncope, angina, and left heart failure. As the disease progresses, systolic BP decreases and pulse pressure narrows.

❑❑ **What are the signs and symptoms of acute aortic regurgitation?**

Dyspnea, tachycardia, tachypnea, and chest pain. Causes include: infectious endocarditis, acute rheumatic fever, trauma, spontaneous rupture of valve leaflets, or aortic dissection.

❑❑ **What physical findings are characteristic of chronic aortic regurgitation?**

Bobbing of the head with systole, bounding carotid pulse (water-hammer), pistol shot sound, the to-and-fro murmur of Duroziez's sign over the femoral arteries, and capillary pulsation of the nailbeds (Quincke's sign).

❑❑ **What is the most common cause of tricuspid stenosis?**

Rheumatic heart disease.

❑❑ **A patient presents to the ED one month after placement of a mechanical prosthetic valve with fever, chills, and a leukocytosis. Endocarditis is suspected. What type of bacterium is most common?**

Staph aureus or *Staph epidermidis.*

❑❑ **Define a hypertensive emergency.**

Increased BP with associated end-organ dysfunction or damage. A controlled drop in BP over one hour should be attempted.

❑❑ **Define a hypertensive urgency.**

BP elevated to dangerous level, typically a diastolic greater than 115 mmHg. Gradually reduce BP over 24 to 48 hours.

❑❑ **Define uncomplicated hypertension.**

Diastolic BP less than 115 mmHg with no symptoms of end-organ damage. Does not require acute treatment.

❑❑ **What lab findings would suggest a hypertensive emergency?**

UA - RBCs, red cell casts, and proteinuria.
BUN and CR - elevated.
X-ray - Aortic dissection, pulmonary edema, or coarctation of the aorta.
ECG - LVH and cardiac ischemia.

❒❒ **What are the signs and symptoms of hypertensive encephalopathy?**

Nausea, vomiting, headache, lethargy, coma, blindness, nerve palsies, hemiparesis, aphasia, retinal hemorrhage, cotton wool spots, exudates, sausage linking, and papilledema. Treat with labetalol or sodium nitroprusside, lower the mean arterial pressure to approximately 120 mmHg.

❒❒ **In general, how quickly should severe elevations in BP (>210/130) be treated?**

Initial diastolic decrease of 20 - 30% over 30 to 60 min.

❒❒ **At what point does magnesium sulfate become toxic?**

Loss of reflexes occurs at levels >8 mEq/L and respiratory arrest at levels >12 mEq/L.

❒❒ **What drugs should be used to lower BP in a patient with thoracic aortic dissection?**

Sodium nitroprusside in combination with propranolol, or labetalol.

❒❒ **A patient presents with a history of episodic elevations in BP. She complains of headache, diarrhea, and skin flushing. Diagnosis?**

Pheochromocytoma.

❒❒ **A patient with a psychiatric history taking a MAO inhibitor, has ingested a 12 pack of beer with a meal of pickled herring and a nice aged cheese. He complains of severe headache. On exam, BP is elevated. A diagnosis of acute hypertension is made secondary to hyperstimulation of the adrenergic receptors. Treatment?**

An α- and ß-adrenergic antagonist such as labetalol.

❒❒ **What drug can be used for all hypertensive emergencies?**

Sodium nitroprusside (not the DOC for eclampsia). Sodium nitroprusside works through production of cGMP which relaxes smooth muscle. This results in decreased preload and afterload, decreased oxygen demand, slight increased heart rate with no change in myocardial blood flow, cardiac output, or renal blood flow. Duration of action is 1 to 2 min. Sometimes, ß-blockade is required to treat rebound tachycardia.

❒❒ **What is the most common complication of nitroprusside?**

Hypotension. Thiocyanate toxicity with blurred vision, tinnitus, change in mental status, muscle weakness, and seizures is seen more often in patients with renal failure and after prolonged infusions. Cyanide toxicity is uncommon, it may occur with hepatic dysfunction, after prolonged infusions, and in rates greater than 10 μg/kg per minute.

❒❒ **A patient presents with sudden onset chest pain and back pain. Further work-up reveals an ischemic right leg. Diagnosis?**

Suspect an acute aortic dissection when chest or back pain is associated with ischemic or neurologic defects.

❒❒ **What physical findings are suspicious for acute aortic dissection?**

BP differences between arms, cardiac tamponade, and aortic insufficiency murmur.
An abnormal ECG may also be present.

❑❑ What CXR findings occur with a thoracic aortic aneurysm?

Change in appearance of aorta, mediastinal widening, hump in the aortic arch, pleural effusion (most common on the left), and extension of the aortic shadow.

❑❑ How are Stanford type A and B aortic dissections defined and treated?

Type A - Ascending, proximal to left subclavian (DeBakey I & II) - surgery.
Type B - Descending, distal to left subclavian (DeBakey III) - usually medical treatment.

❑❑ A 74 year-old male presents with acute onset testicular pain. Ecchymosis is present in the groin and scrotal sac. Diagnosis?

Ruptured aortic or iliac artery aneurysm.

❑❑ In a patient with an abdominal mass and a suspected ruptured AAA, what x-ray study should be ordered?

None. They should go to the OR immediately. About 60% of AAA will have calcification and can be visualized on a supine or lateral abdominal x-ray.

❑❑ What percentage of patients beyond the age of 80 experience CP with an AMI?

50% experience CP. 20% experience diaphoresis, stroke, syncope, and/or acute confusion.

❑❑ In a patient with substantial aortic stenosis, what murmur would be expected?

Prolonged, harsh, loud (grade IV, V, or VI) systolic murmur.

❑❑ What historical findings suggest an embolus vs. a thrombosis in a lower extremity?

Embolus - arrhythmia, valvular disease, MI, no skin changes of chronic arterial insufficiency, and no symptoms in the opposite extremity.
Thrombosis - opposite extremity shows evidence of chronic arterial occlusive disease with history of rest pain claudication, etc.

❑❑ How is thrombus vs. embolus distinguished on arteriogram?

Thrombus - tapering lumen. Embolus - sharp cutoff.

❑❑ What is the risk of PE in a patient with an axillary or subclavian vein thrombus?

The risk of PE is about 15%.

❑❑ Rheumatic heart disease is the <u>most</u> <u>common</u> cause of stenosis of what 3 heart valves?

Mitral, aortic (along with congenital bicuspid valve) and tricuspid.

❑❑ A patient presents to the emergency department with a neurologic deficit and chest pain. Other than MI, what diagnosis must be excluded?

Aortic dissection.

❑❑ What is a mnemonic for absolute contraindications to thrombolytics?

Altered-mental status, Annie-aneurysm, Accidentally-CVA (in the last 6 months), Cut-trauma or surgery (in the last 2 weeks), Surgery to the brain, eye, or spinal cord (in the last 8 weeks), Pregnant-self-explanatory, Perry's-pericarditis, PeT-PT as in protime stands for bleeding disorder, Can-cancer in the brain, Stroke-hemorrhagic stroke (ever), Bleed-active bleeding, Malform-A-V malformation, an Allergist's-allergy to the thrombolytic, Head-head trauma.

❏❏ What are the x-ray findings in ARDS?

Diffuse ground-glass-like infiltrates that do not follow anatomical boundaries, usually bilateral.

❏❏ What complications are associated with ARDS?

Barotrauma leading to pneumothorax, pulmonary infection, pulmonary hypertension, multisystem organ failure.

❏❏ What are the three phases of ARDS?

Acute or exudative (up to 6 days), proliferative phase (4 to 10 days), chronic or fibrotic phase (after 7 days).

❏❏ The treatment of choice for patients with supraventricular tachycardia and cardiovascular compromise?

Adenosine, but in the event that vascular access is not available quickly synchronized cardioversion becomes the treatment of choice.

❏❏ When should atropine be used for the treatment of bradycardia?

Only after adequate ventilation and oxygenation have been established, since hypoxemia is a common cause of bradycardia.

❏❏ What percentage of patients with acute myocardial infarction develop cardiogenic shock?

10%.

❏❏ What percentage of patients who are found to have myocardial infarction by other objective means, such as cardiac enzymes or radionuclide imaging studies, have normal initial ECGs?

10%.

❏❏ A 65 year-old female presents to the hospital with sudden crushing chest discomfort and moderate shortness of breath. Her initial ECG reveals 2mm ST depression in leads V1-V4 with inverted T waves. She has bibasilar rales in the lower half of both lungs on auscultation. CXR reveals moderate pulmonary edema. Serial ECGs and CPKs confirm a non-Q wave myocardial infarction. With diuretics, her pulmonary edema resolves within 24 hours. What is the most appropriate management strategy at this point?

Cardiac catheterization with coronary angiography. A non-Q wave MI that results in pulmonary edema signifies a large amount of myocardium at risk for reinfarction within the next year.

❏❏ What two groups of patients are more likely to present with "silent" myocardial infarction?

Patients with diabetes mellitus and the elderly.

❏❏ Moderate to heavy physical exertion and emotional stress or excitement are temporally related to the onset of symptoms in what percentage of patients with acute myocardial infarction?

About 50%.

❐❐ What percentage of patients with confirmed acute myocardial infarction, determined by other objective means, have a normal initial ECG?

10%.

❐❐ What is the mortality rate of patients under the age of 40 with their first myocardial infarction?

2-4%.

❐❐ What is the mortality rate of patients over age 80 with their first myocardial infarction?

25-35%.

❐❐ Which age group has the greatest reduction in mortality following the administration of thrombolytic therapy in the presence of an acute myocardial infarction?

Patients over the age of 65, and more specifically, those patients over age 75.

❐❐ Previously, there had been concerns over increased likelihood of intracranial hemorrhage following the administration of thrombolytic therapy in patients over age 75. What are the respective incidences of intracranial hemorrhage following the administration of thrombolytic therapy in patients under age 75 and over age 75?

The overall incidence of intracranial hemorrhage in patients under age 75 is 1%, slightly higher with t-PA, as opposed to streptokinase or APSAC. The overall incidence of intracranial hemorrhage in patients over age 75 is 1.3%, again slightly higher with t-PA, as opposed to streptokinase or APSAC.

❐❐ What are the two most common and serious side effects of streptokinase and APSAC?

Hypotension and hypersensitivity reaction, which is antigen mediated and manifested by vomiting, itching and swelling.

❐❐ What is the recurrence rate of thrombosis following administration of t-PA without the concomitant use of intravenous heparin?

20-30%.

❐❐ What is the recurrence rate of thrombosis following administration of streptokinase without intravenous heparin following the completion of streptokinase therapy?

15-20%.

❐❐ What is the rethrombosis rate following the administration of APSAC in the absence of subsequent intravenous heparin use?

10%.

❐❐ What is the rationale for intravenous heparin administration being started concomitantly with t-PA administration?

Because the plasma clearance time of t-PA is 4-8 minutes, the coronary rethrombosis rate in the absence of intravenous heparin is significantly increased and ranges between 20-30%. With concomitant heparin administration and continued heparinization for at least 24 hours following t-PA therapy, the coronary rethrombosis rate is reduced to approximately 5-10%.

❑❑ What is the 90-minute infarct-related coronary artery patency rate following the administration of "front-loaded" or accelerated intravenous t-PA in acute myocardial infarction, assuming concomitant administration of intravenous heparin and oral aspirin?

80-90%.

❑❑ What is the 90-minute infarct-related coronary artery patency rate following the administration of intravenous streptokinase in acute myocardial infarction, assuming concomitant aspirin administration?

55-70%.

❑❑ What is the 90-minute infarct-related coronary artery patency rate following the administration of intravenous APSAC in acute myocardial infarction, assuming concomitant aspirin administration?

70-80%.

❑❑ In the GUSTO-1 trial, what was the percentage of grade TIMI-3 (normal) flow occurring in infarct-related arteries following the administration of accelerated t-PA with intravenous heparin, compared to streptokinase and intravenous heparin?

TIMI-3 flow was present at 90 minutes in 54% of infarct-related arteries with accelerated t-PA, compared to 32% of infarct-related arteries in the streptokinase group.

❑❑ T/F: The frequency of hemorrhagic stroke following the administration of t-PA was statistically similar to the frequency of hemorrhagic stroke following the administration of streptokinase in patients under age 70.

True.

❑❑ T/F: The frequency of hemorrhagic stroke following the administration of t-PA was statistically similar to the frequency of hemorrhagic stroke following the administration of streptokinase in patients over age 75.

False. The incidence of hemorrhagic stroke following the administration of t-PA was statistically higher than that following the administration of streptokinase. The overall incidence of hemorrhagic stroke in patients over age 75 receiving streptokinase is 1.1%, and 1.5% in patients over age 75 receiving t-PA.

❑❑ Which of the thrombolytic agents, administered to patients with acute myocardial infarction, preserves left ventricular function the most?

Except for the GUSTO-1 trial, left ventricular function, measured within the first week, as well as after one month, was similar, regardless of the thrombolytic agent used. In the GUSTO-1 trial, left ventricular function paralleled the patency rates at 90 minutes, and the group that received accelerated t-PA and intravenous heparin had slightly better left ventricular function, post-infarct, than the group that received streptokinase or the combination of streptokinase and standard dose t-PA.

❑❑ Which adjunctive pharmacologic therapies have been shown to improve both short-term and long-term survival following acute myocardial infarction?

Aspirin, beta-blockers and ACE inhibitors, when given within the first 24 hours after the onset of symptoms, have all been shown to improve short-term survival following an acute myocardial infarction. Aspirin, beta-blockers and ACE inhibitors, when started between 24 hours and seven days following an acute myocardial infarction, have been shown to improve long-term survival following an acute myocardial infarction. Intravenous heparin, when administered with or immediately after thrombolytic therapy, has been shown to improve short-term survival following an acute myocardial infarction. Calcium channel blockers, nitroglycerin or nitrates, and intravenous or oral magnesium have not been shown to improve either short-term or long-term survival in acute myocardial infarction.

❑❑ A 57 year-old gentleman with hypertension and diabetes mellitus presents to your hospital's Emergency Department with abrupt onset of crushing substernal chest pressure radiating to the jaw. His blood pressure is 75/40, his pulse is 132, his respiratory rate is 36. His lung exam reveals bibasilar rales in the lower half of both lungs, and he has both severe JVD and an S3 gallop. His electrocardiogram shows 4 mm ST segment elevation in leads V1 through V6. He has never had a myocardial infarction in the past. His symptoms began 45 minutes ago. What should be the favored treatment regimen for this patient?

If your hospital has a catheterization laboratory and it is unoccupied, this patient should undergo immediate coronary angiography with immediate PTCA of the culprit vessel. If your hospital does not have a catheterization lab, thrombolytic therapy should be immediately administered and hemodynamic support with an intra-aortic balloon counterpulsation should be strongly considered.

❑❑ A 63 year-old gentleman presents to your hospital with substernal chest tightness of 45 minutes duration. His electrocardiogram reveals 1.5 mm ST depression in leads I, aVL, and V4-V6. Should you give him thrombolytic therapy if he has no contraindications?

No. Patients with non-Q wave myocardial infarctions and those with unstable angina, who eventually rule out for myocardial infarction, do not appear to benefit from thrombolytic therapy. These patients should be started on intravenous heparin, given aspirin, and if they do not have pulmonary edema on initial presentation, should be started on Diltiazem.

❑❑ What is the acute mortality of patients with non-Q wave myocardial infarction?

2-3%, as opposed to 10% for Q wave infarction.

❑❑ What percentage of patients with acute myocardial infarction will develop transient supraventricular arrhythmias?

33%.

❑❑ What percentage of patients with acute myocardial infarction develop atrial fibrillation?

10-15%.

❑❑ What is the preferred agent of choice in the treatment of atrial fibrillation occurring in the setting of acute myocardial infarction?

Beta-blockers. Alternative agents, such as procainamide or amiodarone, are particularly useful in converting atrial fibrillation to sinus rhythm.

❑❑ A 60 year-old woman presents to your hospital with substernal chest tightness and her electrocardiogram reveals acute ST elevation in the anterior leads, consistent with an acute myocardial infarction. She is given aspirin, t-PA, beta-blockers and heparin. She is hemodynamically stable and not in heart failure. Her cardiac monitor shows 4-6 PVCs per minute with rare couplets. Should she receive lidocaine "prophylactically"?

No. The risk-benefit ratio is unfavorable in this setting, and occasional PVCs are an unreliable predictor of ventricular fibrillation following an acute myocardial infarction. Lidocaine may also block the "escape" rhythm of accelerated idioventricular rhythm that occurs with coronary reperfusion, thus, creating a potentially life-threatening event.

❑❑ What is the percentage of rupture of the free wall of the left ventricle occurring in patients who die as a result of acute myocardial infarction?

10%. This event occurs between 1 and 5 days following infarction and is almost always fatal.

❑❑ A 66 year-old woman has sudden onset of substernal chest pressure and comes to the Emergency Department. Her electrocardiogram and cardiac enzymes confirm an acute anterior myocardial infarction. On admission, she is hemodynamically stable, but on day 3, she develops sudden shortness of breath and she is noted to have a blood pressure of 85/50. On physical exam, she is noted to have an loud apical holosystolic murmur, bibasilar rales and an S3 gallop at the apex. A Swan-Ganz pulmonary artery catheter is placed and the pulmonary capillary wedge pressure tracing shows prominent V waves. What is the diagnosis?

Partial or total rupture of a papillary muscle with severe mitral insufficiency.

❑❑ In the above patient, what is the best way to confirm the diagnosis?

Two-dimensional and color flow Doppler echocardiography.

❑❑ In the above patient, what is the preferred treatment?

Aggressive vasodilator therapy, insertion of an intra-aortic balloon counterpulsation device and then emergent repair of the papillary muscle and mitral valve apparatus. Mortality with medical treatment alone in this setting is 80-90%.

❑❑ What is the treatment of a patient with right ventricular infarction who is hypotensive?

Volume expansion to an optimal LV filling pressure, then cautious administration of intravenous dobutamine.

❑❑ What percentage of patients with acute myocardial infarction develop left ventricular aneurysms?

10%.

❑❑ Where are most left ventricular aneurysms located and what is the cause?

80% of left ventricular aneurysms occur in the anterior-apical segment of the left ventricle. They are discrete, thin, bulging, non-contractile segments of the left ventricle that are akinetic or dyskinetic during systole. Their development is related to ventricular remodeling and they result mostly from occlusion of the left anterior descending coronary artery.

❑❑ What are some of the complications that may arise from the development of left ventricular aneurysms?

Development of mural thrombi occurs in about one-half of patients with acute anterior-apical Q wave infarctions, with the resultant five-fold increase in the likelihood of embolic events. Other complications include congestive heart failure and serious ventricular arrhythmias.

❑❑ What percentage of patients with acute myocardial infarction have a clinically evident embolic event?

About 4%, most often during the first week following infarction.

❑❑ Should anticoagulation be routinely administered to patients with acute myocardial infarction?

For large anterior myocardial infarctions, it is currently recommended to administer intravenous heparin, until discharge, in a dose sufficient to prolong the APPT to 1.5 to 2 times normal. Those patients with a mural thrombus or a large akinetic apical segment should be treated with warfarin for three to six months. Long-term anticoagulation is generally indicated in patients with a dilated, severely hypokinetic left ventricle.

❑❑ **Pericarditis occurs in what percentage of patients with acute myocardial infarction?**

10-20%, as defined by the presence of a friction rub.

❑❑ **What is the significance of infarct-related pericarditis?**

Patients with infarct-related pericarditis usually have larger infarcts, have lower post-MI ejection fractions, and a higher incidence of congestive heart failure and serious ventricular arrhythmias. Patients with infarct-related pericarditis and/or the presence of pericardial effusion have a higher mortality, again related to infarct size.

❑❑ **What is the most important prognostic determinant following acute myocardial infarction?**

Infarct size.

❑❑ **What is the most important post-infarct diagnostic strategy following acute myocardial infarction?**

Pre-discharge non-invasive testing to risk stratify patients into those low-risk and those who are at high risk to develop non-fatal or fatal reinfarction or sudden death from arrhythmias. Many advocate pre-discharge submaximal treadmill testing, particularly in those who received thrombolytic therapy, so long as the patient did not have post-infarct angina, congestive heart failure, hypotension or serious arrhythmias. Those patients with post-infarct angina, congestive heart failure, post-infarct silent ischemia as measured by ST depression and serious arrhythmias, should undergo pre-discharge cardiac catheterization and/or further intervention (e.g., antiarrhythmic therapy, PTCA or CABG). Some advocate symptom-limited treadmill exercise testing, instead of submaximal testing, before discharge, and there is good evidence that this is safe. Symptom-limited stress testing, either on a treadmill, or pharmacologic stress, with supplementary imaging techniques using technetium-99m sestamibi or thallium, or echocardiography, should be carried out between 10 days and 6 weeks following acute myocardial infarction in those patients deemed low-risk at discharge. Those patients with abnormal post-infarct stress tests should be referred for cardiac catheterization and, if warranted, revascularization.

❑❑ **What percentage of patients who received thrombolytic therapy for acute myocardial infarction have single vessel disease and a total occlusion of the infarct-related artery?**

15%.

❑❑ **What percentage of patients who received thrombolytic therapy for acute myocardial infarction have a patent infarct-related artery with a less than 50% stenosis?**

15%.

❑❑ **What percentage of patients who received thrombolytic therapy for acute myocardial infarction have single vessel disease and > 50% stenosis in the infarct-related artery?**

35%.

❑❑ **What percentage of patients who received thrombolytic therapy for acute myocardial infarction have a patent infarct related vessel and 2- or 3-vessel disease?**

30%.

❑❑ **What percentage of patients with acute myocardial infarction, who receive thrombolytic therapy, have left main disease and a patent infarct-related artery?**

5%.

❑❑ **What is the concept of "stunned myocardium"?**

This refers to muscle that is hypocontractile as a result of a brief ischemic insult but is still viable. In this situation, progressive recovery of contractile function following reperfusion may occur several hours to weeks after the ischemic insult. This recovery occurs without revascularization from PTCA or CABG.

❒❒ What is the concept of "hibernating myocardium"?

Hibernating myocardium refers to a chronically hypoperfused and hypocontractile left ventricular segment that improves functionally only after coronary revascularization.

❒❒ Are thrombolytic agents effective in non-Q wave MI?

No, there is no evidence to support their use. In fact, some published data suggest that their use may be detrimental.

❒❒ What is the prognosis of patients presenting with Q wave MI complicated by acute mitral regurgitation?

Prognosis is quite compromised with an approximate one-year survival of only 50%.

❒❒ A 68 year-old man with a history of angina at three blocks exertion presents with onset of chest pain typical of his angina occurring after breakfast. He says this is his usual pain except that it has never occurred at rest. Physical exam is unremarkable, and the ECG reveals only non-specific findings. His pain is relieved with IV nitroglycerine and a dose of metoprolol. Laboratory findings: Total CK 110 (upper limit of normal is 150), CK-MB is 10% (upper limit of normal is 6%). What is the patient's prognosis?

The patient appears to have unstable angina and does not meet the criteria for thrombolytic therapy. However, the CK findings suggest he actually developed a non-Q wave MI. The diagnosis remains unclear in this circumstance. Whatever the diagnosis, the prognosis is <u>worse</u> in these patients compared to that of patients with UA without CK-MB elevation. Thus, these patients are probably better off if evaluated as if the diagnosis is non-Q wave MI.

❒❒ A 77 year-old man presents complaining of chest pain. He states that he was playing racquet-ball, and slipped and hit his head on the wall. After this he noted the onset of chest pain radiating to the arm. A hot shower did not relieve his symptoms. He notes that he has continued to have dull ache in his chest. He also reports an episode of diaphoresis after the shower and mild nausea. ECG reveals acute anterior wall MI. What would you do to treat him?

Administer aspirin immediately. The choice for additional therapy is complicated by the presence of head trauma. In the proper setting, direct PTCA is the treatment of choice, since it produces higher TIMI-3 flow rates and defines the coronary anatomy, with lower stroke risk. The benefits of direct PTCA over thrombolytic therapy, while still debated, required a high volume operator and access to a lab within 60-90 minutes. If direct PTCA was not available for this patient, the decision to give thrombolytic therapy is a difficult one.

❒❒ A 58 year-old woman without past medical history presents with complaints of one day of dull ache in the center of her chest that is unrelieved with aspirin or antacids. She states that the day prior to admission she had about three hours of severe discomfort in the chest associated with sweating which resolved spontaneously and she is now left with the symptoms described. Her blood pressure is 120/80, pulse is 100 and she is mildly diaphoretic. A pan-systolic murmur is heard at the left sternal border. Her lungs are clear. ECG reveals Q-Waves in leads VI-V4. Over the next twelve hours, you note that she becomes cold and clammy to palpation with signs of decreased peripheral perfusion. Her lungs remain clear. What is the diagnosis?

Acute ventricular septal defect. Patients with acute mitral regurgitation usually have pulmonary congestion, making this diagnosis less likely. Risk factors for development of VSD include: female gender and hypertension. Despite pathological reports that VSD most often occurs about day 4 post-myocardial infarction, clinical observations suggest that the risk is higher in the first 24 hours. Definitive treatment is surgical, but operative mortality ranges from 20 to 70%. The diagnosis should be confirmed by echocardiography. Following this, vasodilator therapy with nitroprusside and insertion of an intra-aortic balloon-pump and Swan-Ganz catheter should be performed.

❑❑ What affects ventricular remodeling?

Ventricular remodeling is the change in size, shape and thickness of both the infarcted and non-infarcted regions of myocardium. The primary factors determining remodeling are: infarct size, scar formation and left ventricular filling pressure. The contribution of the latter may be part of the explanation of the effect of ace inhibitors in preserving left ventricular function when administered in the peri-infarct setting.

❑❑ What is infarct expansion?

An increase in the size of the infarct zone unrelated to additional myocardial necrosis. Causes may include slippage of the muscle bundles, disruption of the normal cellular array and tissue loss in the infarct zone. This occurs almost exclusively in transmural MI, is more common in anterior infarction, and the degree of expansion may be related to pre-existing wall thickness (hypertrophy may be protective). Infarct expansion has been shown to be associated with increased mortality and increased incidence of non-fatal complications.

❑❑ What are the major precipitants of AMI?

In over half of patients with AMI, no precipitant can be identified. However, some contributory factors which have been identified include emotional stress, surgical procedures, neurological disturbances and perhaps extreme physical exertion. Circadian changes in plasma catecholamines and cortisol may also play a role.

❑❑ What is the most common presenting symptoms of AMI?

Chest pain. Unlike aortic dissection, this pain often waxes and wanes, and over time will become severe. It usually lasts greater than 30 minutes and is frequently described as crushing, constricting, or as pressure. The pain is typically retrosternal and frequently radiates to the jaw and the ulnar aspect of the left arm. In some patients, particularly the elderly, AMI may present as a symptoms of acute left ventricular failure rather than chest pain.

❑❑ What are the other typical symptoms of AMI?

Diaphoresis, apprehension, sense of doom, nausea and vomiting, which occur in greater than 50% of patients with transmural infarction. These latter symptoms, and perhaps the others to some extent, occur presumably due to the Bezold-Jarisch reflex. Nausea and vomiting occur more frequently in inferior myocardial infarction.

❑❑ What are the chief differential diagnoses of AMI?

Acute pericarditis, aortic dissection and acute GI illness. Acute pulmonary embolism and costochondritis are also frequently considered in the differential.

❑❑ What are the most common atypical presentations of AMI?

Congestive heart failure, angina without a prolonged or severe episode and atypical pain location.

❑❑ What is a silent AMI?

Population studies suggest that 20 to 60% of non-fatal MIs are unrecognized by the patient and are found on subsequent routine ECG. About one-half of these MIs are truly silent with no identifiable symptoms recalled by the patient. Unrecognized or silent infarction occurs more often in patients without previous anginal syndromes and is more common in diabetics and hypertensive patients.

❒❒ What are the most common physical findings in AMI?

There really aren't any, and findings depend upon the absence or presence of acute complications such as congestive heart failure, acute mitral regurgitation or cardiogenic shock. Most patients will appear to be in some distress. Of note, a fourth heart sound is almost universally present in patients with acute MI.

❒❒ Describe the characteristic pattern of creatine phosphokinase (CK-MB) elevation in AMI.

CK exceeds normal levels in 4 to 8 hours after onset of MI. The mean peak for CK is 24 hours, but can range from 8 to 58 hours. Peak levels occur earlier in patients who receive reperfusion therapy, with mean peak CK rise occurring at approximately 12 hours. In general, CK levels normalize 3 to 4 days after onset of pain.

❒❒ What are the main causes of false positive CK elevation?

Muscle disease, alcohol intoxication, diabetes mellitus, skeletal muscle trauma, vigorous exercise, convulsion, PE and thoracic outlet syndrome.

❒❒ Describe the characteristic pattern of lactate dehydrogenase (LDH) elevation after onset of AMI.

Levels exceed normal by 24 to 48 hours after AMI onset, peak 3 to 6 days after onset and normalize 8 to 14 days after onset. Total LDH, while sensitive, is not specific. Fractionation into its isoforms increases specificity, since myocardium contains primarily LDH-1, where other sources contain primarily the other LDH isoforms. Thus, an LDH-1 to LDH-2 ratio of greater than 1.0 is a commonly used cutoff for diagnosing recent MI. Use of LDH analysis should be limited to those patients with normal CK measurements.

❒❒ What other serum markers are important in diagnosing AMI?

Recently, it has been shown that the troponins demonstrate high concordance with CK-MB, and they appear a bit earlier in the course of MI. Also, subsets of the troponins are highly specific for myocardial damage. Lastly, recent published data suggest that the amount of troponin released may be an independent marker of survival.

❒❒ What are the most common findings on chest X-ray in AMI?

The chest X-ray is often normal, but pulmonary vascular congestion and cardiomegaly are the most common abnormalities found.

❒❒ How sensitive is the ECG for detecting AMI?

The initial ECG is 50 to 70% sensitive for AMI. Serial ECGs increase the sensitively to about 80%. The presenting ECG is important in determining the acute treatment. All patients with suspected AMI should receive aspirin. ST-elevation AMI or new left bundle branch block are generally considered for reperfusion therapy.

❒❒ What defines high risk ECG changes in AMI?

Anterior location, previous MI and complex ectopy.

❒❒ What is the differential diagnosis of "ischemia at a distance?"

ST-depression in a territory subtended by a coronary artery other than the one presumed to be responsible for the ST elevation diagnostic of MI is termed ischemia at a distance. The differential diagnosis: true ischemia, reciprocal ECG changes without ischemia or, in the case of anterior ST depression with inferior infarction, posterior wall infarction.

Importantly, differentiation cannot be reliably made by ECG or even vectorcardiography. Surprisingly, regardless of whether the ECG changes represent ischemia in another territory or electrocardiographic changes only, they imply a worse prognosis.

❑❑ Does the use of thrombolytic therapy in the pre-hospital setting result in better reperfusion rates?

Probably not. Although not well studied, data from several trials suggest that a thorough pre-hospital assessment, including 12 lead ECG, which prepares the receiving Emergency Department for the patient, saves enough time that pre-hospital thrombolysis is unnecessary. There are some trials however, which did show some advantage to pre-hospital thrombolytic administration. In addition, where a hospital is greater than 60 minutes away, pre-hospital thrombolysis may be advantageous.

❑❑ What factors contribute to defining patients at high risk for complications from thrombolytic therapy? (This is <u>not</u> the same as contraindications).

Advanced age, systolic blood pressure greater than 200 and/or diastolic blood pressure greater than 110 that is not effectively lowered with medical therapy in the emergency department, history of definite stroke and recent surgery. There are many other factors which add incremental risk, such as CHF, hypotension and anterior locations, to name a few. It should be noted that high risk patients receive the greatest benefits from thrombolytic therapy.

❑❑ What are key findings of the GUSTO-I trial as related to choice of thrombolytic agent?

GUSTO-I showed that accelerated t-PA provided a 14.5% relative risk reduction in 30 day mortality compared with streptokinase. The absolute risk reduction for mortality was 1%. This was seen in patients receiving thrombolytic therapy within 4 hours of onset of chest pain. Stroke occurred slightly less frequently in streptokinase-treated patients, and the difference reached statistical significance in patients greater than 75 years of age.

❑❑ Is routine use of oxygen beneficial in acute MI?

The rationale is that hypoxemia is bad for myocardial necrosis and that ventilation-perfusion mismatch is common in patients with acute MI, particularly after heparin administration. However, the routine use of oxygen in non-hypoxemia patients has not been proven beneficial. Regardless, most centers recommended routine use of oxygen for 6 to 12 hours to ensure adequate oxygenation of the patient.

❑❑ What are the major contraindications to beta-blocker therapy in AMI?

All patients with AMI should be considered for beta-blocker therapy, and only patients with a major contra-indication should be excluded. These contraindications include pulmonary edema with rales greater than one-third of the lung fields, marked hypotension, PR-interval greater than 24 seconds or advanced heart block, bradycardia (heart rate less than 55-60 bpm) or known bronchospasm (active or history of severe bronchospasm). Several studies have repeatedly shown that beta-blocker therapy reduces mortality and recurrent ischemia when administered early in acute myocardial infarction.

❑❑ Which agent for the treatment of AMI has the best cost-benefit ratio with regard to improved survival?

Aspirin. When all MIs are considered, overall acute mortality is about 13 to 14%. Administration of aspirin reduces this to about 10 to 11% (a relative reduction of about 20%). The only thrombolytic agent studied without concomitant aspirin use was streptokinase, which reduced mortality to about 10.4% The combination of aspirin plus thrombolytic agent has reduced overall mortality to 7-8 %.

❑❑ What are the indications for temporary transvenous pacing in AMI?

Temporary pacing is indicated in patients at high risk with developing complete heart block, particularly new bifascicular bundle branch block or LBBB. Patients who develop asystole, Mobitz type II and complete heart block will may also benefit from temporary transvenous pacing. It should be noted, however, that the use of temporary pacing has never been statistically shown to improve prognosis.

❑❑ What is the most common sustained supraventricular arrhythmia in AMI?

Sinus tachycardia. About one-third of patients will develop sinus tachycardia in the first days after acute AMI. The most common causes are anxiety, persistent pain, and left ventricular failure.

❑❑ What is the least common sustained supraventricular arrhythmia AMI?

Atrial flutter, occurring in 1-3%.

❑❑ What is the most common sustained arrhythmia in AMI?

Probably ventricular fibrillation, occurring in up to 10% of patients, and is seen more commonly in transmural infarction. The majority (60%) of VF events in AMI patients occur within 4 to 6 hours, and 80% by 12 hours. This "Primary" VF have been thought not to affect prognosis when treated rapidly, but some investigators have suggested this may indicate a worse prognosis.

❑❑ What is the best treatment for accelerated idioventricular rhythm (AIVR)?

AIVR, characterized by a wide QRS rhythm with a rate faster than the atrial rate and less than 150 bpm, should not be treated, unless associated with a very significant drop in blood pressure. This rhythm is seen frequently in the early stages of AMI and occurs more often in patients with early reperfusion. However, it is neither sensitive nor specific enough to be considered a reliable marker for reperfusion.

❑❑ What is reperfusion injury?

The acceleration of myocardial cell necrosis after reperfusion. It is characterized by rapid cellular swelling and wide spread architectural disruption. It is likely the acceleration of necrosis occurs in cells already destined to die, but it is possible that reperfusion may cause necrosis of reversibly injured myocardial cells as well.

❑❑ What factors predict development of pericarditis in AMI patients?

Pericarditis usually occurs 1 day to 6 weeks after AMI. It is more common in males, Q wave infarction and patients with congestive heart failure. Some reports suggest that pericarditis occurs in 10 to 20% of patients, but pericardial effusion without evidence of pericarditis is far more common.

❑❑ In AMI patients surviving their event, what is the most powerful predictor of long-term survival?

This is still debated, but the degree of increase in end systolic volume may be the strongest. The extent of underlying left ventricular dysfunction (LVEF) and congestive heart failure are also strong predictors.

❑❑ How common is acute myocardial infarction (AMI)?

It is estimated that one and a half million myocardial infarctions occur every year in the U.S. Approximately one third of the patients with these events will die, with one half of deaths occurring prior to institution of medical therapy.

❑❑ What is the pathophysiology of acute MI?

In general, acute occlusion secondary to thrombosis is considered the most common cause of AMI. Most transmural MIs are associated with complete obstruction whereas non-transmural MIs may be done to thrombosis alone, spasm with associated thrombosis, or, in significantly obstructed arteries, may be done to hypoxemia or hypotension.

❏❏ What is the most common cause of acute coronary thrombosis?

Plaque disruption. Not all plaques have the same propensity to rupture. Characteristics rendering plaques "vulnerable" to disruption include: high lipid content, thin (as opposed to thick) fibrous cap, monocyte content and shear forces present.

❏❏ What are the most common non-atherosclerotic causes of AMI?

Embolization, arteritis, trauma, aortic or coronary dissection and congenital anomalies.

❏❏ What is the most common cause of myocardial infarction in patients with angiographically normal coronary arteries?

Approximately 6% of all MI patients, and as many as 25% of MI patients less than age 35 will have normal coronaries by arteriography. Possible explanations for this include oxygen demand supply mismatch, prolonged hypotension, anatomic abnormalities of the coronary arteries and hematologic disorders. It has been theorized that coronary spasm and small vessel disease may also be possible causes.

❏❏ What are the most common metabolic disorders associated with increased risk of myocardial infarction?

Hurler's disease, homocystinuria, Fabry's disease, amyloidosis and pseudoxanthoma elasticum.

❏❏ What is the most common congenital anomaly associated with AMI?

Anomalous origin of the left coronary artery from the pulmonary artery. If the left of right coronary artery originates from the contralateral aortic sinus, aberrant passage of the vessel between the aorta and the right ventricle outflow tract may result in MI, but more often results in sudden death.

❏❏ Describe the difference between "supply" and "demand" ischemia.

Supply ischemia is due to occlusion or critical narrowing of the coronary artery, and it usually occurs in acute transmural MI. Demand ischemia is essentially due to a mismatch in oxygen supply and demand when coronary narrowing does not allow sufficient delivery of oxygen associated with the increased oxygen demand of an active myocardium. This move often occurs in unstable anginal syndromes and clinically defined non-Q wave MI.

❏❏ Why is the difference between supply and demand ischemia important?

While the difference is a bit artificial, and both frequently occur together, the difference is important because different metabolic and mechanical changes occur in the myocardium depending upon the type of ischemia. The consequence of supply ischemia is the simultaneous development of cellular hypoxia and impaired washout of metabolites. As a result, the ischemia tissue becomes flaccid. In demand ischemia, while hypoxia also develops, washout of metabolites is relatively preserved, so contractility (which is related to a balance between calcium and inorganic phosphate and protons) is maintained.

❏❏ List the most common causes of myocardial oxygen supply-demand mismatch.

Severe coronary artery disease, aortic stenosis, aortic insufficiency, carbon monoxide poisoning, thyrotoxicosis and prolonged hypotension.

❏❏ What are the phases of contraction abnormalities seen with acute cessation of blood flow to the myocardium?

They occur sequentially and are generally categorized as dyssynchrony, hypokinesis, akinesia and dyskinesis.

❑❑ **How much of the left ventricle needs to be involved before hemodynamic signs of left ventricular failure are present?**

Clinical congestive heart failure can occur with almost any overall left ventricular dysfunction. In AMI, hemodynamic evidence of left ventricular dysfunction occurs when 20 to 25% of the LV exhibits abnormal wall.

❑❑ **What percentage of arteries successfully opened with thrombolytic therapy for acute myocardial infarction re-occlude?**

15% of arteries successfully opened re-occlude during the first few days following thrombolytic therapy.

❑❑ **What is the mortality benefit from aspirin alone in acute myocardial infarction with thrombolytic therapy and in subsequent reinfarction?**

Aspirin reduced mortality from acute myocardial infarction by 23% and reduced non-fatal reinfarction by 49%. When used with thrombolytic therapy, there was a 40-50% reduction in mortality from acute myocardial infarction.

❑❑ **A 63 year-old gentleman presents to the Emergency Department with moderate substernal chest pressure and lightheadedness for 90 minutes. His BP on admission is 80/40 and his HR is 110/min and regular. Physical exam reveals JVD to the angle of the jaw, a right parasternal S3 gallop, an apical S4 gallop and clear lungs on auscultation. ECG reveals 2 mm ST elevation in leads II, III, and aVF with reciprocal ST depression in V1-V3. What is the most likely diagnosis and what is the most appropriate initial therapy?**

Inferior myocardial infarction with right ventricular infarction. Following 160-325 mg of aspirin administration, thrombolytic therapy and a large bolus of intravenous saline followed by a moderately high infusion rate of saline are indicated. If the patient remains hypotensive despite adequate intravenous saline, as measured by the development of lung congestion on auscultation, intravenous dobutamine is indicated.

❑❑ **A 70 year-old man is admitted to the hospital with chest pain of 3 hours duration. ECG demonstrates anterior ST elevation for which he is given aspirin, r-TPA, heparin and intravenous nitroglycerin. His symptoms resolve. Serum chemistries reveal a peak CPK of 1800 and a CK-MB fraction of 15%. He is eventually transferred out of the CCU and his hospitalization is uneventful until day 5, when he develops sudden, severe shortness of breath. BP is 110/75 and his pulse is 125 and regular. Examination reveals a new systolic murmur. What would the most appropriate therapeutic intervention be?**

Intravenous sodium nitroprusside. This patient is most likely suffering from rupture of the left ventricular septum and subsequent defect, a not uncommon complication of MI. Afterload reduction is key to stabilization until surgical repair of the VSD can be performed, usually in about 8-12 weeks, after the infarct has healed. If nitroprusside fails to stabilize the patient, intra-aortic balloon counterpulsation and intravenous nitroglycerin should be employed.

❑❑ **What are the major complications of left ventricular aneurysms?**

LV thrombus formation (with the subsequent risk of thromboembolic events), CHF and ventricular arrhythmias.

❑❑ **What ECG changes arise in a true posterior infarction?**

Large R wave and ST depression in V1 and V2. V2 is the most ideal lead to examine to identify posterior infarction of the left ventricle.

❑❑ **What conduction defects commonly occur in an anterior wall MI?**

The dangerous kind. Damage to the conducting system results in a Mobitz II second or third degree AV block.

❒❒ **How should PSVT be treated during an AMI?**

Vagal maneuvers, adenosine, or cardioversion. Stable patients may be able to tolerate negative inotropes, such as verapamil or even beta-blockers.

❒❒ **A patient presents one day after discharge for an AMI with a new, harsh systolic murmur along the left sternal border and pulmonary edema. What is the diagnosis?**

Ventricular septal rupture. Diagnosis is confirmed with Swan-Ganz catheterization or echo. The treatment regime includes nitroprusside for afterload reduction, and possibly an intra-aortic balloon pump followed by surgical repair.

❒❒ **When does cardiac rupture usually occur in patients who have suffered acute MIs?**

50% arise within the first 5 days, and 90% occur within the first 14 days post-MI.

❒❒ **Which type of infarct commonly leads to papillary muscle dysfunction?**

Inferior wall MI. Signs and symptoms include a mild transient systolic murmur and pulmonary edema.

❒❒ **A patient presents two weeks post AMI with chest pain, fever and pleuropericarditis. A pleural effusion is detected by on CXR. What is the diagnosis?**

Dressler's (post-myocardial infarction) syndrome. This syndrome is caused by an immunologic reaction to myocardial antigens.

❒❒ **What percentage of patients over age 80 experience chest pain with an AMI?**

Only 50%. 20% experience diaphoresis, stroke, syncope and/or acute confusion.

❒❒ **Which thrombolytic agent is fibrin-specific?**

Tissue plasminogen activator. This agent is a human protein with no antigenic properties.

❒❒ **What is unstable angina (UA)?**

In the presence of ECG or enzyme evidence of AMI, the term UA is usually applied in three historical circumstances: 1) New onset angina of Canadian class III or worse; 2) Angina at rest as well as with minimal exertion; 3) More severe or prolonged angina in the context of a previous stable pain pattern. The more traditional definitions require one or more of these historical features with electrocardiographic changes, but many centers will classify patients as having unstable angina in the absence of ECG findings.

❒❒ **What is the primary pathophysiologic disturbance in UA?**

In general, patients presenting with UA tend to have more severe and/or extensive CAD, and UA may be precipitated by a decrease in oxygen supply or an increase in demand. Typically, reduction in oxygen supply is the primary problem and is usually the result of thrombosis (often with spontaneous recanalization) and less often the result of progression of atherosclerosis or vasoconstriction.

❒❒ **How does one treat unstable angina?**

UA, like AMI, is usually due to plaque rupture followed by platelet aggregation and thrombosis. Thus, the use of aspirin, heparin, or both is essential. Of note, while aspirin and heparin are both effective, there has not been definitive proof that one is better than the other, or that the combination is better than either agent alone. Use of nitroglycerin, beta-blockers and calcium channel blockers are also standard therapy.

❒❒ Are thrombolytic agents affective in non-Q wave MI?

No, there is no evidence to support their use. In fact, some published data suggest that their use may be detrimental.

❒❒ What is the prognosis of patients presenting with Q-wave MI complicated by acute mitral regurgitation?

Prognosis is quite compromised with an approximate one year survival of only 50%.

❒❒ What is the best treatment of cardiogenic shock (SBP <90 and/or evidence of peripheral hypoperfusion)?

The best treatment has not been established. Use of inotropic agents and vasopressor agents is standard. The role of direct PTCA is still unresolved. Although survival remains dismal in patients presenting with shock, meta-analyses suggest there may be some benefit with administration of thrombolytic agents (particularly streptokinase).

❒❒ What is the definition of unstable angina?

Unstable angina is an intermediate coronary syndrome between angina pectoris and acute myocardial infarction. Its presence depends on one or more of the following three historical features: 1) crescendo angina (more severe, prolonged or frequent) superimposed on a pre-existing pattern or relatively stable, exertion-related angina pectoris, 2) angina pectoris of new onset (within one month) which is brought on by minimal exertion or 3) angina pectoris at rest as well as minimal exertion. Variant angina, which is also characterized by angina at rest, has sometimes been considered to be a form of unstable angina, but it is pathophysiologically different from unstable angina.

❒❒ What is the classification of unstable angina?

Class I: New onset, severe or accelerated angina occurring within two months of presentation without rest pain. Also included in this class are patients whose angina is more frequent, severe, longer in duration or precipitated by substantially less exertion than previously.
Class II Patients with angina at rest during the preceding two months but not within the last 48 hours.
Class III Patients with rest angina at least once within the preceding 48 hours.

❒❒ What are some of the clinical circumstances in which unstable angina occurs?

Secondary unstable angina refers to patients, usually with underlying obstructive CAD, in whom the imbalance between myocardial oxygen supply and demand causing the instability results from conditions that are extrinsic to the coronary vascular bed. This includes patients who have anemia or hypoxemia that cause reduced myocardial oxygen supply, as well as patients with fever, infection, aortic stenosis, uncontrolled hypertension, thyrotoxicosis, extreme emotional upset and tachyarrhythmias that cause increased myocardial oxygen demand.

Primary unstable angina, the most common form of unstable angina, occurs in the absence of an identifiable extracoronary condition and in patients who have not suffered an acute myocardial infarction within the preceding two weeks. Post-infarction unstable angina is present in patients who develop unstable angina within two weeks of a documented acute myocardial infarction; it occurs in approximately 20% of patients following infarction.

❒❒ What is the etiology of primary unstable angina?

Atherosclerotic plaque rupture followed by platelet aggregation and thrombus formation. Aggregation of platelets and thrombus formation, usually superimposed on an atherosclerotic plaque, obstructs blood flow to the affected myocardium sufficiently long enough to cause ischemia and clinical symptoms, but not long enough to result in myocardial necrosis and infarction, as recanalization of the affected coronary artery occurs, usually within 20 minutes to one hour after the onset of plaque rupture. Unstable angina is often a precursor of acute myocardial infarction, and the two conditions share a common pathophysiologic link.

❒❒ Among all patients with unstable angina, what percentage of patients have three-vessel coronary artery disease?

Approximately 40%.

❒❒ Among all patients with unstable angina, what percentage of patients have left main coronary artery disease (> 50% stenosis)?

Approximately 20%.

❒❒ Among all patients with unstable angina, what percentage of patients have no critical coronary obstruction on coronary angiogram?

Approximately 10%.

❒❒ Among all patients with unstable angina, what percentage of patients have two-vessel coronary artery disease? Single-vessel CAD?

Approximately 20% have two-vessel CAD and 10% have single-vessel disease.

❒❒ What percentage of patients with unstable angina present with unstable angina as their <u>initial</u> manifestation of CAD?

Approximately 50%.

❒❒ Of patients who present with unstable angina as their <u>initial</u> manifestation of CAD, what percentage have single-vessel CAD? Three-vessel disease?

Approximately 50% have single-vessel disease (the majority have left anterior descending involvement) and less than 20% have three-vessel disease.

❒❒ What is the short-term prognosis of patients with unstable angina and no critical obstruction of a coronary artery on coronary angiogram (no intraluminal stenosis > 60%)?

Excellent.

❒❒ What is the percentage of intracoronary thrombus found on coronary angiography in patients with unstable angina?

50-70%.

❒❒ When a prior angiogram is available, the lesion responsible for an episode of unstable angina with documented ischemia is formerly greater than a 50% stenosis what percentage of the time? Formerly greater than 70% stenosis?

Lesions responsible for acute ischemic episodes are formerly greater than 50% stenotic only 33-50% of the time and formerly greater than 70% less than 25% of the time.

❒❒ What percentage of patients with acute myocardial infarction have a prodrome of unstable angina shortly before infarction?

Approximately 50%.

❐❐ What percentage of patients with unstable angina develop myocardial infarction in the short-term?

Approximately 5%.

❐❐ What is the 5-year survival of patients with unstable angina rendered asymptomatic on medical therapy prior to discharge from the hospital who have a normal resting electrocardiogram and an exercise electrocardiogram negative for ischemia?

Greater than 95%.

❐❐ Can patients with unstable angina, who have been stabilized and rendered asymptomatic on medical therapy prior to discharge from the hospital, be safely evaluated by exercise testing?

Absolutely. However, coronary angiography is indicated for the vast majority of patients with unstable angina as the first diagnostic test, even in patients rendered asymptomatic by medical therapy.

❐❐ What factors portend a worse prognosis and signify a high-risk patient in those with unstable angina?

Older patients, patients with continued rest pain despite medical therapy, and patients with thrombi, complex coronary morphology or multivessel disease on coronary angiography. Patients who have ischemia detected on ambulatory electrocardiographic monitoring and those with significant ST-T wave abnormalities at presentation are also at higher risk and tend to have an unfavorable outcome.

❐❐ What is the most useful diagnostic test in the evaluation of patients with unstable angina?

Coronary angiography.

❐❐ What is the hallmark of drug therapy for patients admitted with unstable angina?

Intravenous low molecular-weight heparin and at least 81 mg of aspirin daily. Intravenous nitroglycerin is strongly recommended for patients with Class II or Class III unstable angina, but one must keep in mind to increase the dose of intravenous heparin during intravenous nitroglycerin administration as nitroglycerin reduces the efficacy of heparin.

❐❐ What is the role of thrombolytic therapy in unstable angina?

None. To date, no clinical trial has shown any benefit of thrombolytic therapy, presumably because thrombi in unstable angina tend to be platelet-rich, not fibrin-rich, and thus resistant to thrombolytic therapy.

❐❐ What are some other highly efficacious drug therapies in patients with unstable angina?

Beta-blockers have been shown to be highly effective in reducing the frequency and duration of both symptomatic and silent myocardial ischemic episodes. Calcium channel antagonists, while not as efficacious as beta-blockers in reducing myocardial oxygen demand, are highly effective in reducing symptoms and ischemic episodes, but should not be used as monotherapy. In fact, monotherapy with nifedipine in unstable angina is associated with an increase in non-fatal myocardial infarctions within the first 48 hours after initiation of therapy.

❐❐ What is the strategy for managing patients with unstable angina?

All patients should receive immediate medical therapy with an eye to stabilization.
Patients who remain unstable and those deemed candidates for invasive management should be referred for cardiac catheterization within 48 hours of presentation, provided there are no contraindications to invasive therapy.

Patients who stabilize easily and who are not at high risk for complications, and those patients who prefer continued medical management, or those who are not candidates for invasive therapy because of contraindications, should continue on intensive medical therapy.

Patients should be strongly considered for cardiac catheterization if they have one or more of the following high-risk indicators: prior revascularization, associated congestive heart failure or depressed LVEF (< 50%) by non-invasive study, malignant ventricular arrhythmias, persistent or recurrent pain/ischemia, and/or a functional study indicating a high risk.

❒❒ What percentage of patients who have sudden cardiac death have a prior history or angina, myocardial infarction or congestive heart failure?

50%.

❒❒ In patients with sudden cardiac death, what percentage of patients are found to have a coronary thrombus on autopsy?

30-75%. It is most commonly found in patients with single-vessel CAD and those with acute myocardial infarction or recent unstable angina. It is less common in patients with previous myocardial infarction or three-vessel CAD.

❒❒ What medical regimen can one use in patients with unstable angina who have a contraindication or a major complication to intravenous heparin?

Ticlopidine, at a dose of 250 mg twice daily, or clopidogrel at 75 mg per day are very suitable alternatives to heparin. Furthermore, unlike intravenous heparin, they can be feasibly continued in the outpatient setting.

❒❒ Among survivors of sudden cardiac death without myocardial infarction, which group of patients are more likely to have complex coronary atherosclerotic lesions: those with inducible ventricular tachycardia or those without inducible ventricular tachycardia on electrophysiologic testing?

Those patients without inducible ventricular tachycardia, suggesting those survivors of sudden cardiac death without inducible ventricular tachycardia on electrophysiologic testing had ischemia as their precipitating event, while those who had inducible ventricular tachycardia had an arrhythmic etiology of their sudden cardiac death episode.

❒❒ Which is the most common type of cardiac failure, high or low output?

Low output failure. Reduced stroke volume, narrowed pulse pressure, and peripheral vasoconstriction are all signs of low output failure.

❒❒ Rales are present on exam in a 50 year-old man with recent anterior wall MI. What can you say about the pulmonary artery occlusion ("wedge") pressure?

It is likely above 20 to 25 mmHg.

❒❒ A 30 year-old woman with long-standing idiopathic cardiomyopathy has faint basilar crackles on lung exam. What would you expect her pulmonary wedge pressure to be?

In chronic heart failure, patients may have elevated wedge pressures (a reflection of elevated left ventricular end diastolic pressure) greater than 30mmHg with only minor findings on lung exam. This is likely due to increased pulmonary lymphatic drainage.

❒❒ Can the chest radiograph show signs of systolic heart failure when the physical exam is negative?

Pulmonary rales develop when there is extravasated fluid within the alveoli. The first site fluid accumulates in hydrostatic pulmonary edema is the interstitial space that surrounds blood vessels and bronchi. This interstitial fluid is visible on X-rays before the exam becomes positive.

❑❑ A 65 year-old man 3 days post an uncomplicated inferior wall MI is noted to have basilar crackles on lung exam that mostly clear with coughing. His creatinine is 2.1 and he weighs 75 kg. Approximately how much furosemide should you administer to promote a diuresis?

Probably none. In the proper clinical context, rales are obviously a useful sign of heart failure, even in its incipient stage. Since most ICU patients are bed-bound and will experience atelectasis of dependent lung tissue, the patient should be reexamined after a few vigorous coughs and gentle pulmonary toilet. Very often rales and diuretics will soon disappear from the bedside.

❑❑ Sustained ventricular tachycardia is well controlled in a 55 year-old man post non-Q wave MI with lidocaine 2 mcg/mL. He has a known history of ischemic cardiomyopathy. On day 3 of his admission, his speech becomes slurred, he is lethargic, and, when aroused, becomes very agitated. What should you do?

This patient has classic findings of lidocaine toxicity, and you should strongly consider stopping this drug. Elderly patients and patients with heart failure of hepatic insufficiency are especially at risk.

❑❑ An elderly man with progressive symptoms of shortness of breath is intubated for respiratory failure. He has a 100 pack/year smoking history. On exam, he is agitated and "bucking the vent." Breath sounds are coarse throughout, heart sounds faint. External jugular veins are prominently distended. His liver edge is palpable; his extremities are dusky with lower extremity pitting edema. EKG shows sinus tachycardia and poor R wave progression. The BUN/creatinine ratio is elevated. You have concluded that the patient has systolic heart failure. What is your next step?

Reconsider your diagnosis! The ICU is fraught with physical exam pitfalls. JVD may be difficult to interpret—especially in a patient who is increasing his intrathoracic pressure by breathing out of synch with the ventilator. Patients with COPD can have dusky extremities. They may have coarse breath sounds throughout their lung fields Pulmonary hypertension and RV dysfunction may lead to peripheral edema. Diaphragmatic or abdominal viscera displacement may alter the axis of the heat and affect EKG interpretation. Under such circumstances, a bedside echo may be very helpful.

❑❑ A 60 year-old man with a recent syncopal episode is hospitalized with congestive heart failure and chest pain. His BP is 165/85 mm Hg; his pulse is 85/min and there is a grade III/VI harsh systolic murmur at the apex and aortic area. An echocardiogram reveals a disproportionately thickened septum and anterior systolic motion of the mitral valve. What is this patient's diagnosis and what physical findings would most likely be present?

Obstructive hypertrophic cardiomyopathy (IHSS). The murmur typically decreases with handgrip and Valsalva, and increases with vasodilators, standing, nitroglycerin, diuretics and digoxin. Mitral regurgitation is frequent as a result of anterior systolic motion of the mitral valve. Congestive heart failure is present because of diastolic dysfunction; thus, an S4 gallop is common.

❑❑ A 72 year-old woman admitted to the ICU with pulmonary edema is much improved after overnight diuresis. Soon after you note that she is 4L negative in fluid balance, she develops polymorphic VT requiring cardioversion. Her regular medications include 80 mg bid of furosemide. What is a likely etiology?

Beware of electrolyte abnormalities (especially hypokalemia) which can induce torsades pointes in CHF patients after vigorous diuresis – especially in patients on chronic diuretics.

❑❑ A 65 year-old man with known severe hypertension, past CHF and COPD is intubated for acute pulmonary edema and suspected pneumonia. BP is 190/110; 92 saturation is 94% on 60% O_2. You successfully lower his blood pressure to 140/80 with intravenous sodium nitroprusside. However, the patient develops chest pressure and you note that his O_2 saturation is now 86%. What happened?

Two effects of nitroprusside are likely culprits. Nonselective dilation of the pulmonary arteriolar bed can worsen ventilation-perfusion mismatch, especially in patients with COPD or pneumonia, and cause desaturation. "Coronary steal" (reduced perfusion to coronary arteries with fixed obstruction in the setting of arteriolar dilation by nitroprusside) may lead to ischemia and chest pain.

❒❒ What are the most common causes of atrial fibrillation?

Hypertension with hypertensive heart disease is very common. Ischemic heart disease, mitral or aortic valvular heart disease, cor pulmonale, dilated cardiomyopathy, hypertrophic cardiomyopathy (particularly the obstructive type), alcohol intoxication ("holiday heart syndrome"), hypo- or hyperthyroidism, pulmonary embolism, sepsis, hypoxia, pre-excitation syndrome and pericarditis are also common causes.

❒❒ How is atrial fibrillation treated?

The treatment of atrial fibrillation consists of three major considerations: 1) control of ventricular rate, 2) conversion, if possible or feasible, to sinus rhythm and 3) prevention of thromboembolic events, particularly CVA. Rate control is best managed with beta-adrenergic blockers or calcium channel blockers (diltiazem or verapamil), or less desirable, digoxin. Digoxin should be used in patients with poor LV systolic function and those with a contraindication to beta-blockers and calcium channel blockers. Digoxin provides good rate control at rest but often suboptimal rate control during exertion. Conversion to sinus rhythm, in the stable patient, is best managed initially with antiarrhythmic agents, such as 1A agents like quinidine or procainamide, 1C agents such as propafenone or Class III agents like amiodarone or sotalol. In the unstable patient or the patient with acute ischemia, hypotension or pulmonary edema, immediate synchronized electrical cardioversion, starting at 200 joules, should be performed. If, in the stable patient, cardioversion with antiarrhythmic agents is unsuccessful, synchronized electrical cardioversion should be performed without interruption of antiarrhythmic therapy. Patients with atrial fibrillation of 1 year duration or longer, or those with left atrial size of >5.0 cm on echocardiography should not be cardioverted because of the extremely low success rate. Patients with recent atrial fibrillation >3 days duration should be started on Warfarin and anticoagulated to an INR between 2-3.5 for at least three weeks before any attempt to cardiovert to sinus rhythm because of the significant risk of embolic CVA. Those patients with chronic atrial fibrillation should be on lifelong Warfarin, unless an absolute contraindication to Warfarin exists or the patient cannot reliably take Warfarin.

❒❒ What percentage of patients with atrial fibrillation converted to sinus rhythm will revert back into atrial fibrillation?

50% will revert back to atrial fibrillation within one year of cardioversion, regardless of medical therapy.

❒❒ What are the common causes of SVT?

Myocardial ischemia, myocardial infarction, congestive heart failure, pericarditis, rheumatic heart disease, mitral valve prolapse, pre-excitation syndromes, COPD, ethanol intoxication, hypoxia, pneumonia, sepsis and digoxin toxicity.

❒❒ What is the treatment of paroxysmal SVT?

In a hemodynamically stable patient, intravenous adenosine. If unsuccessful, then intravenous verapamil, beta-blockers or procainamide. In the unstable patient with hypotension, angina or heart failure, immediate synchronized cardioversion should be performed.

❒❒ What is the most common supraventricular arrhythmia in the perioperative setting?

Atrial fibrillation.

❒❒ **You are called to the CCU to evaluate the sudden onset of hypotension in an 80 year-old woman. She received a porcine aortic valve for severe aortic stenosis less than 24 hours ago. The bedside monitor reveals atrial fibrillation at a rate of 120 bpm. What is the pathophysiology?**

A rapid ventricular response and loss of AV synchrony, as can be seen in new-onset atrial fibrillation, can have devastating hemodynamic consequences, especially in patients with impaired diastolic filling – often including the elderly, and patients with left ventricular hypertrophy, which this patient with long-standing aortic stenosis most likely has.

❒❒ **What pharmacotherapy is most appropriate in the above patient?**

None. Hemodynamically unstable patients with tachyarrhythmias are best treated with electrical cardioversion.

❒❒ **What is the key feature of Mobitz Type I 2° AV block (Wenckebach)?**

A progressive prolongation of the PR interval until the atrial impulse is no longer conducted through to the ventricle, resulting in a dropped QRS. Almost always transient, atropine and transcutaneous/transvenous pacing is required in the rare instances of symptoms or cardiac instability.

❒❒ **What is the primary feature of Mobitz II 2° AV block?**

A constant PR interval until one sinus beat fails to conduct through to the ventricle, resulting in a dropped QRS. Since this rhythm is indicative of His bundle damage, and 85% of patients with this rhythm eventually develop complete heart block, temporary followed by permanent pacing is usually required.

❒❒ **What is the most common cause of Mobitz Type II 2° AV block?**

Coronary artery disease with acute myocardial ischemia. In the absence of coronary artery disease, the most common cause is degenerative AV node and His bundle disease.

❒❒ **What is the appropriate management of the above arrhythmia in a patient on no SA or AV nodal suppressant drugs?**

Temporary transvenous pacemaker insertion followed by permanent pacemaker implantation.

❒❒ **A 57 year-old male is scheduled for a total colectomy for ulcerative colitis. He has stable angina for several years and has hypertension. His pre-op ECG reveals NSR, LVH and 1° AV block. What is the likelihood of high degree AV block occurring in the perioperative period?**

Patients with 1° AV block have an extremely low incidence of developing high degree AV block in the perioperative period or any other period. Thus, no temporary pacing in the perioperative period is required.

❒❒ **What is the treatment of Torsades de Pointes?**

Torsades de Pointes is a polymorphic form of ventricular tachycardia that occurs in the setting of long repolarization. Treatment usually requires removal of the reversible triggers that caused Q-T prolongation, such as hypokalemia and drugs (such as quinidine and other antiarrhythmic agents), pacing the atrium or ventricle to increase cardiac rate and rapidly infusing magnesium sulfate.

❒❒ **Name five useful ECG criteria for identifying VT.**

1. AV dissociation – often best seen in lead V1 and rare in SVT with aberrancy.
2. Capture of fusion beats – often noted as a "narrow" premature beat occurring during a wide complex tachycardia.
3. A QRS with a RBBB morphology greater than 140 ms in duration, or a LBBB morphology greater than 160 ms in duration.
4. Extreme right or left axis deviation ("northwest axis") is seldom seen outside of VT.

5. Positive or negative concordance of QRS complexes in the precordial leads.

❑❑ Which antiarrhythmic agents increase defibrillation threshold (i.e., increase the energy requirement for successful defibrillation)?

Lidocaine, mexiletine, encainide, flecainide, propafenone, amiodarone and verapamil.

❑❑ What are the most common initial rhythms in adults with cardiac arrest?

VF and VT.

❑❑ For VF or unstable VT, what is the most important intervention to optimize chances for successful resuscitation?

Defibrillation.

❑❑ What percentage of individuals successfully resuscitated from sudden cardiac death will succumb to a second episode within 2 years?

60%.

❑❑ What is the primary indication for atropine?

Symptomatic bradycardia.

❑❑ A 28 year-old presents with hemodynamically stable paroxysmal supraventricular tachycardia (PSVT) at a rate of 170. What is the drug of choice?

Vagal maneuvers are tried first. If unsuccessful, adenosine is the drug of choice.

❑❑ What is the treatment of choice for rapid atrial fibrillation in a patient with Wolff-Parkinson-White syndrome?

Cardioversion if the patient is unstable, otherwise procainamide (20 to 30 mg/min up to 17 mg/kg) is the treatment of choice. The infusion should be stopped if further widening of the QRS or hypotension occurs.

❑❑ What percentage of Americans experiencing cardiac arrest are resuscitated? What percentage of these suffer neurological damage?

Up to one-third are resuscitated and survive to discharge. Of this group, 20 to 40% develop permanent brain damage ranging from subtle to severe.

❑❑ Tachycardia occurs after a cardiac arrest and is treated successfully with defibrillation and epinephrine. Would you treat this post-resuscitation rhythm?

If the patient has a pulse and is hemodynamically stable, no treatment may be necessary. If epinephrine is responsible for the tachycardia, it should resolve quickly. Sustained sinus tachycardia should not be allowed to persist, however, as it increases myocardial oxygen consumption.

❑❑ T/F: An AICD (automated implantable cardioverter-defibrillator) is a contraindication to defibrillation.

False. If functioning, the AICD should assess, charge and shock within 30 seconds. If the patient is in ventricular fibrillation (VF) and the device doesn't deliver a shock, proceed with external defibrillation.

TRAUMA PEARLS

"The only missing clotting factor is silk."
Donald Trunkey, M.D.

❒❒ **A radial pulse on exam indicates a BP of at least _____.**

80 mmHg.

❒❒ **A femoral pulse on exam indicates a BP of at least_____.**

70 mm Hg.

❒❒ **A carotid pulse indicates a BP of at least_____.**

60 mm Hg.

❒❒ **What is the most common long bone fractured?**

The tibia.

❒❒ **A trauma patient presents with decreasing level of consciousness and an enlarging right pupil. Diagnosis?**

Probable uncal herniation with oculomotor nerve compression.

❒❒ **The corneal reflex tests?**

Ophthalmic branch (V_1) of the trigeminal (5th) nerve [afferent pathway] and the facial (7th) nerve [efferent pathway].

❒❒ **Name five clinical signs of basilar skull fracture.**

Periorbital ecchymosis (raccoon's eyes), retroauricular ecchymosis (Battle's sign), otorrhea or rhinorrhea, hemotympanum or bloody ear discharge, and 1st, 2nd, 7th, and 8th CN deficits.

❒❒ **A trauma patient presents with anisocoria, neurological deterioration, and/or lateralizing motor findings. Treatment?**

Mannitol 1 g/kg infused rapidly. (Avoid if hypovolemic). Elevate head of bed 30°. Some authors recommend dexamethasone 1 mg/kg, and phenytoin 18 mg/kg at 20 mg/min. If mannitol has been administered in this clinical circumstance, a neurosurgeon must be summoned immediately. Mannitol "shrinks" the brain and may promote rapid expansion of an intracranial hematoma (especially an epidural hematoma).

❒❒ **How is posterior column function tested and why is it significant?**

Position and vibration sensation are carried in the posterior columns and are usually spared in anterior cord syndrome. Light touch sensation may also be spared. Pain and temperature sensation cross near the level of entry and are carried in the more posterior spinothalamic tract.

❑❑ At what point of airway obstruction will inspiratory stridor become evident?

70% occlusion.

❑❑ What is the most common cause of shock in patients with blunt chest trauma?

Pelvic or extremity fractures.

❑❑ What nerve should be avoided during pericardiotomy?

Open the pericardium vertically, anterior (medial) to the phrenic nerve. The nerve runs along the superolateral aspect of the pericardium.

❑❑ Differential diagnosis of distended neck veins in a trauma patient?

Tension pneumothorax, pericardial tamponade, air embolism, and cardiac failure. Neck vein distention may not be present until hypovolemia has been corrected.

❑❑ A trauma patient presents with a "rocking-horse" type of ventilation. Diagnosis?

Probable high spinal cord injury with intercostal muscle paralysis.

❑❑ What should be checked prior to inserting a chest tube in an intubated patient with respiratory distress and decreased breath sounds on one side?

Position of the distal tip of the ET tube. Most of the time this can be accomplished clinically by immediate auscultation after withdrawing the ET tube 1-2 cm.

❑❑ Should a chest tube be placed into a bullet hole apparent in the 4th lateral interspace?

No. The tube might follow the bullet track into the diaphragm or lung. A chest tube should never be inserted through any traumatic wound.

❑❑ A trauma patient presents with subcutaneous emphysema. Diagnosis?

Pneumothorax or pneumomediastinum; if emphysema is severe, consider a major bronchial injury.

❑❑ A pneumothorax is suspected but does not show up on PA and Lat CXR. What other x-rays should be considered?

Expiratory films. A pneumothorax is usually best seen on expiratory films.

❑❑ What rib fracture has the worst prognosis?

First rib. First and second rib fractures are associated with bronchial tears, vascular injury, and myocardial contusions.

❑❑ What cardiovascular injury is commonly associated with sternal fractures?

Myocardial contusions (blunt myocardial injury).

❑❑ How much fluid needs to collect in the chest to be seen on decubitus or upright chest x-rays?

200 to 300 mL; if supine, greater than 1 liter may be necessary to be seen on AP CXR.

❑❑ Describe Beck's triad.

Muffled heart tones, hypotension, and distended neck veins. Causes include: myocardial contusion, AMI, pericardial tamponade, and tension pneumothorax. Tamponade may also cause pulsus paradoxus and distention of neck veins during inspiration. Total electrical alternans is highly specific for pericardial tamponade.

❒❒ **Which valve is most commonly injured with blunt trauma?**

Aortic valve.

❒❒ **What is the most likely cause of a new systolic murmur and ECG infarct pattern observed in a patient with chest trauma?**

Ventricular septal defect.

❒❒ **With a myocardial contusion (blunt myocardial injury), when should the CPK-MB peak?**

About 18 to 24 h.

❒❒ **What is the most accurate plain film x-ray finding indicating traumatic rupture of the aorta?**

Deviation of the esophagus > 2 cm to the right of the spinous process of T4.

❒❒ **What is the basic disorder contributing to the pathophysiology of compartment syndrome?**

Increased pressure within closed tissue spaces compromising blood flow to muscle & nerve tissue. There are three prerequisites to the development of compartment syndrome:

1) Limiting space.
2) Increased tissue pressure.
3) Decreased tissue perfusion.

❒❒ **What are the two basic mechanisms for elevated compartment pressure?**

1) External compression -- by burn eschar, circumferential casts, dressings, or pneumatic pressure garments.
2) Volume increase within the compartment -- hemorrhage into the compartment, IV infiltration, or edema due to post-ischemic swelling.

❒❒ **Which two fractures are most commonly associated with compartment syndrome?**

Tibia (resulting most often in anterior compartment involvement) and supracondylar humerus fractures.

❒❒ **What are the early general signs & symptoms of compartment syndrome?**

Early findings: 1. Tenderness and pain out of proportion to the injury, 2. Pain with active and passive motion, and 3. Hypesthesia (paresthesia) -- abnormal 2-point discrimination. Late findings: 1. Compartment tense, indurated, and erythematous, 2. Slow capillary refill, and 3. Pallor and pulselessness.

❒❒ **What are the four compartments of the leg?**

Anterior, lateral, deep posterior, and superficial posterior compartments.

❒❒ **What signs & symptoms would be noted for a compartment syndrome involving the superficial posterior compartment of the leg?**

Pain on active and passive foot dorsi-flexion and plantar-flexion and hypesthesia of the lateral aspect of the foot (sural nerve).

❑❑ **What signs & symptoms would be noted for a compartment syndrome involving the deep posterior compartment of the leg?**

Pain on foot eversion or toe dorsiflexion and hypesthesia of plantar surface of foot.

❑❑ **What intracompartmental pressure raises concern?**

Normal pressure is less than 10 mm Hg. It is generally agreed that > 30 mm Hg mandates emergent fasciotomy. The treatment for compartment pressures between 20 and 30 mm Hg is controversial and may require surgical consultation especially if the patient is unreliable (i. e. with altered level of consciousness).

❑❑ **What are the two major wounding mechanisms of ballistic injuries?**

Tissue crush and tissue stretch. Crush creates a permanent cavity; the degree of crush is largely determined by the missile. Stretch is primarily determined by the tissue itself.

❑❑ **What bullet characteristics determine the degree of tissue crushing?**

Yaw, deformation, & fragmentation (of missile and bone). These three factors determine the surface area of the missile(s) and subsequent tissue damage.

❑❑ **Why are civilian bullets usually more damaging than military bullets?**

Military bullets are usually jacketed and are less prone to fragmentation/"mushrooming" than hollow/soft point civilian bullets.

❑❑ **Which tissues are more prone to significant wounding due to temporary cavitation?**

Less elastic tissues such as brain, spleen & liver; fluid-filled organs such as bladder, bowel, and heart; and dense tissue such as bone.

❑❑ **Why do simple through-and-through wounds of the extremities fare well regardless of velocity of bullet?**

The short path in the tissue results in:
1) little or no deformation of slower bullets,
2) less time for higher velocity bullet to yaw, thereby resulting in a lesser degree of tissue damage.

❑❑ **Is the heat of firing significant enough to sterilize a bullet and its wound?**

No, contaminants from body surface & from viscera can be carried along the bullet's path.

❑❑ **What features of the brain/skull result in higher severity of head wounds?**

The brain is highly sensitive to cavitation due to poor elasticity & cohesiveness, enclosure of calvarium contains the cavitation forces. Also, the brain is really important in most people and causes a lot of problems when it is shot.

❑❑ **What anatomic locations of bullets/pellets are associated with lead intoxication?**

Within bursa, joints, or disc spaces.

❑❑ **Other than lead intoxication, why should intraarticular bullets be removed?**

Potential for lead synovitis leading to severe damage of articular cartilage.

❑❑ **What causes a boutonnière deformity?**

A disruption of the extensor hood at the PIP joint of the finger.

❒❒ Describe a Gamekeeper's thumb.

Disruption of the ulnar collateral ligament of the MP joint of the thumb (stress testing showing > 20° opening indicates need for surgical repair).

❒❒ For which condition does Finkelstein's test test?

Tenosynovitis of the extensor pollicis brevis & abductor pollicis (DeQuervan's stenosing tenosynovitis). To perform the Finkelstein test, the patient places the flexed thumb in the palm of the hand and closes the fist around it. The wrist is then actively deviated to the ulnar side. If this produces pain along the flexor aspect of the thumb, the test is positive.

❒❒ What is the treatment of a felon?

10-12 years with time-off for good behavior. A felon is a subcutaneous infection of the pulp space of the fingertip, usually *S. aureus*; treat by incising the pulp space.

❒❒ What is a paronychia?

An infection of the lateral nail fold. Usually from *S. aureus* or *Streptococcus*. Treat with I&D followed by warm soaks.

❒❒ Describe Tinel's and Phalen's tests.

Tinel's - Tapping the volar aspect of the wrist over the median nerve produces paresthesias that extend along the index & long finger.

Phalen's - Full flexion at the wrist for one minute leads to paresthesia along distribution of median nerve. Both test for carpal tunnel syndrome.

❒❒ What are the three most common carpal fractures?

The scaphoid, dorsal chip (triquetrum), and the lunate. All may be 2° to falls on an outstretched hand. Radiographs may initially be normal. <u>The scaphoid is the most common</u>.

❒❒ What is Kienböck's disease?

Avascular necrosis of the lunate with collapse of the lunate secondary to fracture. As with a navicular (scaphoid) fracture, initial wrist x-rays may not demonstrate the fracture. Therefore, tenderness over the lunate warrants immobilization.

❒❒ Which bone is most commonly fractured at birth?

The clavicle.

❒❒ Most common shoulder dislocation?

Anterior (95%).

❒❒ A patient cannot actively abduct her shoulder. What injury does this suggest?

Rotator cuff tear. The cuff is comprised of the supraspinatus, infraspinatus, subscapularis, and the teres minor muscles and their tendons.

❒❒ Why is a displaced supracondylar fracture (of the distal humerus) in a child considered a true emergency?

The injury often results in injury to brachial artery or median nerve. It can also cause compartment syndrome.

❐❐ What is the significance of the fat pad sign with an elbow injury?

Fat pad sign or radiolucency just anterior to the distal humerus is indicative of effusion or hemarthrosis of the elbow joint; this suggests an occult fracture of the radial head. The most significant fat pad sign is visualization of the posterior fat pad of the distal humerus. It is virtually never visualized unless there is a fracture. In that circumstance, hematoma then displaces the posterior fat pad out of the olecranon fossa. The posterior fat pad is not visible on a normal film.

❐❐ Define increased intracranial pressure.

ICP > than 15 mmHg.

❐❐ What is the most common site of a basilar skull fracture?

Petrous portion of the temporal bone.

❐❐ What is the most common artery involved with an epidural hematoma?

Meningeal artery, specifically the middle.

❐❐ Where are epidural hematomas located?

Between the dura and inner table of the skull.

❐❐ Where are subdural hematomas located?

Beneath the dura and over the brain and arachnoid. Caused by tears of pial arteries or of bridging veins. Subdurals typically become symptomatic within 24 h to 2 wk after injury.

❐❐ For a trauma victim, which test is most helpful for evaluating retroperitoneal organs and spaces?

CT.

❐❐ How should a DPL be performed in a trauma victim with a fractured pelvis?

Supraumbilical incision to avoid pelvic hematoma.

❐❐ Absolute contraindication to DPL?

None. Relative contraindications: clear indication for laparotomy, previous abdominal surgery and gravid uterus (use open technique).

❐❐ What findings represent a positive DPL in blunt trauma?

RBC > 100,000 cells/mm^3, WBC > 500 cells/mm^3, bile, bacteria, or vegetable material.

❐❐ What clues are evident with duodenal injury?

Increased serum amylase and retroperitoneal free air.

❐❐ What is the most frequently injured organ after blunt abdominal trauma?

Spleen.

❑❑ What is Kehr's sign?

Left shoulder pain after splenic rupture.

❑❑ What type of injury most commonly damages the pancreas?

Penetrating.

❑❑ Inability to pass a nasogastric tube in a trauma victim suggests damage to what organ?

Diaphragm, usually on the left.

❑❑ What type of contrast medium should be used to evaluate the esophagus if traumatic injury is suspected?

Gastrografin.

❑❑ Describe the 3 zones of the neck and their evaluation?

I - Below the cricoid cartilage - Arteriogram.
II- Between the cricoid and the mandible - Surgery. "2 surgery!"
III - Above the angle of the mandible - Arteriogram.

❑❑ A stress fracture is suspected of the 2nd or 3rd metatarsal, but none is found on initial x-rays. How long before a 2nd set of x-rays will likely be positive?

14-21 days.

❑❑ The three steps of bone healing after a fracture are:

Union - consolidation - remodeling.

❑❑ How long after a fracture does callus start to form?

5 - 7 days.

❑❑ The most common Salter-Harris class fracture?

Type II. A triangular fracture involving the metaphysis and an epiphyseal separation.

❑❑ What tarsal bone is most commonly fractured?

Calcaneus (60%). Calcaneal fractures are commonly associated with lumbar compression injuries (10%).

❑❑ The tarsal-metatarsal joint is also called:

Lisfranc's joint.

❑❑ The second metatarsal is the locking mechanism of the mid-part of the foot. A fracture at the base of the second metatarsal should raise suspicion of:

A disrupted joint - treatment may require ORIF.

❑❑ What is a ballet fracture?

An avulsion fracture at the base of the 5th metatarsal usually secondary to plantar flexion and inversion.

❑❑ What is the 2nd most common tarsal fracture?

Talus.

❑❑ What is the most common metatarsal fracture?

5th.

❑❑ What is the most common foot fracture?

Calcaneus.

❑❑ Which patellar fracture requires orthopedic consultation?

Displaced transverse fracture, comminuted fractures, and open fractures.

❑❑ What is the most common mechanism for fractures of the femoral condyles?

Direct trauma, fall or blow to the distal femur.

❑❑ Of tibial plateau fractures, where is the most common site?

Lateral, more common in the older population, usually presenting with swollen painful knee and limited range of motion.

❑❑ With complete rupture of medial or collateral ligaments, how much laxity is expected on exam?

>1 cm without endpoint as compared to uninjured knee.

❑❑ What is the most common ligamentous injury to the knee?

Anterior cruciate ligament, usually from non-contact injury.

❑❑ Why 'tap' a knee with an acute hemarthrosis?

Relieve pressure and pain and see if fat globules are present indicating a fracture.

❑❑ How would you 'un-lock' a 'locked' knee?

Hang leg over table at 90 degree flexion, allow relaxation and apply longitudinal traction with internal and external rotation.

❑❑ Where is the most common site of compartment syndrome?

Anterior compartment of the leg - contains tibialis anterioris, extensor digitorum longus, extensor hallucis longus, and peroneus muscles, as well as anterior tibial artery and deep peroneal nerve.

❑❑ Who gets Achilles' tendon rupture?

Middle aged men most commonly on the left side.

❑❑ Where is the most common site for a palpable defect of Achilles' tendon?

2 - 6 cm proximal to its insertion.

❑❑ What are the most common lower extremity injuries to bone in children?

Tibial and fibular shaft fractures, usually secondary to twist forces.

❑❑ What radiograph would one order with suspected patellar fracture in a child?

Standard radiographs including patellar or "sunrise" views, plus comparison radiographs of uninvolved knee.

❑❑ What are the differences between Osgood-Schlatter disease and avulsion of tibial tubercle?

Both occur at tibial tubercle, avulsion presents with acute inability to walk, lateral view of the knee is most diagnostic, treatment is surgical. Osgood-Schlatter's has vague history of intermittent pain, is bilateral in 25% of cases, has pain with range of motion but not with rest; treatment is symptomatic and not surgical.

❑❑ What is a toddler fracture?

Common cause of limp or refusal to walk in this age group is a spiral fracture of the tibia without fibular involvement.

❑❑ What is the most common cause of a painful hip joint in infants?

Septic arthritis. *Staphylococcus* is the most common cause in infancy. Hip usually abducted, flexed, and externally rotated.

❑❑ Most common cause of painful hip in older children?

Transient synovitis. It can be difficult to distinguish from septic arthritis.

❑❑ 8 year-old male presents with a limp. On exam, hip range of motion is decreased. What rare disease should be considered?

Children 5-9 year-old may get idiopathic avascular necrosis of the femoral heal (Legg-Calvé-Perthes Disease).

❑❑ Describe a typical patient with a slipped capital femoral epiphysis?

Obese boy, age 10 to 16 year-old. Groin or knee discomfort increases with activity; may have a limp. Often bilateral. The slip is best seen on a lateral view.

❑❑ What is the most important complication of a proximal tibial metaphyseal fracture?

Arterial involvement, especially when there is a valgus deformity.

❑❑ What is the most common ankle injury?

75% of ankle injuries are sprains with 90% of these involving the lateral complex. 90% of lateral ligament injuries are <u>anterior talofibular</u>.

❑❑ What is the most helpful physical exam test for anterior talofibular ligament injury?

Anterior drawer test, >3 mm of excursion might be significant (compare sides), >1 cm is always significant.

❑❑ How are sprains classified?

1st° - <u>stretching</u> of ligament, normal x-ray.

2nd° - severe stretching with partial tear, marked tenderness, swelling, pain, normal x-ray (now stressed).
3rd° - complete ligament rupture, marked tenderness, swelling and obviously deformed joint. X-ray may show an abnormal joint.

❑❑ What is unique about avulsion fractures at the base of the fifth metatarsal?

It is one of the most commonly missed fractures, history is of ankle injury from plantar flexion and inversion.

❑❑ A 21 year-old female complains of pain and 'clicking' sound located at the posterior lateral malleolus. You sense a 'fullness' beneath the lateral malleolus. Dx?

Peroneal tendon subluxation, with associated tenosynovitis.

❑❑ What percentage of distal tibial (medial malleolus) fractures treated closed result in non-union?

10 - 15%.

❑❑ Traumatic arthritis occurs in what percentage of ankle fractures?

20 - 40%.

❑❑ Name the function of, and spinal level innervating, the biceps, triceps, flexor digitorum, interossei, quadriceps, extensor hallucis, biceps femoris, soleus and gastrocnemius, and rectal sphincter.

Muscle	Action	Spinal Level
Biceps	Forearm flexion	C 5,6
Triceps	Forearm extensors	C7
Flexor digitorum	Finger flexion	C8
Interossei	Finger Add/Abd	T1
Quadriceps	Knee extension	L3,4
Extensor hallucis	Great toe dorsiflexion	L5
Biceps femoris	Knee Flexion	S1
Soleus and gastrocnemius	Foot plantar flexion	S1,2
Rectal sphincter	Sphincter tone	S2-4

❑❑ What is the dose of methylprednisolone used to treat acute spinal cord injury?

30 mg/kg load over 15 min in the 1st h followed by 5.4 mg/kg per h over the next 23 h.

❑❑ Sensory innervation to the nipple, umbilicus, and perianal region?

Nipple - T4
Umbilicus - T10.
Perianal - S2-4.

❑❑ What percent of fractures are seen on lateral, odontoid, AP films of the neck?

Lateral 90%
Odontoid 10%.
AP just a few.

❑❑ On lateral Csp, how much soft tissue prevertebral swelling is normal from C1-4?

Up to 4 mm is normal; >5 mm suggests fracture.

❑❑ How much anterior subluxation is normal on an adult lateral Csp?

3.5 mm.

❑❑ How much angulation is normal in an adult lateral Csp, measured across a single interspace?

Up to 10°; greater is abnormal.

❑❑ On lateral Csp, what does "fanning" of the spinous processes suggest?

Posterior ligamentous disruption.

❑❑ What are the three most unstable cervical spine injuries?

1 - Transverse atlantal ligament rupture.
2 - Dens fracture.
3 - Burst fracture with posterior ligament disruption.

❑❑ Describe a Jefferson fracture.

Burst of ring of C1, usually from vertical compression force. Best seen on odontoid view.

❑❑ Describe a Hangman's fracture?

C2 bilateral pedicle fracture. Usually caused by hyperextension.

❑❑ What is a clay - shoveler's fracture?

In order of frequency C7, C6, or T1 avulsion fracture of the spinous process. Flexion or direct blow.

❑❑ Most common thoracolumbar wedge fracture in the elderly?

L1. Wedge > 50% usually requires admit for pain control and observation for ileus.

❑❑ Describe the key features of spinal shock.

Sudden areflexia which is transient and distal which lasts hours to weeks. BP is usually 80 to 100 mmHg with paradoxical bradycardia.

❑❑ A 34 year-old female patient presents to the ED with complaints of pain in the jaw, she also has a burning sensation in the roof of her mouth, pain when opening the mouth, and an earache. On exam, crepitus is present as well as tenderness over the joint capsule. Diagnosis?

TMJ syndrome.

❑❑ A trauma patient has blood at the urinary meatus. What test should be ordered?

Retrograde urethrogram. 10 mL of radiocontrast solution is injected into the urinary meatus.

❑❑ What are the 2 most commonly injured genitourinary organs?

1) Kidney.
2) Bladder (associated with pelvic fracture).

❑❑ In blunt trauma, what is the most common renal pedicle injury?

Renal artery thrombosis.

❑❑ **Describe the leg position in a patient with a femoral neck fracture.**

Shortened, abducted, and slightly externally rotated.

❑❑ **Describe the leg position in a patient with an anterior dislocation.**

Hip is abducted and externally rotated. 10% of hip dislocations. Mechanism is forced abduction. If anterior superior, hip is extended. If anterior inferior, hip is flexed.

❑❑ **Describe the leg position in a patient with a posterior hip dislocation.**

Shortened, adducted, and internally rotated. 90% of hip dislocations. Force applied to a flexed knee directed posteriorly. Associated with sciatic nerve injury (10%) and avascular necrosis of the femoral head.

❑❑ **A pneumatic tourniquet can be inflated on an extremity to more than a patient's systolic blood pressure for how long?**

2 hours without damage to underlying vessels or nerves.

❑❑ **For how long can wound care be delayed before proliferation of bacteria that may result in infection?**

3 hours.

❑❑ **What mechanisms of injury create wounds that are most susceptible to infection?**

Compression or tension injuries. They are 100 times more susceptible to infection.

❑❑ **What are the 3 anatomic subdivisions of the body created by composition of skin microflora?**

Moist areas: axilla & peritoneum - 10^4 to $10^6/cm^2$.
Dry areas: trunk, upper arms & legs - 10^1 to $10^3/cm^2$.
Exposed areas: head, face, hands, feet - 10^4 to $10^6/cm^2$.

❑❑ **What is the dose of bacteria necessary to cause wound infection without a foreign body & with a foreign body?**

Without foreign body - > 10^6 bacteria/gm of tissue.
With foreign body - 100 bacteria.

❑❑ **What 2 factors determine the ultimate appearance of a scar?**

Static & dynamic skin tension on surrounding skin.

❑❑ **What has been proven to decrease the pain of local anesthetic administration?**

Buffering the solution with sodium bicarbonate, decreasing the speed of injection and use of a subdermal injection instead of superficial or intradermal injections.

❑❑ **Why is epinephrine added to local anesthesia?**

To increase the duration of the anesthesia. Epinephrine also causes vasoconstriction & decreased bleeding, which weakens tissue defenses and increases the incidence of wound infection.

❑❑ **Where does one inject local anesthesia for an ulnar nerve block?**

On the anterior wrist, proximal volar skin crease, between the ulnar artery & the flexor carpi ulnaris.

❒❒ Where does one inject local anesthesia for a median nerve block?

On the anterior wrist, proximal volar skin crease, between the tendon of the palmaris longus & the flexor carpi radialis.

❒❒ What nerve block is used for anesthesia of the sole of the foot?

Tibial nerve block. Tibial nerve block does not provide anesthesia to the lateral aspect of the heel and foot.

❒❒ What is the preferred route for anesthesia for deep lacerations of the anterior tongue?

Lingual nerve block.

❒❒ What local anesthetic, ester or amide, is responsible for most allergic reactions?

Esters - procaine.

❒❒ How should hair be removed prior to wound repair?

By clipping the hair around the wound, not by using razor preparation which increases infection rates.

❒❒ What are the 4 C's in determining muscle viability?

Color, Consistency, Contraction, and Circulation.

❒❒ How long should one wait before delayed primary closure?

4 days. This will decrease the infection rate and is used for severely contaminated wounds.

❒❒ Bacterial endocarditis secondary to soft tissue infections may be caused by which two organisms?

Staphylococcus aureus and *Staphylococcus epidermidis*.

❒❒ What factors increase the likelihood of wound infection?

Dirty or contaminated wounds, stellate or crushing wounds, wounds longer than 5 cm, wounds older than 6 h, and infection prone anatomic sites.

❒❒ Gabriella Sabatini, the famous tennis star, presents to your "fast-track" after stepping on a nail that went right through her favorite, oldest pair of tennis shoes. What organism might infect her puncture wound?

Pseudomonas aeruginosa.

❒❒ What is the common bacteria seen in cat bite wounds which can also occur with dog bites?

Pasteurella multocida.

❒❒ Which has greater resistance to infection, sutures or staples?

Staples.

❒❒ What types of wounds result in the majority of tetanus cases?

Lacerations, punctures, & crush injuries.

❏❏ Characterize tetanus prone wounds.

Age of wound:	> 6 h.
Configuration:	Stellate wound.
Depth:	> 1 cm.
Mechanism of injury:	Missile, crush, burn, frostbite.
Signs of infection:	Present.
Devitalized tissue:	Present.
Contaminants:	Present.
Denervated &/or ischemic tissue:	Present.

❏❏ T/F- It is acceptable to clip or shave an eyebrow if needed to repair the skin.

False. Eyebrows are valuable landmarks. 15% will not regrow.

❏❏ When is a scar considered mature so that scar revision can be performed?

6 - 12 months.

❏❏ What is the risk associated with not treating a septal hematoma of the nose?

Absorption of the septal cartilage resulting in septal perforation.

❏❏ What are the important structures to be considered when repairing lacerations of the cheek?

Facial nerve, and parotid duct & gland.

❏❏ What is the resultant deformity if an auricular hematoma is not properly treated?

Cauliflower ear.

❏❏ What percent of nailbed injuries have associated fracture of the distal phalanx?

50%.

❏❏ How are tattoos and teeth related to trauma frequency?

The frequency of trauma is directly proportional to the number of tattoos and inversely proportional to the number of teeth. In addition, the more distal the tattoos, the worse the injury.

❏❏ Following blunt trauma to the chest, what type of injury is implied by the presence of pneumomediastinum, subcutaneous emphysema and a large air leak following tube thoracostomy?

Tracheobronchial tear or disruption.

❏❏ What are the early general signs & symptoms of compartment syndrome?

Early findings:
- Tenderness and pain out of proportion to the injury
- Pain with active and passive motion
- Hypesthesia (paresthesia)

Late findings:
- Compartment tense, indurated and erythematous
- Slow capillary refill
- Pallor and pulselessness

NOTE: A PULSE MAY STILL BE PRESENT IN FULLY DEVELOPED COMPARTMENT SYNDROME!

❑❑ What is the incidence of developing a compartment syndrome after an open tibial fracture?

10%. It is more common with the more severe injuries, such as open fractures.

❑❑ What associated injuries must be considered in the presence of calcaneal fractures?

Vertebral compression or burst fractures.

❑❑ What are typical clinical findings of a compartment syndrome?

Tenseness of the involved compartment to palpation, pain with passive motion, paresis and intact distal pulses. Loss of distal pulses is a late sign.

❑❑ T/F: There is an absolute value for a compartment pressure which is diagnostic of a compartment syndrome.

False. There is no specific value. In general an abnormal compartment pressure is > 25 mmHg, but this does not take into account systemic pressures. Some have suggested that when the difference between the mean arterial pressure and the compartment pressure is less than 40 mmHg a compartment syndrome should be suspected. Normal compartment pressure is between 0-8 mmHg.

❑❑ The majority of neurologic deficits associated with penetrating trauma to the brachial artery involve which nerve?

The median nerve. (The brachial artery and the median nerve are immediately adjacent in the elbow.)

❑❑ Which joint dislocation is associated with the highest rate of arterial injury?

Knee dislocation has the highest incidence of arterial injury. As many as 30% of high energy knee dislocations injure the popliteal artery.

❑❑ Among venous injuries the most commonly injured vein is in which anatomic location?

The superficial femoral vein.

❑❑ Humeral shaft fractures are associated with injury to which upper extremity nerve?

Radial nerve.

❑❑ T/F: Neural injury associated with fractures have a good chance of spontaneous recovery.

True. Recovery is much less common with injuries associated with dislocations.

EENT PEARLS

"But facts are facts and flinch not."
Robert Browning 1812-1889.

❑❑ **Define Ellis Class I, II, and III.**

I - Enamel.
II - Enamel plus dentin exposure (pink). Complain of sensitivity to heat and cold.
III - Enamel, dentin, and pulp. Complain of pain or no pain depending on nerve involvement. Treat by application of tinfoil, analgesics, and immediate referral. Avoid topical analgesics which may cause sterile abscesses.

❑❑ **How is a Schiøtz tonometer interpreted?**

Low scale readings suggest high pressure and high scale readings suggest low pressure. A scale of 4 or greater is equal to 20 mmHg or less (normal).

❑❑ **A patient is seen with herpetic lesions on the tip of the nose. Why is this a problem?**

The tip of the nose and the cornea are both supplied by the nasociliary nerve (a branch of the ophthalmic division of cranial nerve V). Thus, the cornea may also be involved.

❑❑ **A patient presents with an itching, tearing, right eye. On exam huge cobblestone papillae are found under the upper lid. Diagnosis?**

Allergic conjunctivitis.

❑❑ **A patient presents with inflammation of the conjunctiva and lid margins. Slit-lamp exam reveals a "greasy" appearance of lid margins with scaling, especially around the base of the lashes. Diagnosis?**

Blepharitis. Often caused by staphylococcal infection of the oil glands and skin next to the lash follicles. Treatment consists of scrubbing with baby shampoo and, in consultation with an ophthalmologist, sulfacetamide drops and steroid.

❑❑ **A patient presents with a painful red eye. On slit-lamp exam, a localized white flocculent infiltrate is seen in the anterior chamber. Diagnosis?**

Hypopyon is an accumulation of white inflammatory exudate in the anterior chamber. Obtain cultures, consult an ophthalmologist immediately, and admit the patient.

❑❑ **A welder presents with severe eye pain. What would be the expected finding on slit-lamp exam?**

Diffuse punctate keratopathy. Multiple pinpoint areas of fluorescein uptake representing ruptured corneal epithelial cells.

❑❑ **A patient presents with a pustular vesicle at the lid margin. Diagnosis and treatment?**

Hordeolum (Stye). Acute inflammation of the Meibomian gland most commonly of the upper lid. Treat with topical antibiotics and warm compresses. Surgical drainage may be necessary.

❒❒ A patient presents with a chronic nontender non-inflamed nodule of the upper lid. Diagnosis?

Chalazion. Treat with surgical curettage with the lid everted.

❒❒ A patient presents with blurred vision, photophobia, and dull pain in the temporal area. Exam reveals a red eye, constricted pupil, ciliary flush, and red sclera at the limbus. Visual acuity is decreased and intraocular pressure is decreased in the affected eye. What would be expected on slit-lamp exam?

Flare and cells are expected with uveitis. Treatment consists of cycloplegics (cyclopentolate or homatropine) and topical steroids in consultation with an ophthalmologist.

❒❒ A patient presents with a history of dull eye pain which developed shortly after entering a dark, sleazy bar. They also have nausea and vomiting, blurred vision, and see "halos" around lights. Exam reveals a red congested eye with decreased visual acuity. The cornea is hazy and pupil is mid-dilated and fixed to light. What reading is expected on the Schiøtz tonometer?

Usually 50 mmHg or greater. Treatment of acute angle closure glaucoma consists of acetazolamide (Diamox) 500 mg and topical timolol 0.5% (Timoptic) 1 drop repeated in 10 min. Avoid timolol in patients with COPD or heart disease. Give oral glycerol or IV mannitol. Pilocarpine 1% q 15 min for 1st h followed by one drop every 30 to 60 min.

❒❒ A patient presents with the sensation of a foreign body in the eye. Slit-lamp exam reveals a dendritic figure which has a Christmas tree pattern. Treatment?

Herpes simplex keratitis is treated with antiviral agents and cycloplegics. Steroids spell disaster!

❒❒ A patient presents with sudden, painless, loss of vision in one eye. What physical findings would be expected?

Central retinal artery occlusion typically results in a pale retina and a small pink dot near the fovea. Digital massage and immediate ophthalmic consultation for possible anterior chamber paracentesis is the treatment of choice.

❒❒ A patient presents with a physical finding of a chaotically blood-streaked retina with congested and dilated veins. Diagnosis?

Central retinal vein occlusion. Patients often complain of painless decrease in vision in one eye.

❒❒ A patient presents with loss of vision in one eye. Physical exam demonstrates a loss of central vision, peripheral vision is preserved. Diagnosis?

Retrobulbar neuritis. Twenty-five percent of cases of retrobulbar neuritis are associated with MS. The clinical presentation of MS is delayed for several years in this circumstance.

❒❒ A patient presents with sudden loss of vision is one eye which returned quickly. Diagnosis?

Amaurosis fugax. Usually caused by central retinal artery embolism from extracranial atherosclerosis.

❒❒ A patient presents with the sensation of painless loss of vision in one eye described as a wall slowly developing in the visual field. Findings expected on exam?

Gray detached retina. Patient may also complain of flashing lights in the peripheral visual field or "spider webs" in the visual field. Inferior detachment is treated with the patient sitting up. Superior detachment is treated with the patient lying flat.

❒❒ What five lid lacerations should be referred to an ophthalmologist?

1. Near the lacrimal canaliculi (between the medial canthus and the punctum).

2. Near the levator (transverse lacerations of the upper lid).
3. Near the orbital septum (upper lid deep wounds, between the tarsus and the superior orbital rim).
4. Canthal tendons (wounds penetrating the lateral and medial canthi).
5. Lid Margins (wounds through the tarsal plate and lid margins).

❏❏ **A patient presents with a history of being struck in the eye with a tennis ball. On exam, no abnormalities are evident. What should the discharge instructions state?**

Return to ED if ocular pain or blurred vision develop. Repeat exam within 24 h. Hyphemas caused by blunt eye trauma may not be present on initial exam.

❏❏ **A patient presents to the ED with a history of blunt trauma to the orbit. On exam, the patient is found to have diplopia and pain on upward gaze. What x-ray should be ordered?**

Modified stereo (Water's view) will show a blowout fracture of the orbit.
Some clinicians prefer the "Caldwell" view - the orbital floor is projected above petrous ridges.

❏❏ **A patient presents with a history of trauma to the orbit with a dull ocular pain, decreased visual acuity, and photophobia. Exam reveals a constricted pupil and ciliary flush. What will be found on slit-lamp exam?**

Flare and cells in the anterior chamber are present with traumatic iritis.

❏❏ **An anxious 24 year-old female presents with a complaint of blurred vision made worse when looking at objects far away. On exam, the eyes are convergent, the pupils are constricted, and accommodation is at a maximum. Diagnosis?**

Spasm of accommodation. Treat anxiety. A short-acting cycloplegic may stop the cycle.

❏❏ **A very anxious 16 year-old male presents stating that his vision is like "looking down a gun barrel". How should physiologic versus hysterical scotoma be differentiated?**

Physiologic -double the distance between the patient and tangent screen (visual screen test) results in a doubling of the size of the central visual field.
Hysterical - Visual field size remains the same.

❏❏ **Which anesthetic works the fastest and which lasts the longest: proparacaine or tetracaine?**

Proparacaine - Rapid onset, duration 20 min.
Tetracaine - Delayed onset, duration 1 h.

❏❏ **Place the following mydriatic-cycloplegic medications in order of duration of activity: tropicamide, homatropine, atropine, and cyclopentolate?**

Tropicamide - Onset 15-20 min, brief duration.
Cyclopentolate - Onset 30-60 min, duration < 24 h.
Homatropine - Long lasting, 2-3 d.
Atropine - Very long lasting, 2 wk.

❏❏ **What are miotics used to treat?**

Glaucoma. Pilocarpine is the most common, instilled 4 times daily.

❏❏ **Function of acetazolamide and glycerol?**

Acetazolamide - carbonic anhydrase inhibitor. Decreases ciliary body aqueous output.
Glycerol - hyperosmotic agent. Decreases intraocular pressure by making plasma hypertonic to aqueous humor.

❒❒ A 48 year-old diabetic male presents with pain, itching, and discharge from the right ear. On exam, the drum is intact. Diagnosis?

Otitis externa. Treat by suctioning ear and treating for one week with an antibiotic-steroid otic solution. May use an ear wick to improve delivery of antibiotic. Suspect necrotizing external otitis (NEO) in the diabetic patient. NEO requires hospitalization, IV antibiotics and surgical consultation.

❒❒ A patient presents with ear pain. On exam, the tympanic membrane has blisters which appear to contain fluid. Diagnosis?

Bullous myringitis, commonly caused by Mycoplasma or viruses. Treat with erythromycin.

❒❒ A 16 year-old former "Golden Gloves" champ presents with right ear pain and swelling after receiving a blow to the ear. Treatment?

If the ear is not treated appropriately, cauliflower deformity may result. As such, the ear should be aseptically drained by incision or aspiration and a mastoid-conforming dressing should be applied. ENT follow-up is mandatory.

❒❒ A patient presents with a swollen, tender, red left auricle. Diagnosis?

Perichondritis caused by *Pseudomonas*.

❒❒ A distal airway foreign body is suspected. What will plain films show?

Plain films may show air trapping on the affected side. Inspiration and expiration views demonstrate mediastinal shift away from the affected side. Lack of dependent atelectasis on a lateral decubitus film is a highly specific sign for hyperinflation (air trapping) 2° to a foreign body.

❒❒ A patient presents with trismus, painful swallowing, a stiff neck, altered voice, and fever. On exam, pharyngeal swelling and tonsillar displacement is present as well as external swelling in the parotid regions. Diagnosis?

Parapharyngeal abscess. Usually treated by a lateral approach I & D through the neck.

❒❒ What potential complication of a nasal fracture should always be considered on physical exam?

Septal hematoma. If not drained, aseptic necrosis of the septal cartilage or septal abscess may develop.

❒❒ In what age group is retropharyngeal abscess most common?

Children less than three. Symptoms may include difficulty breathing, fever, enlarged cervical nodes, difficulty swallowing, and a stiff neck. Exam may reveal a mass or fullness in the posterior pharyngeal area.

❒❒ In what age group are peritonsillar abscesses most common?

Adolescents and young adults. Symptoms may include ear pain, trismus, drooling, and alteration of voice.

❒❒ A 5 year-old child presents with a history of sinus infection. On exam, the child's eyelid is red and swollen, the globe is displaced laterally and inferiorly, and proptosis is present. Diagnosis?

The child may have orbital cellulitis and an abscess associated with ethmoid sinusitis.

❒❒ A patient with a history of frontal sinusitis presents with a large forehead abscess. Diagnosis?

Pott's puffy tumor.

❒❒ A patient presents 3 d after tooth extraction with severe pain and a foul mouth odor and taste. Diagnosis?

Alveolar osteitis (dry socket). Treat by irrigation of the socket, medicated dental packing, or iodoform with Campho-Phenique™ or eugenol.

❒❒ A patient presents with gingival pain and foul odor and taste in the mouth. On exam, fever and lymphadenopathy are present. The gingiva is bright red and the papillae are ulcerated and covered with a gray membrane. Diagnosis?

Acute necrotizing ulcerative gingivitis.

❒❒ A 47 year-old female presents to the ED with a complaint of excruciating sudden waxing and waning pain in the right cheek. She says it feels like an electric shock. Diagnosis and treatment?

Tic douloureux. Carbamazepine (100 mg bid starting dose and increase to 1200 mg daily if needed). Referral to neurologist and dentist. Rule out cerebellopontine angle tumor, MS, nasopharyngeal carcinoma, cluster headache, polymyalgia rheumatica, temporal arteritis, and oral pathology.

❒❒ What are the signs and symptoms of a mandibular fracture?

Malocclusion, pain, decreased range of motion, bony deformity, swelling, ecchymosis, and mental nerve anesthesia.

❒❒ What is the most common type of mandibular fracture?

Alveolar (tooth-bearing segment of the mandible). Numbness of the lower lip suggests a mandibular fracture.

❒❒ Signs and symptoms of fracture of the zygomaticomaxillary complex?

Emphysema of the tissue, edema, ecchymosis, facial flattening, unilateral epistaxis, anesthesia, step deformity, decreased mandibular movement and diplopia.

❒❒ What are the two most common findings with an orbital floor injury?

Diplopia and globe lowering.

❒❒ Describe a Le Fort I fracture.

Fracture line starting at the nasal apertures to the wall of the maxillary sinuses bilaterally, across the pterygomaxillary tissue, and involving the lateral pterygoid plates. X-rays often miss this fracture.

❒❒ Describe the physical findings of a Le Fort II fracture.

Swelling of the nose, lips, eyes, and midface. Subconjunctival hemorrhage may be present with blood in the nares. Suspect cerebrospinal involvement and check for rhinorrhea. Water's view and bilateral tomograms should be ordered. Fracture involves facial aspects of the maxillae extending to the nasal and ethmoid bones. Fracture also involves the maxillary sinuses and infraorbital rims bilaterally across the bridge of the nose.

❒❒ Describe the fracture line in a Le Fort III fracture.

Runs through the frontozygomatic suture lines bilaterally, through the orbits, and through the base of the nose and ethmoid region. Also called a "Dishface" fracture. Movement of the zygoma and midface is suggestive. Water's view and bilateral orbital tomograms confirm the diagnosis.

❑❑ Is cerebrospinal rhinorrhea most common with Le Fort I, II, or III?

III.

❑❑ A 42 year-old female presents with dull jaw and ear pain and a burning sensation in the roof of her mouth. The pain is worse in the evening. She also hears a "popping" sound when she opens and closes her mouth. Exam reveals tenderness of the joint capsule. Diagnosis?

TMJ syndrome. Treat with physiotherapy, analgesics, soft diet, muscle relaxants, and occlusive therapy. Apply warm moist compresses 4 to 5 times daily for 15 min for 7 to 10 d.

❑❑ A 48 year-old male presents with a history of high fever and swelling of the inferior borders of the mandible and lateral neck. Pain is severe. The patient has increased pain with swallowing and trismus. Diagnosis?

Parapharyngeal space infection.

❑❑ What is the most common site associated with Ludwig's angina?

Lower 2nd and 3rd molars. It is a boardlike swelling in the region of the submandibular, sublingual, and submental spaces. The most common organisms are hemolytic *Streptococci*, *Staphylococcus*, and mixed anaerobes and aerobes.

❑❑ What is the most feared complication of an infection in the retropharyngeal space?

Mediastinitis.

❑❑ What fascial space is involved in Ludwig's angina?

The submandibular space.

❑❑ What is the most common origin of infection in patients with Ludwig's angina?

Dental abscesses.

❑❑ What are the most common local findings in patients with Ludwig's angina?

Swelling of the floor of the mouth and tongue.

❑❑ What is the most common cause of death in Ludwig's angina?

Asphyxiation.

❑❑ What is the most common indication for surgical drainage in patients with Ludwig's angina?

Failure of antibiotic therapy.

❑❑ What are the most important organisms in Ludwig's angina?

Oral anaerobes.

❑❑ What are the antibiotics of choice for Ludwig's angina?

Penicillin and metronidazole.

❑❑ What are the most common presenting signs of lateral pharyngeal space infections?

Trismus, swelling at the angle of the mandible and medial bulging of the pharyngeal wall.

❑❑ What is the most feared complication of lateral pharyngeal space infections?

Septic thrombophlebitis of the jugular vein.

❑❑ What are the most common findings on lateral neck x-ray in patients with a retropharyngeal abscess?

Prevertebral soft tissue widening, air-fluid levels and loss of cervical lordosis.

❑❑ What is Lemierre's syndrome?

Septic thrombophlebitis of the internal jugular vein with septic pulmonary emboli associated with anaerobic oropharyngeal infection.

❑❑ What is the most common site of bleeding in posterior nosebleeds?

The sphenopalatine artery's lateral nasal branch.

❑❑ What are the findings in a pseudotumor cerebri patient?

An obese, young, female patient complaining of chronic headaches, transient visual changes, who on examination has papilledema, an enlarged blind spot on visual field testing and has a normal brain CT scan, except for smaller ventricles. Pseudotumor cerebri is a classic example of the idiopathic intracranial hypertension. A high opening pressure during lumbar puncture is both diagnostic as well as therapeutic. Treatment consists of acetazolamide and repeat lumbar puncture.

PULMONARY PEARLS

"We rarely gain a higher or larger view except when it is forced upon us through struggles which we would avoid if we could."
Charles Cooney

❑❑ **What is the most common cause of bacterial pneumonia?**

Pneumococcus.

❑❑ **What percentage of upper respiratory infectious agents are non-bacterial?**

Non-bacterial agents account for over 90% of pharyngitis, laryngitis, tracheal bronchitis, and bronchitis.

❑❑ **Name two anti-viral medications that are useful for viral pneumonia.**

Amantadine for influenza A and aerosolized Ribavirin for RSV.

❑❑ **If a patient has a patchy infiltrate on a chest x-ray and bullous myringitis, what antibiotic should be given.**

Erythromycin for Mycoplasma. Newer macrolides may also be utilized.

❑❑ **What kind of pneumonia occurs in alcoholics and other persons who develop aspiration pneumonia?**

Anaerobic and gram-negative pneumonia.

❑❑ **What secondary bacterial pneumonia often occurs following a viral pneumonia?**

Staph. aureus pneumonia.

❑❑ **What 3 findings should be present to consider a sputum sample adequate?**

There should be > 25 PMN and <10 squamous epithelial cells per low powered field along with a predominant bacterial organism.

❑❑ **A 40 year-old alcoholic presents with rigors and shortness of breath. Currant jelly sputum shows short, plump gram-negative bacilli. Chest x-ray shows a necrotizing lobar pneumonia in the right upper lobe. What is the etiologic agent?**

Klebsiella pneumonia.

❑❑ Legionella pneumoniae **occurs in summer or winter?**

Predominantly in the summer. *Staph* pneumonia also occurs more frequently in summer.

❑❑ **An older patient with GI symptoms, hyponatremia, and a relative bradycardia most likely has what type of pneumonia?**

Legionella.

❑❑ **What is the treatment for** Legionella **pneumonia?**

IV erythromycin. Rifampin is a second-live agent.

❑❑ **Should steroids be used in aspiration pneumonia?**

No.

❑❑ **Who will benefit from pentamidine prophylactic therapy for PCP?**

People with previous history of PCP and those with CD4 counts less than 200.
Criteria for pentamidine prophylaxis are becoming more relaxed.

❑❑ **Are aspirated foreign bodies more likely to be found in the right or left bronchus?**

Right.

❑❑ **T/F: Flora of lung abscesses are usually polymicrobial.**

True.

❑❑ **What are some common organisms of empyema?**

Staph, gram negatives, and anaerobes.

❑❑ **Describe the classic chest x-ray of Mycoplasma pneumonia.**

Patchy diffuse densities involving the entire lung are most common. Pneumatoceles, cavities, abscesses and pleural effusions can occur, but are uncommon. Rx. Erythromycin.

❑❑ **What are the classic signs and symptoms of TB?**

Night sweats, fever, weight loss, malaise, cough, and a green/yellow sputum most commonly seen in the mornings.

❑❑ **Why does an initial tubercle bacillus infection develop in the apical and posterior segments of the upper lobe and the superior segments of the lower lobe?**

The tubercle bacillus requires a relatively high oxygen tension for survival.

❑❑ **What are some common extrapulmonary TB sites?**

Lymph node, bone, GI tract, GU tract, meninges, liver and the pericardium.

❑❑ **Right upper lobe cavitation with parenchymal involvement is classic for:**

TB. Lower lung infiltrates, hilar adenopathy, atelectasis, and pleural effusion are also common.

❑❑ **T/F: People under 35 year of age with positive TB skin tests should have at least six months of isoniazid chemoprophylaxis.**

True.

❑❑ **Is there a higher incidence of spontaneous pneumothorax among males or females?**

Males.

❑❑ **What accessory x-rays may be obtained to diagnose a pneumothorax?**

1) Expiratory film and 2) Lateral decubitus film on the affected side.

❑❑ **What kind of pneumonias are commonly associated with a pneumothorax?**

Staph, TB, Klebsiella, and PCP. (Any pneumonic that can produce an abscess.)

❑❑ **What diagnostic test is helpful in subclinical PCP infection?**

Exertional pulse oximetry is positive for PCP if after 3 minutes of exercise the O_2 saturation decreases by 3% or the A-a gradient increases by 10mmHg from rest.

❑❑ **What laboratory tests aid in the diagnosis of PCP?**

A rising LDH or LDH > 450 and an ESR > 50. A low albumin implies a worse prognosis.

❑❑ **Most common radiographic finding of PCP?**

A reticulonodular pattern.

❑❑ **When are corticosteroids recommended for severe PCP?**

$pO_2 < 70$ mmHg or an A-a gradient > 35 mmHg.

❑❑ **List two drugs that can cause ARDS.**

Heroin and aspirin.

❑❑ **How long after an initial insult does ARDS usually occur?**

12 to 72 hours.Q: Are sedatives beneficial in acutely asthmatic patients?

No. They are dangerous!

❑❑ **Discuss some agents that may be used to induce unconsciousness.**

AGENT	AKA	CLASS	ONSET	DURATION	DOSE
Thiopental	Pentothal	Barbiturate	≈ 30 s	2-30 min. d	2.0-5.0 mg/kg @
ep. on source	40 mg/min.				
Methohexital	Brevital	B			
a					
rbiturate	Fast	Very short	5-12 mL of 1%		
					solution @ 1 mL/5 sec.
Fentanyl	Sublimaze	Opiate	2 min.	≈ 20 min.	20-150 mg/kg

❑❑ **T/F: Pulse oximetry provides a reliable means of estimating oxyhemoglobin saturation in a patient suffering CO poisoning.**

False. COHb has light absorbance that can lead to a falsely elevated pulse oximeter transduced saturation level. The calculated value from a standard ABG may also be falsely elevated. The oxygen saturation should be measured using a co-oximeter that measures the amounts of unsaturated O_2Hb, of COHb and of metHb.

❑❑ **What is the half-life of COHb for a patient breathing room air, breathing 100% oxygen and breathing 100% oxygen @ 3 atm pressure?**

Source	$FIO_2 = 0.21$	$FIO_2 = 1.0$	$FIO_2 = 1.0$ @ 3 atm
Tintinalli, 4th. Ed., pg 918.	4 - 5.3 h	50 - 80 min	23 min
Harwood-Nuss, 2nd Ed., pg 1280.	4 - 5 h	40 - 80 min	20 min
Rosen, 3rd Ed., pg 2675	4 - 6 h	90 min	30 min

Using weighted averages and throwing out the outlying values it seems safe to try to remember these values as ≈6 h, 1.5 h and 0.5 h.

❑❑ **What is the cause of hypoxemia in ARDS?**

An increase in alveolar fluid that causes a reduction in the diffusion of oxygen into the capillaries, increasing the shunt.

❑❑ **What is the mortality of ARDS?**

40 to 60%.

❑❑ **What are the major risk factors for ARDS?**

Sepsis, trauma, aspiration, multiple transfusions, shock and pulmonary contusions. Many other systemic and local insults may trigger ARDS.

❑❑ **Why is the pulmonary artery wedge pressure an important feature in the diagnosis of ARDS?**

The presence of a significantly elevated wedge pressure implies that the pulmonary edema is due to left ventricular dysfunction rather than alveolar dysfunction.

❑❑ **Does PEEP improve ARDS?**

PEEP commonly improves oxygenation. However, it does not reduce the amount of total lung water.

❑❑ **What is the distribution of pulmonary edema in ARDS?**

Routine chest x-ray appears to show a diffuse distribution. However, CT scan studies reveal an increased involvement in the dependent portions of the lung fields.

❑❑ **What are the x-ray findings in ARDS?**

Commonly, patchy bilateral peripheral infiltrates. Cardiogenic pulmonary edema typically demonstrates an enlarged heart, pleural effusions and peribronchial cuffing with septal lines.

❑❑ **What complications are associated with ARDS?**

Pneumothorax, pulmonary infection, pulmonary hypertension and multisystem organ failure.

❑❑ **What is the advantage of pressure controlled ventilation in ARDS?**

It often allows for higher mean airway pressure with a lower peak airway pressure. Oxygenation often improves with an increase in the mean airway pressure.

❑❑ **T/F: Any cause of shock can cause ARDS.**

True.

❑❑ **T/F: Too much oxygen can cause ARDS.**

True.

❒❒ **What is a safe level of oxygen for prolonged use?**

An FiO_2 of 0.50 is safe and 0.60 is probably safe.

❒❒ **What does normal ventilation with mismatched decreased lung perfusion suggest?**

Pulmonary embolus.

❒❒ **Can a patient with a PE have a pO_2 greater than 90 mmHg?**

Yes, but rarely (5%).

❒❒ **What are two relatively specific CXR findings in PE?**

Hampton's hump: a wedge shaped infiltrate abutting the pleura.
Westermark's sign: decreased lung vasculature markings on the side with a PE.
However, these findings are relatively uncommon.
.

❒❒ **What is the classical ECG finding in pulmonary embolism?**

$S_1Q_3T_3$ pattern. (This is also relatively uncommon.)

❒❒ **A 48 year-old woman is transferred from another hospital a week and a half after sustaining a left upper extremity fracture, a complex pelvic fracture, bilateral lower extremity femur fractures and a left tibial fracture. While sitting in bed, she experiences severe dyspnea, tachypnea and tachycardia. Pulse oximetry reveals an oxygen saturation of 88% on room air. She is given supplemental oxygen and transferred to the ICU. What is your diagnosis**?

Pulmonary embolism secondary to deep vein thrombosis.

❒❒ **What tests can be used to diagnosis pulmonary embolism?**

Pulmonary angiogram is still the gold standard. V/Q (ventilation/perfusion) scans are the best non-invasive tests to establish or exclude the diagnosis of PE. A high probability scan in a clinical scenario of high likelihood for PE is an indication to treat. An intermediate or low probability scan necessitates further studies. Duplex ultrasound is used to detect DVT not to diagnose PE. However, if the duplex ultrasound is positive, then therapy for DVT will also treat PE. Spiral CT, MRI and newer methods for detecting D-dimers are recent diagnostic advances that may help improve the diagnostic evaluation for pulmonary embolism

❒❒ **What are the indications for pulmonary angiography?**

Non-diagnostic non-invasive lower extremity venous study with a non-diagnostic ventilation-perfusion scan or anticipated embolectomy.

❒❒ **What is the diagnostic test of choice for documenting DVT?**

Duplex ultrasound. The accuracy of physical examination for DVT is generally quoted to be 50%.

❒❒ **What are the risk factors for DVT?**

Surgery (knee and hip greater than abdominal and urological)
Pregnancy
Cardiac disease, especially post-MI
Age greater than 50 years
Prior DVT
Immobilization
Acute paraplegia (but not chronic paraplegia)
Oral contraceptives (but not hormonal replacement therapy)

Major trauma
Malignancy, especially adenocarcinoma
Factor deficiency state
Antiphospholipid antibodies
Nephrotic syndrome
Paroxysmal nocturnal hemoglobinuria
Protein losing enteropathy

❒❒ **What is the most common CXR finding in PE?**

Atelectasis (an elevated hemidiaphragm) or pulmonary parenchymal defect.

❒❒ **What are other CXR findings in PE?**

Pleural effusion, pleural based opacity, elevated diaphragm, Westermark's sign and normal.

❒❒ **What are the two most common ECG finding in PE?**

Sinus tachycardia and nonspecific ST-T wave changes.

❒❒ **What are other ECG findings in PE?**

Normal, left axis deviation, RBBB, atrial fibrillation, pseudo-infarction pattern and S1Q3T3.

❒❒ **What is the primary utility in getting an ECG and CXR in a patient suspected of having a PE?**

To rule out other causes for their respiratory symptoms.

❒❒ **In a patient with a high probability V/Q scan and a high clinical risk for PE, are any other studies needed?**

No.

❒❒ **In a patient with a normal V/Q scan and a low clinical risk for PE, are any other studies needed?**

No.

❒❒ **What is the probability of a PE in all patients with a low probability V/Q scan?**

14%. This varies from 4% to 40%, depending on the clinical likelihood of a PE.

❒❒ **In a patient with high clinical and V/Q scan probabilities for pulmonary embolism and being considered for thrombolysis, is an angiogram necessary prior to thrombolysis?**

No. The prevalence of PE in patients with high clinical and V/Q scan probabilities for PE is 96%.

❒❒ **What can be performed in a patient whose post V/Q test probability is still uncertain?**

A lower extremity ultrasound can be performed. If positive, the patient will be treated the same as for a PE. If negative, a pulmonary angiogram can be performed.

Some support the use of serial lower extremity ultrasounds in patients with adequate cardiopulmonary reserve. For those with limited reserve, an angiogram is recommended. The use of serial lower extremity ultrasound in such a setting has not been commonly practiced in the United States.

The role of D-dimers in the setting of suspected PE has yet to be clarified.

❑❑ **What are the accepted indications for the use of thrombolytics in PE?**

Definitely accepted: hemodynamic instability.
Controversial: 40% or more of pulmonary vasculature involved with PE, obstruction of blood flow to one lobe or multiple pulmonary segments, severe hypoxia and right heart failure seen echocardiographically.

❑❑ **What is the advantage of using thrombolytic agents for PE?**

The only proven benefits have been short-term hemodynamic parameters. No randomized study has been performed with a large enough sample size to assess the impact on mortality.

❑❑ **Which drugs prolong the effect of coumadin?**

Alcohol (with liver disease), amiodarone, cimetidine, erythromycin, fluconazole, INH, metronidazole, omeprazole, phenylbutazone, propafenone and propranolol.

❑❑ **Which drugs shorten the effect of coumadin?**

Barbiturates, carbamazepine, griseofulvin, nafcillin, rifampin, sucralfate and vitamin K.

❑❑ **What are the modified PIOPED criteria for a high probability V/Q scan?**

2 large V/Q mismatches
1 large and 2 or more moderate mismatches
4 or more moderate mismatches
(Large = >75% of a segment)

❑❑ **What are the modified PIOPED criteria for an intermediate probability V/Q scan?**

1 large V/Q mismatch, with or without 1 moderate mismatch
1-3 moderate mismatches
1 matched defect with a normal CXR
(Moderate = 25% to 75% of a segment)

❑❑ **What are the modified PIOPED criteria for a low probability V/Q scan?**

1 or more perfusion defect that is smaller than the CXR defect
2 or more matches with a normal CXR and some areas of normal perfusion in lung
1 or more small perfusion defect with a normal CXR
Perfusion defects thought to be caused by effusions, cardiomegaly, aortic dilatation, hila, mediastinum and elevated hemidiaphragms
(Small = <25% of a segment)

❑❑ **Do calf vein thrombi embolize to the lung?**

Generally no, but they may propagate to the popliteal vein. Popliteal vein thrombi can embolize to the lung.

❑❑ **What are the ultrasonographic findings in acute DVT?**

Presence of echogenic material in vein lumen, noncompressibility of vein, venous distention, free-floating thrombus and absence of Doppler tracing.

❑❑ **What is the best initial method for localizing hemoptysis in a patient who is actively bleeding?**

Bronchoscopy.

❑❑ **What is the location for aspiration pneumonias?**

In the supine patient, it is in the posterior segment of the upper lobe and in the superior segment of the lower lobe. In the upright patient, it is in the basilar segments of the lower lobes. The right lung is favored over the left because of the straighter takeoff of the right mainstem bronchus.

❑❑ **What are the common directly toxic (non-infected) respiratory tract aspirates?**

Gastric contents, alcohol, hydrocarbons, mineral oil, animal and vegetable fats. All of these produce an inflammatory response and pneumonia. Gastric contents are the most common offender.

❑❑ **What are the consequences of aspirating acid?**

The response is rapid, with near immediate bronchitis, bronchiolitis, atelectasis, shunting and hypoxemia. Pulmonary edema may occur within 4 hours. The clinical manifestations are dyspnea, wheezing, cough, cyanosis, fever and shock.

❑❑ **What is the bacteriology of inpatient acquired infectious aspiration pneumonia?**

Mixed aerobic and anaerobic organisms. Unlike outpatients, *Staphylococcus aureus*, *Escherichia coli*, *Pseudomonas aeruginosa* and *Proteus* species are common.

❑❑ **What are the major causes of massive hemoptysis?**

Tuberculosis, bronchiectasis and lung cancer.

❑❑ **What causes hemoptysis in patients with tuberculosis (either active or healed)?**

Pulmonary artery (Rasmussen's) aneurysm, bronchiolar ulceration and necrosis, bronchiectasis, broncholithiasis and mycetoma (fungus ball).

❑❑ **What is the purpose of bronchoscopy in hemoptysis?**

Localization and diagnosis.

❑❑ **What is the frequency of hemoptysis in pulmonary embolism?**

20%.

❑❑ **What are the most common causes of hemoptysis in non-hospitalized patients?**

Bronchitis, bronchogenic carcinoma and idiopathic.

❑❑ **What systemic illnesses cause hemoptysis?**

Amyloidosis, CHF, mitral stenosis, sarcoidosis, SLE, vasculitis, coagulation disorders and pulmonary-renal syndromes.

❑❑ **What are the expected blood gas findings of a near-drowning victim?**

Metabolic acidosis from poor perfusion and hypoxia.

❑❑ **Can drowning occur without aspiration of water?**

Yes. 10% of victims die from intense laryngospasm.

❑❑ **How does hemoptysis differ from hematemesis?**

Blood in hemoptysis is often frothy and bright red. Alveolar macrophages may be seen on microscopy. Hematemesis is often acidic with a pH less than 2.5

❑❑ An asthmatic patient suddenly develops a supraventricular tachycardia. Blood pressure is normal and the QRS complex is also narrow. What therapy is most appropriate?

Verapamil. Avoid the use of adenosine as it is relatively contraindicated and may exacerbate bronchospasm in asthmatic patients. Also avoid ß-blockers.

❑❑ What is the predominant auscultatory finding in a patient with a foreign body lodged in the right mainstem bronchus?

Expiratory wheezing.

❑❑ Which diseases are associated with pneumothorax?

COPD, asthma, eosinophilic granuloma and lymphangioleiomyomatosis.

❑❑ Which types of pneumonia are commonly associated with pneumothorax?

Staphylococcus, TB, *Klebsiella* and PCP

❑❑ What is the indication for a tube thoracostomy in patients with a pneumothorax?

Over 20% pneumothorax or a clinical indication such as respiratory distress or enlarging pneumothorax.

❑❑ What special chest x-ray may be useful for diagnosing pneumothorax?

An expiratory film.

❑❑ What is a hemothorax?

It is when the pleural fluid hematocrit is at least 50% of that in the blood. All traumatic hemothoraces should have chest tube drainage. Thoracotomy is necessary for ongoing bleeding. Nontraumatic hemothorax is usually due to metastatic disease or as a complication to anticoagulation.

❑❑ What is the typical time period during which acute radiation pneumonitis develops?

Within the first eight weeks after radiation.

❑❑ What are the classic chest x-ray findings in a patient with sarcoidosis?

Bilateral hilar and paratracheal adenopathy with diffuse nodular appearing infiltrates. Sarcoidosis can be staged by the chest x-ray:
Stage 0: Normal
Stage 1: Hilar adenopathy
Stage 2: Hilar adenopathy and parenchymal infiltrates
Stage 3: Parenchymal infiltrates only
Stage 4: Pulmonary fibrosis

GI PEARLS

"Victory at all costs, victory in spite of all terror, victory however long and hard the road may be; for without victory there is no survival."
Sir Winston Leonard Churchill, Speech, House of Commons, 13 May, 1940.

❒❒ A patient has trouble swallowing cold liquids because they "end up in my nose." The likely condition(s)?

Motor disorders such as CVA, bulbar palsies, polio and myositis.

❒❒ After a week, an ill-appearing patient says her sore throat got worse and she complains of spiking fevers and central chest burning. What is your concern?

Retro- or parapharyngeal abscess with extension to superior mediastinitis.

❒❒ A child presents with odynophagia and drooling. What should you expect on examination of the oropharynx?

Trouble, if you look with a tongue blade! A patient with suspected epiglottitis is at high risk for upper airway compromise; intubation with direct visualization, typically in the OR, is best. This dogma may be evolving.

❒❒ A patient says food gets stuck in his mid-chest, then is regurgitated as a putrid, undigested mess. A barium study shows a dilated esophagus with a distal "beak." Diagnosis?

Achalasia.

❒❒ A woman with telangiectasias, "tight knuckles," and "acid indigestion" might have what findings on an upper GI series?

Aperistalsis, characteristic of scleroderma.

❒❒ A 40 year-old smoker describes acute, crescendo substernal chest tightness going to his back, unrelieved by antacids. An ECG shows ST changes, and his pain resolves 7-10 minutes after a nitroglycerin tablet. Is this angina?

Maybe, though the delayed response to nitrates characterizes "esophageal colic" caused by segmental esophageal spasm, often triggered by reflux.

❒❒ An elderly woman has progressive trouble swallowing first solids, then liquids. She presents with sudden drooling after dinner. Your concern?

A peptic stricture or esophageal cancer complicated by bolus obstruction.

❒❒ A patient with an "acid stomach" develops melena and vomits bright red blood. Is esophagitis a likely cause?

No. Capillary bleeding rarely causes impressive acute blood loss. Arterial bleeding (from a complicated ulcer, foreign body, or Mallory-Weiss tear) or variceal bleeding are much more likely.

❑❑ A cirrhotic patient vomits bright red blood. He has a systolic blood pressure of 90 mmHg. After an aggressive fluid resuscitation, 4 units of PRBC, and gastric lavage, his pressure is 90 mmHg. What is next?

Assume a coagulopathy and transfuse fresh frozen plasma; start a vasopressin drip; and arrange for emergent endoscopic intervention for sclerotherapy or banding.

❑❑ Recurrent pneumonias, especially in the right middle lobe or the superior segments of the bilateral upper lobes, suggests what syndrome?

Aspiration, associated with motor diseases and gastroesophageal reflux.

❑❑ List 4 contraindications to introduction of a nasogastric tube.

1) Suspected esophageal laceration or perforation.
2) Near obstruction due to stricture.
3) Esophageal foreign body.
4) Severe head trauma with rhinorrhea.

❑❑ Repeated, violent bouts of vomiting can result in both Mallory-Weiss tears and Boerhaave's syndrome. Differentiate the two.

Mallory-Weiss tears involve the submucosa and mucosa, typically in the right posterolateral wall of the GE junction.
Boerhaave's is a full-thickness tear, usually in the unsupported left posterolateral wall of the abdominal esophagus.

❑❑ After a high-speed MVA, an unrestrained driver develops abdominal and chest pain radiating to the neck. An upper chest film shows left pleural fluid. What gastroesophageal catastrophe might have occurred?

Impact against a steering wheel, can result in Boerhaave's syndrome with esophageal perforation and mediastinitis.

❑❑ You suspect a perforated esophagus; what's the next test to order?

A water-soluble contrast study. In the mean time, start broad-spectrum antibiotics and call the surgeons ASAP.

❑❑ Pediatric foreign bodies lodge at what esophageal levels?

Typically at levels of the cricopharyngeus muscles (most usual), thoracic inlet, aortic arch, tracheal bifurcation, and lower esophageal sphincter.

❑❑ When is removing a button battery lodged in the esophagus indicated?

Always. If this corrosive foreign body was swallowed <u>less than 2 hours</u> ago, and endoscopy is <u>not</u> available, consider attempting Foley balloon removal. More wisely, find a scope doc for immediate endoscopic removal.

❑❑ X-rays are crucial in the search for a suspected swallowed foreign body. In kids, what physical findings can tip you off?

Besides a child's distress, you may also find a red or scratched oropharynx, dysphagia, a high fever, or peritoneal signs. Subcutaneous air suggests perforation.

❑❑ Most objects, even sharp ones, pass thorough the GI tract without incident. What objects should be removed?

Any object that obstructs or perforates, that is > 5 cm long and >2 cm wide (won't make it past the GE junction), or is toxic (batteries) should be removed, either endoscopically or surgically. Sharp or pointed objects (sewing needles and razor blades) should be removed if they haven't passed the pylorus.

❒❒ An obstructing meat bolus should be removed within 12 hours. What's the best approach?

Endoscopy, through a trial of IV glucagon (given as 1 mg push after a small test dose, then repeated as a 2 mg dose at 20 min if no relief), or sublingual nifedipine, 10 mg, may work. Both relax esophageal smooth muscle. Meat tenderizer is best avoided, since perforation has occurred.

❒❒ Which test is mandatory after the food bolus is cleared?

A barium study or endoscopy to both confirm the passage/removal of the foreign body and to look for underlying pathology (present in virtually all adults with obstructing food boluses).

❒❒ Are there clinical findings that reliably distinguish duodenal ulcer from gastric ulcer?

No. Some findings are suggestive: A typical DU causes pain 2 h after a meal that may radiate to the back, and wake a patient from sleep, while GU often causes immediate postprandial pain and is more often due to ethanol or NSAID use.

❒❒ Name two endocrine problems that cause peptic ulcer.

Zollinger-Ellison syndrome and hyperparathyroidism (hypercalcemia).

❒❒ Postprandial midabdominal pain might suggest what ectopic syndrome?

Peptic ulcer in a Meckel's diverticulum.

❒❒ T/F: H_2 blockers decrease the risk of perforation and rebleeding in peptic ulcer disease.

False. However, cimetidine has reduced the need for surgery, improved rates of ulcer healing, and reduced the mortality from the initial bleeding episode.

❒❒ Any worries in giving cimetidine to a wheezing, anticoagulated patient with a seizure disorder?

Maybe. By decreasing blood flow to the liver and competing with the drug-eliminating cytochrome p450 system, cimetidine can increase the levels of theophylline, warfarin, and phenytoin, not to mention diazepam, propranolol, and lidocaine.

❒❒ A patient with "half a stomach" after surgery for a bleeding ulcer presents with weight loss, epigastric burning, and diarrhea. Potential reasons?

An obstructed afferent loop (Billroth II), bile reflux gastritis, dumping syndrome, malabsorption (poor mixing, of gastric/pancreatic juices, bacterial overgrowth), or gastric remnant carcinoma. Anemia (from B_{12}, iron, and folate malabsorption) and osteoporosis (from vitamin D and calcium malabsorption) are common.

❒❒ Is a person with massive upper GI bleeding likely to have a perforated ulcer?

No.

❒❒ After fluid and blood resuscitation for a bleeding ulcer, the most useful diagnostic test?

Endoscopy, which can also be therapeutic, with cryo- or electrocautery of an arterial bleeder.

❒❒ In a patient with early satiety and ulcer symptoms, what clinical finding essentially rules out a gastric outlet obstruction?

Bilious vomitus.

❒❒ T/F: Upright abdominal, left lateral decubitus, or upright chest films show free air in most perforations.

True, but just barely. Some 49% of cases show no free air (typically they are walled off). Insufflate 300-500 cc of air through a nasogastric tube, then clamp it, and have the patient sit up for 10 min to up the yield.

❒❒ Are "stress ulcers" a surgical problem?

Not usually. The diffuse gastric bleeding that results from CNS tumors, head trauma, burns, sepsis, shock, steroids, aspirin, or alcohol is usually mucosal, can be life-threatening, and can most often be managed medically. Endoscopic diagnosis is key.

❒❒ Burning epigastric pain shooting to the back, hypovolemic shock, and a high amylase suggests . . .

Posterior perforation of a duodenal ulcer.

❒❒ Can non-gallstone cholecystitis perforate?

Yes. Up to 40% of gallbladder perforations are associated with acalculous cholecystitis.

❒❒ Who gets acalculous cholecystitis?

Dehydrated post-op, post-trauma, and burn patients, as well as those with transfusion related hemolysis or narcotic use (illicit or prescribed).

❒❒ Enteric coated potassium tablets, typhoid, tuberculosis, tumors, and strangulated hernia may cause what rare process?

Non-traumatic small-bowel perforation.

❒❒ The most common cause of lower GI perforation?

Diverticulitis, followed by tumor, colitis, foreign bodies, and instrumentation.

❒❒ A pregnant woman with right upper quadrant pain should be assumed to have what intraabdominal pathology until proven otherwise?

Acute appendicitis.

❒❒ Rovsing's, psoas, and obturator signs can all indicate an inflamed posterior appendix. Please describe these signs.

Rovsing's sign - right lower quadrant pain on left lower quadrant palpation.
Psoas sign - right lower quadrant pain on right thigh extension.
Obturator sign - right lower quadrant pain on internal rotation of the flexed right thigh.

❒❒ What does ultrasound show in acute appendicitis?

A fixed, tender, non-compressible mass, but only in 75 to 90% of cases.

❒❒ What does abdominal CT scanning show in acute appendicitis?

Not much in early appendicitis; the study is useful to distinguish the causes of a right lower quadrant mass (late appendicitis, perforation/abscess, carcinoma, and pseudomyxoma).

❐❐ What does laparoscopy show in acute appendicitis?

Appendicitis, if you're lucky. Unfortunately, just seeing an inflamed appendix does not prove appendicitis; finding another cause of abdominal pain does not rule out appendicitis.

❐❐ What about blood tests?

An elevated WBC or a left shift are seen in 95 to 99% of cases; this is a sensitive test (helps rule out appendicitis), but nonspecific (can't rule it in).

❐❐ So what's the point of the last four questions?

Don't rely on diagnostic studies to diagnose acute abdominal pain. Rely instead on an exam by an experienced clinician, hospital admission, serial exams, and surgical consultation.

❐❐ The most common cause of small bowel obstruction?

Adhesions are the most common causes of extraluminal obstruction, followed by incarcerated hernia, while gallstones and bezoars are the most common causes of intraluminal obstruction.

❐❐ Recurrent small bowel obstruction in an elderly woman associated with unilateral pain into one thigh suggests what occult process?

Obturator hernia incarceration. May often present with pain down medial thigh to knee.

❐❐ The most common causes of colonic obstruction?

Cancer, then diverticulitis followed by volvulus.

❐❐ An elderly man presents with new constipation without tenesmus, abdominal pain, nausea or vomiting. He has hard stool in the vault on rectal exam. A KUB shows a colon "full of stool." Is an enema all he needs?

No. Fecal impaction with "obstipation" is both common and benign, but it is usually associated with tenesmus. He needs a workup for a colorectal tumor.

❐❐ A KUB is suspicious for a large bowel obstruction. The next step(s) in evaluation?

Unprepared sigmoidoscopy to confirm obstruction, then a barium study to determine the cause. If you suspect pseudo-obstruction (typically due to medications), **don't** order a barium study (for fear of concretion and obstruction). Colonoscopy can be diagnostic and therapeutic.

❐❐ List three classes of drugs that cause pseudo-obstruction.

Anticholinergics, antiparkinsonian drugs, and tricyclic antidepressants.

❐❐ While you're at it, list three types of internal hernias.

Diaphragmatic hernia, lesser sac hernia (through the foramen of Winslow), and omental or mesenteric hernia.

❐❐ Which is more dangerous, a small hernia or a large one?

Incarceration is more likely with small hernias.

❒❒ Is a hernia in Hesselbach's triangle (between the inguinal ligament, inferior epigastric vessels, and lateral border of the rectus abdominis) likely to incarcerate?

Direct hernias rarely incarcerate.

❒❒ What about a hernia that is lateral to the epigastric vessels?

Indirect hernias are much more likely to incarcerate.

❒❒ Which is the most common hernia in women, inguinal or femoral?

Inguinal, not femoral. While it's true that femoral hernias are more common in women than in men, inguinal hernias remain the most common hernia in women.

❒❒ Distinguish between a groin hernia, a hydrocele and a lymph node.

Hydroceles transilluminate and are non-tender. Lymph nodes tend to be freely moving, firm, and multiple. Hernias don't transilluminate and may have bowel sounds.

❒❒ A patient tells you that 2 d ago his groin bulged and he developed severe pain with progressive nausea and vomiting. He has a tender mass in his groin. What shouldn't you do?

Don't try to reduce a long-standing, tender incarcerated hernia! The abdomen is no place for dead bowel.

❒❒ How does the pathology of Crohn's disease differ from that of ulcerative colitis?

Crohn's is a trans-mucosal, segmental, granulomatous process, while ulcerative colitis is a mucosal, juxtapositional, ulcerative process.

❒❒ A young man with atraumatic chronic back pain, eye trouble, and painful red lumps on his shins develops bloody diarrhea. What is the point of this question?

To remind you of extraintestinal manifestations of inflammatory bowel disease, such as ankylosing spondylitis, uveitis, and erythema nodosum, not to mention kidney stones.

❒❒ At least a third of patients with Crohn's disease have kidney stones. Why?

Dietary oxalate is usually bound to calcium and excreted. When terminal ileal disease leads to decreased bile salt absorption, the resulting fattier intestinal contents bind calcium by saponification. Free oxalate is "hyper-absorbed" in the colon, resulting in hyperoxaluria and calcium oxalate nephrolithiasis.

❒❒ Complications of Crohn's include perirectal abscesses, anal fissures, rectovaginal fistulas, and rectal prolapse. How often is perirectal disease present?

Approximately 90 percent of patients.

❒❒ A patient with chronic, occasionally bloody diarrhea develops severe diarrhea and abdominal pain with marked distention. What "can't-miss" diagnosis does this suggest?

Toxic megacolon, a life-threatening complication of ulcerative colitis.

❒❒ What are the odds that a patient with severe ileal disease will be cured by surgery?

Virtually zero. Crohn's almost invariably recurs in the remaining GI tract. In contrast, total proctocolectomy with ileostomy is curative in ulcerative colitis.

❒❒ A patient with new diarrhea and abdominal pain tells you she took antibiotics for sinusitis two weeks ago. Sigmoidoscopy might reveal what?

Yellowish superficial plaques suggestive of pseudomembranous colitis. Stool studies would show *C. difficile* toxin.

❒❒ What's the treatment?

Oral vancomycin, 125 mg qid or oral metronidazole, 500 mg qid. Either regimen should be given for 7 to 10 days. Cholestyramine, which binds the toxin, can help limit the diarrhea. Follow-up stool studies should confirm clearance of the toxin.

❒❒ Is diverticulitis the likely diagnosis in a patient with low abdominal pain and bright red blood per rectum?

No. Typically diverticulosis bleeds, while diverticulitis doesn't. Diverticular bleeding is typically painless.

❒❒ Is sigmoidoscopy or contrast x-ray study indicated in acute diverticulitis?

A controversial topic. The conventional wisdom says wait until the acute inflammation resolves.

❒❒ Crampy abdominal pain with mucus in the stool suggests what syndrome?

The irritable bowel one. Patients are afebrile, and often improve after passing flatus.

❒❒ What barium findings distinguish colonic obstruction due to acute diverticulitis from that due to colon cancer?

Diverticulitis is extraluminal, so the mucosa appears intact and involved bowel segments are longer. Adenocarcinoma distorts the mucosa, involves a short segment of bowel, and has overhanging edges.

❒❒ Abdominal pain in a gray-haired patient should always suggest _____ ______, until proven otherwise.

Mesenteric ischemia.

❒❒ Prescribe an outpatient antibiotic regimen for uncomplicated diverticulitis.

Ciprofloxacin plus metronidazole.

❒❒ Which is more sensitive for locating the source of GI bleeding, a radioactive Tc-labeled red cell scan, or angiography?

A bleeding scan can find a site bleeding at a rate as low as 0.12 mL/min, while angiography requires rapid bleeding (greater than 0.5 mL/min).

❒❒ A patient known to have gallstones presents with acute, postprandial right upper quadrant pain. What's the KUB likely to show?

Nothing specific. Only around 10% of gallstones are radiopaque. Complications of cholelithiasis - emphysematous cholecystitis, perforation, and pneumobilia - are uncommon but useful findings.

❒❒ A child with sickle cell disease presents with fever, right upper quadrant pain, and jaundice. The likely diagnosis?

Charcot's triad suggests ascending cholangitis. The precipitating cause is most likely pigment stones resulting from chronic hemolysis.

❒❒ A post-surgical patient develops right upper quadrant pain, nausea, and low-grade fevers. According to his surgeon, the gallbladder was normal intraoperatively. What's a probable diagnosis?

Acalculous cholecystitis.

❒❒ Eight years after her cholecystectomy, a woman develops right upper quadrant pain and jaundice. What's the chance of developing recurrent biliary tract stones after cholecystectomy?

At least 10%, due either to retained stones or *in-situ* formation by biliary epithelium.

❒❒ List the ultrasound findings suggestive of acute cholecystitis.

Presence of gall stones (or sludge, in acalculous cholecystitis), gall bladder wall thickening > 5 mm, and pericholecystic fluid. A dilated common bile duct (>10 mm) suggests common duct obstruction.

❒❒ Name two findings in acute cholecystitis that mandate emergent laparotomy.

Emphysematous cholecystitis and perforation. Otherwise, timing of surgery is somewhat institution- and surgeon-dependent.

❒❒ What simple test can distinguish between conjugated and unconjugated hyperbilirubinemia?

A dipstick test for urobilinogen, which reflects conjugated (water soluble) hyperbilirubinemia.

❒❒ In addition to conjugated hyperbilirubinemia, what liver function abnormalities suggest biliary tract disease?

Elevated alkaline phosphatase out of proportion to transaminases.

❒❒ Which two LFT abnormalities reflect a poor prognosis in acute viral hepatitis?

A total bilirubin > 20 mg/dL, and prolongation of the prothrombin time > 3 seconds. The extent of transaminase elevation is not a useful marker.

❒❒ Match the following hepatitis serologies with the right clinical description:

(1) HBsAg (-), antiHBs(+)	___ongoing viral replication; highly infectious.
(2) IgM HBcAg (+), antiHBs(-)	___remote infection; not infectious.
(3) IgG HBcAg (+), antiHBs(-)	___recent or ongoing infection; a high titer means high infectivity, while a low titer suggests chronic, active infection.
(4) HBeAg (+)	___prior infection or vaccination; not infectious.

Answers: 4,3,2,1.

HBeAg (+):	"e" = "eeeek! I'm infectious!", for e ANTIGEN, anti-HBe implies decreased infectivity.
IgG HBcAg (+):	"G" = Gone.
IgM HBcAg (+):	"M" = Might be contagious still.
ANTIHBs (+):	"s" = Stopped, Pt. has antibodies to surface antigen.

WARNING! YOU MUST SPECIFY WHETHER THE ANTIGEN OR THE ANTIBODY IS PRESENT WHEN LEARNING THESE LETTER CODES, OTHERWISE YOU WILL LEARN THESE THINGS THE WRONG WAY AROUND!! Go over it ten times or so in the text of your choice, then it will make sense and remembering the letters won't be necessary.

❒❒ T/F: The "delta agent" can cause hepatitis D in a patient without active hepatitis B.

False. The d-agent is an incomplete, "defective," RNA virus responsible for hepatitis D. It is an obligate covirus and requires hepatitis B for replication.

❑❑ You stick yourself with a needle from a chronic hepatitis B carrier. You've been vaccinated, but never had your antibody status checked. What would be the appropriate post-exposure prophylaxis?

Have your anti-HBs titer measured. If it's adequate (>10 mIU), you need no treatment. If it's inadequate, you need a single dose of HBIG as soon as possible and a vaccine booster.

❑❑ Match the following hepatotoxic drugs with the correct toxic syndrome:

(1) Halothane, methyldopa, isoniazid.	___chronic active hepatitis and cirrhosis.
(2) Anabolic steroids, oral contraceptives, oral hypoglycemics, erythromycin estolate.	___massive hepatic necrosis.
(3) Carbon tetrachloride, phosphorus, acetaminophen, *Amanita* mushrooms.	___acute hepatitis.
(4) Vinyl chloride, arsenic.	___steatosis, hepatocellular necrosis.
(5) Ethanol.	___cholestatic jaundice.

(Answer: 4, 3, 1, 5, 2)

❑❑ A high fever and leukocytosis accompanying acute alcoholic hepatitis is worrisome. Why?

Alcohol is marrow toxic, so leukocytosis often reflects serious associated infection. Get a chest x-ray, and obtain blood cultures, a urinalysis, and ascitic fluid for cell count and culture.

❑❑ A cirrhotic presents with weakness and edema. What electrolyte imbalances might be present?

Hyponatremia (dilutional or diuretic-induced), hypokalemia (from GI losses, secondary hyperaldosteronism, or diuretics), and hypomagnesemia.

❑❑ The best diuretic choice for most cirrhotics with ascites?

Potassium-sparing agents (treat the hyperaldosterone state specifically).

❑❑ A confused cirrhotic presents to the ED. She is afebrile and has asterixis. What should your exam consist of as you look for the precipitant of hepatic encephalopathy?

Give thiamine and folate. Assess her mental status and search for localizing neurologic signs (occult head injury); look for dry mucous membranes and a low jugular venous pressure (hypovolemia and azotemia); check a stool guaiac (GI bleeding). Focused lab testing can pinpoint other causes (diuretic overuse and hypokalemia, hypoglycemia, anemia, hypoxia, and infection).

❑❑ Aside from fixing the above, what therapy is useful?

Lactulose, which produces an acidic diarrhea that traps nitrogenous wastes in the gut.

❑❑ Are there any useful therapies for the rapid renal failure that can complicate cirrhosis?

Unfortunately not. The hepatorenal syndrome still has a mortality that approaches 100%.

❑❑ An ascitic patient presents with fever but no localizing signs or symptoms of infection, and a normal WBC. Because you know that spontaneous bacterial peritonitis can be an occult disease, you perform an abdominal paracentesis. What WBC in ascitic fluid suggests SBP?

Greater than 250/mm^3. You should also Gram stain the fluid and send at least 10 cc in blood culture bottles for aerobic and anaerobic culture.

❑❑ The most common organism responsible for SBP?

E. coli, followed by *S. pneumoniae*.

❑❑ So the best therapy is . . .?

Intravenous Ampicillin **plus** an aminoglycoside is reasonable empiric therapy pending culture results.

❑❑ What two therapies can reduce the risk of recurrent SBP?

Diuretics decrease ascitic fluid, and nonabsorbable oral antibiotics decrease the gut bacterial load, limiting bacterial translocation. Both treatments have cut the risk of recurrence in compliant patients.

❑❑ A non-drinker presents with acute pancreatitis. What conditions may underlie this acute process?

Biliary tract disease, trauma (blunt or penetrating), ulcers (posterior penetrating duodenal ulcer), diabetes (ketoacidosis), and hypertriglyceridemia.

❑❑ Which is a more sensitive test for pancreatitis, serum amylase or lipase?

Amylase elevation is 70-90% sensitive for pancreatitis; lipase is 75-100% sensitive; the combination is up to 95-97% sensitive. Remember that up to 10% of patients with severe acute pancreatitis may have a normal amylase. In chronic pancreatitis, up to 30% may have a normal amylase.

❑❑ What are Ranson's five predictors of complications from acute pancreatitis upon admission?

Age over 55, blood glucose >200 mg/dl, WBC > 16,000/mm^3, SGOT (AST) >250 U/l, and LDH > 350 IU/l.

❑❑ Forty-eight h after admission, what six findings predict poor outcome?

Hematocrit drop > 10%, rise in BUN > 5 gm/dl, calcium lower than 8 mg/dl, PaO_2 < 60 mmHg, over 6 liter third-space fluid accumulation, and base deficit > 4 mEq/l.

❑❑ Is a nasogastric tube always indicated in acute pancreatitis?

Only if nausea and vomiting are severe. One trial showed a worse outcome with NG tubes because of complications, including aspiration.

❑❑ When are antibiotics useful in acute pancreatitis?

Pancreatitis is a chemical disease, and antibiotics are only useful for treating complications such as abscess or sepsis. The only exception is in pancreatitis associated with choledocholithiasis, when antibiotics are indicated.

❑❑ Symptoms that last longer than a week or **the presence of an abdominal mass, hyperamylasemia, and leukocytosis suggest what potentially disastrous complications of pancreatitis?**

Pancreatic abscess or pseudocyst.

❑❑ Are there any useful plain film findings in pancreatitis?

Right upper quadrant calcifications suggests gallstone pancreatitis, air in the region of the pancreas suggests abscess, and calcific stippling in the epigastrium suggests chronic pancreatitis.

❑❑ Portal hypertension produces internal hemorrhoids through which veins?

Internal hemorrhoids are proximal to the fabled dentate line in the **2**-, **5**-, and **9**-o'clock position in the prone patient, and are typically not palpable on rectal exam. They occur in the superior rectal and inferior mesenteric veins.

❐❐ Are painful hemorrhoids always external hemorrhoids?

No. Though hemorrhoidal pain is more likely to be due to thrombosed external hemorrhoids, be on the lookout for prolapsed and/or incarcerated internal hemorrhoids.

❐❐ Distinguish, by location, the following: anal cryptitis, anal fissure, anorectal abscess, and fistula in ano.

Cryptitis, fissures and perianal abscess typically occur in the posterior midline; deep abscesses can point to areas far from the anus. Goodsall's rule on fistulas: those that open anteriorly go straight to the anal canal, while those that open posteriorly may follow a circuitous route.

❐❐ T/F: Antibiotics are unnecessary after an uncomplicated perirectal abscess is incised and drained.

True, assuming the patient has no underlying immunoincompetence (HIV, diabetes, malignancy). Sitz baths beginning the next day are the primary after-care.

❐❐ Distinguish anal chancres and herpetic ulcers.

Anal chancres of primary syphilis are painless, symmetric, indurated, and diagnosed by dark-field microscopy. Herpes simplex produces perianal paresthesias and pruritus, followed by red-haloed vesicles and apthous ulcers (ruptured vesicles); a Tzanck smear is diagnostic. Both cause painful inguinal adenopathy.

❐❐ A patient presents with proctitis, and a Gram stain of a rectal swab reveals neutrophils with Gram-negative intracellular diplococci. The treatment?

Ceftriaxone, 250 mg IM, once, with tetracycline, 500 mg qid (or doxycycline 100 mg bid) for 10 days to cover possible Chlamydia co-infection (send a Chlamydia swab and a serologic test for syphilis to the lab, as well). Sexual partners should be notified, and follow-up cultures obtained after therapy. (Note: some authors suggest empiric treatment for Chlamydia in women only, since Chlamydial proctitis is less common in men).

❐❐ Procidentia in adults mandates what intervention?

Rectal prolapse can be manually reduced in children with good results; adults typically require proctosigmoidoscopy and surgical repair.

❐❐ Is it better to have cancer of the anal margin or of the anal canal?

Anal margin cancer is usually low-grade, and late to metastasize, while anal canal cancers (i.e., more proximal tumors) are more aggressive and metastasize early.

❐❐ Watery diarrhea with profuse rectal discharge and weakness might suggest what uncommon tumor?

Villous adenoma, with watery diarrhea and hypokalemia.

❐❐ Do pilonidal abscesses communicate with the anal canal?

No. They are virtually always midline and overlie the lower sacrum. Posterior-opening, horseshoe-type anorectal fistulas can find their way to the lower sacrum, but are rarely in the midline. Remember Goodsall's rule.

❑❑ **Should pilonidal cysts be excised in the emergency department?**

Probably not. Incision and drainage is OK, followed by a bulky dressing, analgesics, and hot sitz baths beginning the next day; antibiotics are not typically necessary. Excision should be completed in the OR once the acute infection clears up.

❑❑ **In adults, pruritus ani is seen with dietary factors contributing to liquid stool (caffeine, mineral oil), sexually transmitted infections, fecal contamination, overzealous hygiene, and vitamin deficiencies. The most common cause in children?**

Enterobius vermicularis, or pinworm. A cheap and diagnostic test: apply a piece of scotch tape sticky-side down to the perineal area, than smooth it out (with a cotton swab) on a glass slide and examine under low power for eggs. Treatment is mebendazole, 100 mg in a single dose, repeated at 2 weeks.

❑❑ **What stool studies are crucial in evaluating acute diarrhea?**

Statistically speaking, acute diarrhea is so common and typically self-limited that most cases need no testing, just oral rehydration. In sick patients or those at risk for complications (at the extremes of age, recently hospitalized, immunocompromised), enteroinvasive infection should be ruled out with a stool guaiac and test for fecal leukocytes (Gram or methylene blue stains are comparable). Also consider checking for ova and parasites.

❑❑ **Which diarrheal illnesses cause fecal leukocytes?**

Usual culprits:
- Shigella.
- *Campylobacter*.
- Enteroinvasive *E. coli.*

Others:
- *Salmonella*, *Yersinia*, *Vibrio parahaemolyticus*, and *C. difficile*.

Fecal WBCs are absent in toxigenic and enteropathogenic infection, even with such a virulent organism as *Vibrio cholera*; viral and parasitic infections rarely produce fecal WBCs.

❑❑ **Name the most likely cause of diarrhea in a 6-mo old in day-care.**

Viral diarrhea is most common, with Rotavirus the most common virus; be on the lookout for Giardia and Cryptosporidia, recently added to the list of day-care-associated diarrheal illnesses.

❑❑ **The most common cause of bacterial diarrhea?**

E. coli (enteroinvasive, enteropathogenic, enterotoxigenic).

❑❑ **A former IV drug user with sickle-cell disease and a history of splenectomy presents with unremitting fever, crampy abdominal pain, and meningismus after recently acquiring a pet turtle. He has no diarrhea. What bacteria may be the culprit?**

Salmonella typhi, the causative agent of typhoid fever. The attack rate is remarkably high in patients with HIV, in asplenic patients, and in those with sickle cell disease. Rose spots occur in 10-20%; relative bradycardia in the face of a high fever, and a low or normal WBC with a pronounced left shift are suggestive findings.

❑❑ **The treatment?**

Intravenous Fluoroquinolone, Ceftriaxone, or Chloramphenicol. Make sure to check blood cultures, which may suggest metastatic infection. Avoid antimotility agents.

❐❐ Match the diarrheal syndrome with the culprit:

(1) *Aeromonas hydrophilia*	___Diarrhea on the way to the car after eating fried rice at a Chinese buffet.
(2) *Bacillus cereus*	___Diarrhea followed by thigh myalgias, perioral dysesthesias, and pruritus.
(3) *Campylobacter*	___Profuse, foul-smelling diarrhea with bloating and cramps after a fishing trip.
(4) *Clostridium difficile*	___Bloody diarrhea and fever in a child.
(5) *Clostridium perfringens*	___Acute dysentery, fever, and pseudoappendicitis after getting a new puppy.
(6) *Vibrio parahaemolyticus*	___Rice water diarrhea without fever or constitutional symptoms.
(7) *Staph. aureus*	___Diarrhea from raw seafood.
(8) *Yersinia*	___Diarrhea from contaminated meat; no nausea or vomiting.
(9) *Giardia*	___Diarrhea from antibiotic-associated enterocolitis.
(10) Ciguatera toxin	___Diarrhea (enterocolitis) associated with either antibiotics *or* food.

(Answers: 2, 10, 9, 3, 8, 1, 6, 5, 4, 7)

Diarrhea on the way to the car after eating fried rice at a Chinese buffet - *Bacillus cereus*; treatment is symptomatic.
Diarrhea followed by thigh myalgias, perioral dysesthesias, and pruritus - Ciguatera toxin; no treatment.
Profuse, foul-smelling diarrhea with bloating and cramps after a fishing trip - Giardia; quinacrine or metronidazole.
Bloody diarrhea and fever in a child - *Campylobacter*; erythromycin; doxycycline or fluoroquinolone in adults.
Acute dysentery, fever, and pseudoappendicitis - *Yersinia*; optimal tx unknown, chloramphenicol, tetracycline, TMP/SMX.
Rice water diarrhea without fever or constitutional symptoms - *Aeromonas hydrophilia* with sx due to enterotoxin; tx primarily symptomatic.
Diarrhea from raw seafood - *Vibrio parahaemolyticus*; treat symptoms.
Diarrhea from contaminated meat; no nausea or vomiting - *Clostridium perfringens*; usually no therapy, rarely antitoxin antibodies.
Diarrhea from antibiotic-associated enterocolitis - *Clostridium difficile*; vancomycin or metronidazole.
Diarrhea (enterocolitis) associated with either antibiotics or food - *Staph. aureus*; treat symptoms.

❐❐ What are the symptoms most commonly associated with neuromuscular associated dysphagia?

Nasopharyngeal regurgitation and hoarseness.

❐❐ The most common causes of dysphagia in the elderly population include?

Hiatal hernia, reflux esophagitis, webs/rings, and cancer.

❐❐ The most common symptom of esophageal disease is?

Pyrosis - heartburn.

❐❐ What are the classical features which distinguish chest pain of esophageal origin from cardiac ischemia?

There are no classical clinical features which distinguish between these two entities. Exertional pain and palliation with rest or NTG occur in both groups. Pain relief in the GI group usually takes 7-10 min while ischemic pain usually responds in 2-3 minutes.

❐❐ Radiographs should be performed in all patients suspected of swallowing coins to determine the presence and location of the FB. How will the coin appear on the X-ray in the AP view?

Coins in the esophagus lie in the frontal plane. Coins in the trachea lie in the sagittal plane.

❐❐ What is the management of button battery ingestion?

Button batteries must be removed from the esophagus by endoscopy. One may consider a Foley catheter technique if the battery has been present less that 2 hours.

❒❒ What is the management of button batteries that have passed the esophagus?

In the asymptomatic patient - repeat radiographs. The symptomatic patient and those patients where the battery has not passed the pylorus after 48 hours require endoscopic retrieval.

❒❒ What medical conditions are associated with an increase incidence of PUD?

COPD, Cirrhosis, and chronic renal failure.

❒❒ What is the most common location of a perforated peptic ulcer?

Anterior surface of the duodenum or pylorus and the lesser curvature of the stomach.

❒❒ What types of patients are at risk for gallbladder perforation?

Elderly, diabetics, and those with recurrent cholecystitis.

❒❒ What percentage of patients with a perforated viscus have radiographic evidence of a pneumoperitoneum?

Sixty to seventy percent will have this finding. Therefore, one-third of patients will not have this sign. Keep the patient in either the upright or left lateral decubitus position for at least 10 minutes prior to performing X-rays.

❒❒ What are the indications for the surgical removal of a GI foreign body?

GI obstruction; GI perforation; toxic properties of the material, and length, size, and shape that will prevent the object from passing safely.

❒❒ What size objects rarely pass the stomach?

Objects longer than 5 cm and wider than 2 cm.

❒❒ Are gastric and duodenal perforations more common in malignant or benign ulcers?

Benign ulcerations.

❒❒ Does significant UGIB accompany perforated ulcers?

Massive GI bleeding almost rules out the presence of a perforated ulcer. One should consider a secondary penetrating ulcer.

❒❒ Acalculous cholecystitis commonly occurs in which conditions?

Postoperative, post-trauma; burn patients secondary to dehydration, and hemolysis secondary to blood transfusions.

❒❒ What are the most common causes of non-traumatic perforations of the lower GI tract?

Diverticulitis, carcinoma, colitis, foreign bodies, barium enemas, and endoscopy.

❒❒ The hallmark of a perforated viscus is?

Abdominal pain.

❑❑ Which is one of the earliest signs of sepsis?

Respiratory alkalosis on an ABG.

❑❑ What are the more common processes that mimic acute appendicitis?

Mesenteric lymphadenitis, PID, Mittleshmertz, Gastroenteritis, and Crohn's disease.

❑❑ What conditions are associated with an atypical presentation of acute appendicitis?

Situs inversus viscerum, malrotation, hypermobile cecum, long pelvic appendix, and pregnancy (1/2200).

❑❑ What are the most frequent symptoms of acute appendicitis?

Anorexia and pain. The classical presentation: anorexia, periumbilical pain with progression to constant RLQ pain is present in only 60% of cases.

❑❑ What clinical maneuvers may aid in the diagnosis of acute appendicitis?

The psoas sign and the obturator sign may aid in the diagnosis of an inflamed posteriorly located appendix.

❑❑ What percentage of acute appendicitis cases have an elevated WBC count?

An elevated leukocyte count and an elevated absolute neutrophil count are present in 86% and 89% respectively.

❑❑ If blood is recovered from the stomach after an NG tube is inserted, where is the most likely location of the bleed?

Above the ligament of Treitz.

❑❑ How much blood must be lost in the GI tract to cause melena?

50 mL. Healthy patients normally lose 2.5 mL/day.

❑❑ A 24 year-old male complains that he has endured two days of rice-water stools, muscle cramps and extreme fatigue. He looks pale, dehydrated and very ill. The patient states that he has just returned from India. What is the diagnosis?

Cholera. The incidence of cholera in the US is 1/10,000,000. This disease usually develops in persons that have traveled to endemic areas, such as India, Africa, Southeast Asia, southern Europe, Central and South America and the Middle East. Infection occurs by consuming unpurified water, raw fruits and vegetables and undercooked seafood.

❑❑ Is diverticulitis the probable diagnosis for a patient with lower abdominal pain and bright red blood per rectum?

No. Typically diverticulosis bleeds, while diverticulitis doesn't. Diverticular bleeding is usually painless.

❑❑ A 40 year-old smoker describes an acute crescendo substernal chest tightness penetrating to his back. Antacids do not relieve the pain. An ECG shows ST changes and his pain resolves 7 to 10 minutes after a nitroglycerin tablet. Is this angina?

Maybe, although the delayed response to nitrates characterizes "esophageal colic" which is caused by segmental esophageal spasm and is often triggered by reflux.

❑❑ Which type of hepatitis is characterized by an SPGT greater than the SGOT?

Viral hepatitis. The SGPT is usually greater than 1,000.

❑❑ Which type of hepatitis is usually contracted through blood transfusions?

Hepatitis C accounts for 85% of hepatitis infections via this route.

❑❑ List four contraindications to the introduction of a nasogastric tube.

1) Suspected esophageal laceration or perforation
2) Near obstruction due to stricture
3) Esophageal foreign body
4) Severe head trauma with rhinorrhea

❑❑ What test should be performed when an elderly patient is suffering from pain that is out of proportion to the physical examination?

Angiography. This test is the gold standard for diagnosing mesenteric ischemia.

❑❑ A KUB suggests a large bowel obstruction. What are the next steps?

An unprepared sigmoidoscopy to confirm obstruction followed by a barium study to determine the cause. If a pseudo-obstruction is suspected, don't order a barium study because of the possibility of concretion and obstruction. Colonoscopy can be diagnostic as well as therapeutic.

❑❑ Pseudo-obstruction is typically caused by medications. What are four classes of drugs that give rise to pseudo-obstruction?

Anticholinergics, anti-parkinsonian drugs, tricyclic antidepressants and especially, opiates.

❑❑ What is the most frequent cause of small bowel obstruction?

Adhesions, followed by incarcerated hernias, are the most common causes of extraluminal obstruction. Gallstones and bezoars are the most common causes of intraluminal obstruction.

❑❑ Is a serum amylase test or a lipase test more specific for pancreatitis?

Lipase.

❑❑ Is a nasogastric tube always required for acute pancreatitis?

No, only if nausea and vomiting are severe. In fact, one study showed that NG tubes contributed to more complications, including aspiration.

❑❑ When are antibiotics useful in acute pancreatitis?

Because pancreatitis is a chemical disease, antibiotics are only useful for treating complications, such as an abscess or sepsis and those cases that are associated with choledocholithiasis.

❑❑ What is the most common cause of lower GI perforation?

Diverticulitis, followed by tumor, colitis, foreign bodies and instrumentation.

❑❑ A patient with chronic and occasionally bloody diarrhea develops severe diarrhea and abdominal pain with marked distention. What "can't miss" diagnosis do these signs suggest?

Toxic megacolon. This condition is a life threatening complication of ulcerative colitis.

❑❑ What is the most common cause of pancreatitis?

Alcohol and gallstones.

❑❑ What are some other causes of pancreatitis?

Surgery, trauma, post-ERCP, viral and mycoplasma infections, hypertriglyceridemia, vasculitis, drugs, penetrating peptic ulcer, anatomic abnormalities about the ampulla of Vater, hyperparathyroidism, end stage renal disease and organ transplantation.

❑❑ What are some of the drugs known to cause pancreatitis?

Sulfonamides, estrogens, tetracyclines, pentamidine, azathioprine, thiazides, furosemide and valproic acid.

❑❑ What are some of the infectious causes of pancreatitis?

Mumps, viral hepatitis, Coxsackie virus group B and mycoplasma.

❑❑ What are the most common causes of colonic obstruction?

Cancer, then diverticulitis followed by volvulus.

❑❑ What is abdominal compartment syndrome?

Increased pressure within the confined anatomical space of the abdomen that may impair end organ perfusion and physiologic function.

❑❑ Forty eight hours post-operatively, a patient develops severe pain about his midline wound, skin bullae, crepitus and irregular blanching at the wound margins with a fever of 104°F. What is the most likely diagnosis?

Clostridial gas gangrene.

❑❑ What is the treatment for patients who present with the sudden onset of inability to swallow food, liquids or saliva?

Esophagoscopy to confirm esophageal obstruction, with endoscopic removal of the impacted food or foreign body. Food is the most common obstructing foreign body in the esophagus.

❑❑ What are the common radiographic signs suggestive of esophageal perforation?

Mediastinal air, pneumothorax, pleural effusion and subcutaneous emphysema.

❑❑ What is the most appropriate initial therapy for a patient with bleeding esophageal varices?

Octreotide (somatostatin analogue) infusion. Vasopressin along with nitroglycerin (to offset the coronary vasoconstriction caused by vasopressin) can be used if this is unavailable. Any coagulation defect must be corrected.

❑❑ What are the other non-surgical options for bleeding esophageal varices that do not respond to somatostatin infusion?

Placement of Sengstaken-Blakemore tube, sclerotherapy or banding of varices and transjugular intrahepatic portosystemic shunting.

❑❑ Four days following placement of a percutaneous endoscopic gastrostomy tube a patient develops sudden onset of fever, chills, tachycardia and hypotension. Physical exam shows abdominal distention and plain films show a large amount of free air. The most likely cause is?

Gastric leakage due to necrosis.

❒❒ What is the most common cause of toxic megacolon?

The most common cause is ulcerative colitis, although other causes include Crohn's disease, amebic colitis, shigella or salmonella infection, pseudomembranous colitis, ischemic bowel disease, mucosal ulcerative colitis, cytomegalovirus infection and anti-cancer chemotherapy.

❒❒ What are the most common causes of lower GI hemorrhage?

Diverticulosis and angiodysplasia.

❒❒ What is the most common colonic site for massive lower GI bleeding?

The right colon.

❒❒ What percentage of fulminant hepatic failure is due to acetaminophen?

In the U.S., about 10% are due to acetaminophen ingestion and another 10% are due to other drugs such as isoniazid, halogenated anesthetics, phenytoin, propylthiouracil and sulfonamides.

❒❒ What disease is suggested by Grey-Turner's sign (flank ecchymosis) and Cullen's sign (periumbilical ecchymosis)?

Severe necrotizing pancreatitis with retroperitoneal hemorrhage.

❒❒ A patient admitted to the ICU for shock describes terrible abdominal pain out of proportion to their physical exam. What is the most likely diagnosis?

Intestinal infarction.

❒❒ What are the common symptoms of acute pancreatitis?

Epigastric abdominal pain radiating to the back associated with nausea and vomiting.

❒❒ T/F: Normal amylase levels rule out pancreatitis.

False.

❒❒ How does retrocecal appendicitis most commonly present?

Dysuria, poorly localized abdominal pain, anorexia, nausea, vomiting, diarrhea and mild fever.

❒❒ Is mesenteric ischemia more serious in the small or large bowel?

The small bowel. Embolization in the superior mesenteric artery effects the entire small bowel. Embolization to the large bowel may not be as serious due to collateral circulation to the large bowel.

METABOLIC AND ENDOCRINE PEARLS

"...I don't want to live-I want to love first, and live incidentally..."
Zelda Fitzgerald, 1919.

❑❑ A 36 year-old female presents with a history of being difficult to arouse in the morning. Her husband says, "After she's had breakfast, she perks right up." Diagnosis?

Fasting hypoglycemia. Fasting hypoglycemia may reflect serious organic disease. As a consequence, evaluation of this disorder typically requires hospitalization.

❑❑ How do you distinguish between endogenously produced and exogenously administered insulin?

Endogenous - Insulin and C peptide levels corresponds.
Exogenously - Insulin level elevated, C peptide level low.

❑❑ In the first two years of life, what is the most common cause of <u>drug-induced</u> hypoglycemia?

Salicylates. In the 2-8 year-old group, alcohol is the most likely cause, and in the 11 to 30 year-old group, insulin and sulfonylureas are the most likely cause.

❑❑ What is the principle hormone protecting the human body against hypoglycemia?

Glucagon.

❑❑ What drugs potentiate the hypoglycemic effects of sulfonylurea?

Salicylates, alcohol, sulfonamides, phenylbutazone, and bis-hydroxycoumarin. Chlorpropamide is the sulfonylurea compound most likely to cause hypoglycemic events. It also causes the most prolonged hypoglycemia.

❑❑ How is sulfonylurea-induced hypoglycemia treated?

IV glucose alone may be insufficient. It may require diazoxide 300 mg slow IV over 30 min repeated every four h.

❑❑ What effect does propranolol have on blood sugar in diabetic patients?

Propranolol is thought to precipitate hypoglycemia.

❑❑ What is the most common cause of hypoglycemia in a child?

Ketotic hypoglycemia. Attacks usually occur when the child is stressed with caloric deprivation. Most common in boys, typically between 18 mo and 5 year of age. Attacks may be episodic, vomiting may occur, and are more frequent in the morning or during periods of illness.

❑❑ What are the neurologic signs and symptoms of hypoglycemia?

Hypoglycemia may produce mental and neurologic dysfunction. Neurologic manifestations may include paresthesias, cranial nerve palsies, transient hemiplegia, diplopia, decerebrate posturing, and clonus.

❒❒ What lab findings are expected with diabetic ketoacidosis?

Elevated ß-hydroxybutyrate, acetoacetate, acetone and glucose. Ketonuria and glucosuria are present. Serum bicarbonate level, PCO_2, and pH are decreased. Potassium may be initially elevated but falls if the acidosis is corrected.

❒❒ What is the treatment of DKA?

Fluids, approximately 5-10 liters of normal saline alternating with 1/2 normal saline. Potassium 100-200 mEq in the first 12-24 h. Insulin 20 unit bolus followed by 5-10 U/h. Add glucose to the IV fluid when glucose levels fall below 250 mg/dl. Phosphate supplement when level drops below 1.0 mg/dL (unlikely to occur before 6-12 hours have elapsed after initial Tx for DKA has begun).
Peds : NS 20 mL/kg/h for 1-2 h.
Insulin 0.1 U/kg bolus followed by 0.1 U/kg/h drip.

❒❒ A 42 year-old female presents with a history of palpitations, sweating, diplopia, blurred vision, and weakness. The family indicates she has been confused. Symptoms usually occur before breakfast. Diagnosis?

Islet cell tumor of the pancreas can be a cause of a fasting hypoglycemia.

❒❒ What sulfonylurea compound most commonly causes severe and sustained hypoglycemia?

Chlorpropamide. (This can occur when the patient is taking standard doses as well as in overdose.)

❒❒ What are the key features of nonketotic hyperosmolar coma?

Hyperosmolality, hyperglycemia, and dehydration. Blood sugar should be greater than 800 mg/dl, serum osmolality should be greater than 350 mOsm/kg, and serum ketones should be negative.

❒❒ What is the treatment of nonketotic hyperosmolar coma?

Fluids (normal saline), potassium 10-20 mEq/h. Insulin 5-10 U/h, and glucose should be added to the IV when the blood sugar drops below 250 mg/dl.

❒❒ What is the most consistent finding with lactic acidosis?

Kussmaul's respirations or hyperventilation.

❒❒ Distinguish between type A and type B lactic acidosis?

Type A lactic acidosis is often seen in the Emergency Department. It is most commonly due to shock. Type A lactic acidosis is associated with inadequate tissue perfusion and resultant anoxia, with subsequent lactate and hydrogen ion accumulation. Type B lactic acidosis includes all forms of acidosis in which there is no evidence of tissue anoxia.

❒❒ What are the pathognomonic findings as well as confirmatory lab tests diagnostic of thyroid storm?

Trick question. Thyroid storm is based on clinical impression. There are no findings or confirmatory tests available.

❒❒ What is the most common cause of thyroid storm?

Infections, typically pulmonary infections, are the most common precipitating event.

❒❒ **What clinical clues might help in the diagnosis of thyroid storm?**

Eye signs of Graves' disease, a history of hyperthyroidism, widened pulse pressure, and a palpable goiter.

❒❒ **What are the diagnostic criteria for thyroid storm?**

Tachycardia, CNS dysfunction, cardiovascular dysfunction, GI system dysfunction, and temperature greater than 37.8° C (100° F).

❒❒ **What are the signs and symptoms of thyroid storm?**

Tachycardia, fever, diaphoresis, increased CNS activity, emotional lability, heart failure, coma, and death.

❒❒ **What are the complications of bicarbonate therapy in DKA?**

Paradoxical CSF acidosis, cardiac arrhythmias, decreased oxygen delivery to tissue, and fluid and sodium overload.

❒❒ **What is the approximate overall mortality of nonketotic hyperosmolar coma?**

Approximately 50%.

❒❒ **What is the most common cause of hypothyroidism?**

Primary thyroid failure. The most common etiology of hypothyroidism in adults is the use of radioactive iodine or subtotal thyroidectomy in the treatment of Graves' disease. The second most common cause is autoimmune thyroid disorders.

❒❒ **In a patient receiving anticoagulation therapy with heparin, when is adrenal hemorrhage most likely to strike?**

Typically between the 3rd and 18th d of anticoagulation. Patients present with sudden hypotension and flank or epigastric pain. Nausea, vomiting, fever, and a change in sensorium may be associated.

❒❒ **What is the most common cause of secondary adrenal insufficiency and adrenal crisis?**

Iatrogenic adrenal suppression from prolonged steroid use. Rapid withdrawal of steroids may lead to collapse and death.

❒❒ **An increase of PCO_2 of 10 mmHg will lead to an expected decrease in pH of about:**

pH increases 0.08.

❒❒ **A decrease of PCO_2 of 10 mmHg will lead to an expected increase in pH of about:**

pH increases 0.13.

❒❒ **What is the expected increase in pH associated with a rise in HCO_3 of 5.0 mEq/l?**

pH increases 0.08.

❒❒ **What is the expected decrease in pH associated with a decrease in HCO_3 of 5.0 mEq/l?**

pH decreases 0.10.

❒❒ **How is the anion gap calculated from electrolyte values?**

Anion gap = Na - Cl - CO_2 The normal gap is 12 $^{+}$/- 4 mEq/l.

❒❒ Acidosis is closely related to anion gap measurement. Name the causes of an increased anion gap acidosis.

A MUDPILE CAT

A = alcohol,

M = methanol,
U = uremia,
D = DKA,
P = paraldehyde,
I = iron and isoniazid,
L = lactic acidosis,
E = ethylene glycol,

C = carbon monoxide,
A = aspirin,
T = toluene.

❒❒ That's a pretty big differential. History and physical can go a long way in narrowing this list down. The magnitude of the anion gap can also be useful; discuss.

Anion gap > 35 mEq/L is usually caused by ethylene glycol, methanol or lactic acidosis.
Anion gap 23 - 30 mEq/L usually also because of increased organic acids.
Anion gap 16 - 22 mEq/L may be due to uremia, which must be quite advanced before it causes an increased gap.

❒❒ There is another "gap" that can aid in diagnosing the cause of an anion gap acidosis - the osmolar gap. Let's distract ourselves for a momentary discussion of the osmolar gap and how it may be useful.

Uh-oh. Osmolality is a measure of the concentration of particles in a solution, its units are osmoles per kg water. Osmolarity is a measure of osmoles per liter of solution - for dilute solutions, like body fluids, these two measures are roughly equivalent. An osmolar gap is a difference between measured osmolality and calculated osmolarity. The osmolar gap is calculated as follows:

Measured osmolality - calculated osmolarity = osmolar gap.

$$CalculatedOsmol(mOsm/l) = 2(Na) + \frac{glucose}{18} + \frac{BUN}{2.8}$$

(Normal = 275 - 285 mOsm/l)

❒❒ Different substances contribute to varying degrees to the osmolar gap, these are listed below:

Substance	mg/dL to increase serum osmol mOsm/L	# mOsm/L increase due to each mg/dL
Methanol	2.6	0.38
Ethanol	4.3	0.23
Ethylene glycol	5.0	0.20
Acetone	5.5	0.18
Isopropyl alcohol	5.9	0.17
Salicylate	14.0	0.07

Thus, small amounts of methanol cause greater increases in osmolality. Large amounts of salicylate will eventually increase osmolar gap. Note also that the contribution to an osmolar gap due to EtOH may be calculated; this can be useful in when a mixed alcohol ingestion is suspected (and your IM colleagues in the ED will be impressed!). The contribution from EtOH is added to the calculated value by adding the following: EtOH/4.6 or add 23 mOsm/L for an EtOH level of 100 mg/dL.

❒❒ O.K., with that distraction now behind us, review some other pearls that can help narrow the d/dx of an anion gap acidosis.

Methanol- visual disturbances and headache common. Can produce quite wide gaps as discussed above.

Uremia- advanced before it causes an anion gap.

Diabetic Ketoacidosis-usually has both hyperglycemia and glucosuria.

Alcoholic Ketoacidosis (AKA)-often has a lower blood sugar and mild or absent glucosuria.

Salicylates-high levels required to contribute to gap.

Lactic Acidosis-can check serum level. Itself has broad differential to be discussed in a question in the random section.

Ethylene glycol- causes calcium oxalate or hippurate crystals in urine.

❒❒ What are the causes of the oxygen saturation curve shift to the right?

A shift to the right delivers more O_2 to the tissue.
Right = Release to tissues.

"CADET! Right face!!"

Hyper	Carbia,
	Acidemia,
2,3	DPG,
	Exercise,
increased	Temperature.

The mnemonic CADET helps in remembering causes of an O_2 shift to the right.

❒❒ When body waste materials (urine & stool) are enterally recycled, they can cause a normal anion gap metabolic acidosis. Thus, USED CRAP does **in fact cause a normal anion gap (hyperchloremic) metabolic acidosis; discuss.**

U = ureteroenterostomy
S = small bowel fistula
E = extra chloride (NH_4Cl or amino acid chlorides 2° TPN)
D = diarrhea

C = carbonic anhydrase inhibitors
R = renal tubular acidosis
A = adrenal insufficiency
P = pancreatic fistula

❒❒ What are the two primary causes of metabolic alkalosis?

Loss of hydrogen and chloride from the stomach.
Overzealous diuresis with loss of hydrogen, potassium and chloride.

❒❒ What is central pontine myelinolysis, aka osmotic demyelination syndrome?

The complication of brain dehydration following too rapid correction of severe hyponatremia. Correct hyponatremia slowly, less than 12 mEq/d in chronic hyponatremia.

❒❒ What causes SIADH?

1. Malignancies (pulmonary, hematologic, pancreatic)
2. Pulmonary disease (tumor, tuberculosis, pneumonia, asthma)
3. CNS disorders (meningitis, trauma, tumors)
4. Drugs (chlorpropamide, oxytocin, vincristine, Cytoxan)
5. Postoperative period (pain)

❒❒ What findings are diagnostic of diabetes insipidus?

Large urinary volumes (usually greater than 3L/day), dilute urine (osmolality < 300 mOsm/L) specific gravity < 1.010 and hypernatremia.

❒❒ How fast should hyponatremia be corrected?

No faster than 0.5 to 1.0 mEq/L/hour of sodium. The initial goal is to correct to sodium level no higher than 120 to 125 mEq/L

❒❒ What is the complication if hyponatremia is corrected too rapidly?

Central pontine myelinolysis or osmotic demyelinating syndrome. This syndrome can present several days after the treatment of hyponatremia. Symptoms include quadriparesis with swallowing dysfunction, pseudobulbar palsy and inability to speak.

❒❒ What is normal plasma osmolality?

Normal plasma osmolality is 285 to 295 mOsm/kg.

❒❒ What are the symptoms of hypernatremia?

Dehydration of brain cells causes lethargy, fatigue, mental status changes, coma, seizures and death.
Most adults do not develop symptoms until serum sodium reaches 160 mEq/L.

❒❒ What are some causes of hypernatremia?

1. Diabetes insipidus (central, nephrogenic)
2. Insensible losses (burns, sweating)
3. Osmotic diuresis (mannitol, hyperglycemia)
4. Hypertonic fluid administration

❒❒ What mechanism causes hypovolemia to result in a metabolic alkalosis?

The kidney will resorb sodium and excrete hydrogen ion to maintain intravascular volume. This is under the influence of aldosterone.

❒❒ What are the muscular manifestations of hyperkalemia?

Hyperkalemia partially depolarizes the cell membrane. Patients may present with neuromuscular weakness that may progress to flaccid paralysis and hypoventilation.

❒❒ How much potassium is contained in extracellular fluid?

Approximately 70 mEq.

❒❒ What hormones regulate potassium balance?

Insulin (promotes tissue uptake)
Catecholamines
- via beta-receptors (increased cellular uptake)
- via alpha-receptors (decreased cellular uptake; hepatic release)

Aldosterone (renal excretion)

❒❒ How does acute metabolic acidosis affect serum potassium? Is there a difference between organic and inorganic acidosis?

Acute inorganic acidosis: plasma potassium increases by 0.8 mEq/L (range 0.5-0.8 mEq/L) for each 0.1 decline in pH.

Organic acidosis: does not affect potassium.

❒❒ How does acute metabolic alkalosis affect serum potassium?

Plasma potassium falls by 0.3 mEq/L for every 0.1 unit rise in pH.

❒❒ How do respiratory acid-base disorders affect plasma potassium?

Respiratory acid-base imbalances are usually not associated with significant changes in plasma potassium.

❒❒ What therapy is available for severe hyperkalemia?

Calcium - protects against depolarizing effects of hyperkalemia (avoid in simultaneous digitalis toxicity)
Sodium bicarbonate - results in cellular potassium uptake
Beta-adrenergic agonists - promotes cellular uptake
Cation exchange resin - binds potassium in bowel
Loop diuretics - enhance potassium secretion in nephrons
Insulin/glucose - promotes cellular uptake
Dialysis – removes potassium from blood directly

❒❒ List some medications that may cause hyperkalemia.

Non-steroidal anti-inflammatory drugs
Angiotensin converting enzyme inhibitors
Heparin - inhibits adrenal steroidogenesis
Spironolactone - blocks renal mineralocorticoid receptor
Triamterene, amiloride – aldosterone independent effects in tubular potassium secretion

❒❒ Succinylcholine is a rapid onset depolarizing neuromuscular blocking agent. How does it affect plasma potassium?

Muscle membrane depolarization results in leakage of potassium producing an average increase of 0.5 to 1.0 mEq/L in serum potassium. However, when succinylcholine depolarizes muscle that has been previously traumatized or denervated (e.g., stroke), large increases in serum potassium can occur causing arrhythmias and cardiac arrest.

❒❒ Non-depolarizing neuromuscular blocking agents are frequently used in intensive care units. What is their effect on plasma potassium?

Non-depolarizing neuromuscular blocking agents do not affect plasma potassium levels.

❒❒ What is the cause of hyperkalemia in diabetics?

Cellular uptake of potassium is decreased because of hypoinsulinism. These patients often have hyporeninemic hypoaldosteronism (type IV renal tubular acidosis).

❒❒ **What mechanism causes hypokalemia to induce a metabolic alkalosis?**

The kidney to will attempt to absorb additional potassium in exchange for hydrogen (lost from blood) in response to hypokalemia.

❒❒ **How much sodium is in normal saline?**

154 mEq/L.

2500 mL/d.

❒❒ **What are the clinical manifestations of hyponatremia?**

Weakness, fatigue, muscle cramps, confusion, anorexia, nausea, vomiting, headache, delirium, seizures and coma.

❒❒ **At what serum sodium level would one expect to see clinical signs and symptoms of acute hyponatremia?**

Approximately 125 mEq/L.

❒❒ **At what sodium level would one expect signs and symptoms of hypernatremia?**

Approximately 160 mEq/L.

❒❒ **What are the signs and symptoms of hypernatremia?**

Restlessness, irritability, ataxia, fever, spasms and seizure.

❒❒ **T/F: Elderly patients may have urine sodium levels that are inappropriately high in the face of decreased renal blood flow.**

True.

❒❒ **What is the urine sodium level and plasma osmolality in SIADH?**

Urine sodium greater than 20 mEq/L and plasma osmolality less than 290 mOsm/L. The urine osmolality is typically greater than 200 mOsm/L.

❒❒ **What signs are associated with hypocalcemia?**

Decreased contractility, hypotension, ventricular arrhythmias, muscle spasms, laryngospasm, paresthesias and tetany.

❒❒ **What are the most common causes of hypernatremia?**

Diabetes insipidus, insensible losses, osmotic diuresis and hypertonic fluid administration.

❒❒ **What therapy is available for severe hyperkalemia?**

Calcium, sodium bicarbonate, β-adrenergic agonists, cation exchange resins, loop diuretics, insulin and glucose and dialysis. Calcium is contraindicated in cases of hyperkalemia related to digitalis toxicity.

❒❒ **Are the T wave amplitudes heightened or diminished in hyperkalemia? What about the QRS duration?**

The T waves are taller and the QRS is prolonged. The "wrist" (bottom) of the T wave is relatively narrow in hyperkalemia.

❒❒ What ECG abnormalities are associated with hypercalcemia?

Shortened Q-T interval, bradycardia and heart block.

❒❒ What are the clinical manifestations of hypokalemia?

Arrhythmias, muscle weakness, mental status changes, impaired intestinal peristalsis and predisposition to digitalis toxicity.

❒❒ What is the quickest way to treat hyperkalemia?

Calcium gluconate (10%) IV.

❒❒ What are the causes of hyperkalemia?

Acidosis, tissue necrosis, hemolysis, blood transfusions, GI bleed, renal failure, Addison's disease, primary hypoaldosteronism, excess oral K^+ intake, RTA Type IV and medications as succinylcholine, beta-blockers, captopril, spironolactone, triamterene, amiloride and high dose penicillin.

❒❒ What are the causes of hypocalcemia?

Shock, sepsis, multiple blood transfusions, hypoparathyroidism, vitamin D deficiency, pancreatitis, hypomagnesemia, alkalosis, fat embolism syndrome, phosphate overload, chronic renal failure, loop diuretics, hypoalbuminemia, tumor lysis syndrome and medications as calcitonin and mithramycin.

❒❒ What is the most common cause of hyperkalemia?

Hemolysis (of lab error variety). Chronic renal failure is the most common cause of "true" hyperkalemia.

❒❒ In order of prevalence, what are the three most common causes of hypercalcemia?

Malignancy, primary hyperparathyroidism and thiazide diuretics.

❒❒ What are the signs and symptoms of hypercalcemia?

The most common gastrointestinal symptoms are anorexia and constipation. Remember:

Stones:	Renal calculi
Bones:	Osteolysis
Abdominal groans:	Peptic ulcer disease and pancreatitis
Psychic overtones:	Psychiatric disorders

❒❒ What is the initial treatment for hypercalcemia?

Restoration of the extracellular fluid with 5 to 10 L of normal saline within 24 hours. After the patient is rehydrated, administer furosemide. Patients with hypercalcemia are dehydrated because high calcium levels interfere with ADH and the ability of the kidney to concentrate urine.

❒❒ A patient with a history of alcohol abuse presents after a recent tonic-clonic seizure. What particular electrolyte abnormality should be considered and treated during evaluation?

Hypomagnesemia.

❒❒ What is the most common cause of hyperphosphatemia?

Acute and chronic renal failure.

❑❑ What are normal and abnormal blood gas values?

VALUE	NORMAL	DECREASED	INCREASED
ARTERIAL BLOOD			
pH	7.35-7.45	<7.35 acidemia	>7.45 alkalemia
$PaCO_2$, mmHg	40	<36 respiratory alkalosis, hyperventilation	>44 respiratory acidosis, hypoventilation
HCO_3^-a, mEq/L	24	<24 metabolic acidosis	>24 metabolic alkalosis
VENOUS BLOOD			
pHv	7.30-7.35		
$PvCO_2$, mmHg	45		
HCO_3v, mEq/L	20-22		

❑❑ What are the normal compensatory responses to alkalosis and acidosis?

The goal of homeostasis is to maintain constancy of the blood pH by maintaining a constant ratio between PCO_2 and HCO_3^-, which is accomplished as follows:

PRIMARY ACID/BASE DISORDER	COMPENSATORY RESPONSE
Increased PCO_2 (respiratory acidosis)	Increased HCO_3^- (metabolic alkalosis)
Decreased PCO_2 (respiratory alkalosis)	Decreased HCO_3^- (metabolic acidosis)
Increased HCO_3^- (metabolic alkalosis)	Increased PCO_2 (respiratory acidosis)
Decreased HCO_3^- (metabolic acidosis)	Decreased PCO_2 (respiratory alkalosis)

❑❑ How does alteration of arterial CO_2 correspond to changes in arterial pH?

DISORDER	PRIMARY DISORDER	SECONDARY COMPENSATION
Metabolic Acidosis	Decreased $HCO3^-$	Expected $PCO_2 = 1.5 * HCO3^- + 8\ (\pm 2)$ PCO_2 = last 2 digits of pH * 100
Metabolic Alkalosis	Increased $HCO3^-$	Expected $PCO_2 = 0.7 * HCO3^- + 20\ (\pm 1.5)$
Respiratory Acidosis Acute (1-2 hr)	Increased CO_2	$pH = 0.005$ to $0.008 * PCO_2$ and $HCO3 = 0.1 * PCO_2$
Chronic (<12-24 hr)	Increased CO_2	$pH = 0.003 * PCO_2$ and $HCO3 = 0.35 * PCO_2$
Respiratory Alkalosis Acute (1-2 hr)	Decrease CO_2	$pH = 0.008$ to $0.01 * PCO_2$ and $HCO3 = 0.2 * PCO_2$
Chronic (<12-24 hr)	Decrease CO_2	$pH = 0.002 * PCO_2$ and $HCO3 = 0.5 * PCO_2$

❑❑ What is a better index of tissue CO_2, arterial or venous CO_2?

Venous CO_2.

❐❐ Is it possible to have the identical PCO_2 in arterial and mixed venous blood?

During respiratory arrest, pulmonary arterial blood and systemic arterial blood have the same PCO_2. However, at the tissue level, the arteriolar PCO_2 is less than that of the tissue venous PCO_2.

❐❐ What is the normal arterial-venous PCO_2 gradient and how would this gradient be affected by decreased cardiac output?

The normal arterial-venous PCO_2 gradient is 4 to 6 mmHg. The arterial-venous PCO_2 gradient is increased by low cardiac output.

❐❐ What is the affect of decreased cardiac output on the arterial PO_2?

In most circumstances, cardiac output has no/minimal influence on arterial blood gas tensions.

Low cardiac output may decrease PaO_2 when there is a high pulmonary shunt fraction (Qs/Qt > 20%). In this case, the decreased cardiac output causes a sufficient reduction in mixed venous saturation such that the venous blood cannot be fully oxygenated during passage through the alveolar capillaries because of the presence of shunting.

❐❐ What are the indications for $NaHCO_3$ administration?

To replace gastroenteric bicarbonate losses, e.g., duodenal fistula.
To replace renal bicarbonate losses, e.g. renal tubular acidosis.
Treatment of acute hyperkalemia.
Treatment of tricyclic antidepressant overdose.
To correct severe metabolic acidosis only in the presence of adequate tissue perfusion and pulmonary ventilation (controversial).

❐❐ For every ampule of $NaHCO_3$, how much CO_2 is generated?

One 50 mL ampule of adult $NaHCO_3$ solution has the following properties, pH = 7.8, pK = 6.1, PCO_2 = 85, 1800 mOsm/L, Na = 892 mmol/L and it contains 44.6 mEq of bicarbonate.

Acutely about 10 to 15% of the administered $NaHCO_3$ is converted to CO_2 gas. Thus, a 44.6 mEq dose of bicarbonate generates 4.5 to 6.7 mEq of CO_2 that corresponds to about 100 to 150 mL of CO_2 gas. To prevent hypercapnia, the drug should be given slowly and necessitates a transient increase in the alveolar ventilation.

Eventually, most/all of the HCO_3^- is converted to CO_2 and 44.6 mEq of CO_2 corresponds to 1,000 mL of CO_2 gas.

❐❐ How much sodium bicarbonate would you administer to correct a respiratory acidosis with the pH=7.21 and PCO_2=90?

None, its a (partially compensated) respiratory acidosis.

❐❐ What are treatments for respiratory acidosis?

Intubation
Increase minute ventilation
Decrease dead space ventilation
Correct auto-PEEP (air-trapping), e.g., bronchospasm, endotracheal tube obstruction.
Treat (prevent) pulmonary embolism
Reverse muscle weakness
Reverse sedatives and narcotics
Decrease CO_2 production (shivering, hyperthermia and excess glucose load due to hyperalimentation)
Nasal CPAP or BiPAP

❑❑ What are the causes of normal anion gap metabolic acidosis?

A normal anion gap acidosis is associated with a relatively high chloride, i.e. hyperchloremic metabolic acidosis.

Gastrointestinal
Diarrhea
Following bowel preparation
High output ileal fistula or external pancreatic fistula
Ingestion of substances that bind $NaHCO_3$: e.g., cholestyramine

Renal
Proximal (Type II) renal tubular acidosis: bicarbonate wasting due to impaired HCO_3^- reabsorption; distal acidification is intact; associated with hypokalemia
Distal (Type I) renal tubular acidosis: failure of distal nephron urinary acidification; associated with hypokalemia
Distal (Type IV) renal tubular acidosis: major problem is hyperkalemia

Other
Mineralocorticoid deficiency: i.e., hypoaldosteronism
Addition of HCl acid or one of its precursors: e.g., NH_4Cl
Post-hyperventilation metabolic acidosis
Dilutional acidosis: volume infusion with high chloride containing fluids (normal saline)

❑❑ How are ketones detected?

Ketones in urine can be assayed with the Acetest (employs the nitroprusside colorimetric reaction). This test, however, only detects acetoacetate (AcAc) and acetone. If beta-hydroxybutyrate is the predominate species the level of AcAc may be too low to be detected by the Acetest and the test result is falsely negative.

❑❑ What is the treatment of alcoholic ketoacidosis (AKA)?

Saline infusion, glucose and thiamine. By the way, the arterial pH may be low, normal, or high in AKA.

❑❑ What are the different kinds of metabolic alkalosis, how are they diagnosed and treated?

Chloride responsive, urine chloride < 10 mmol/L
Volume contraction: e.g., diuretics
Loss of gastric acid: e.g., nasogastric suction
Post-hypercapnia

Chloride resistant, urine chloride > 20 mmol/L
High blood pressure: renovascular hypertension, renin producing tumor, hyperaldosteronism (tumor, licorice), Cushing syndrome and exogenous steroid use
Normal blood pressure: laxative abuse, Bartter's syndrome, severe hypokalemia and magnesium deficiency

❑❑ What are the causes of respiratory alkalosis (hyperventilation)?

Hypoxemia or tissue hypoxia
Pulmonary edema
Pulmonary embolism (air, fat, thromboembolism, amniotic fluid, etc).
Shock
Cyanide toxicity
Carboxyhemoglobin
Methemoglobin
Any pulmonary parenchymal disease

Any obstructive pulmonary process

Central
Agitation, anxiety, pain
CNS infection
Central hyperventilation associated with injury to midbrain and upper pons

Metabolic acidosis
DKA
Lactic acidosis
Ingestion of acids: aspirin and alcohol

Other
Sepsis
Pregnancy
Hepatic failure
Respiratory stimulants: progesterone

❒❒ In a spontaneous ventilating patient, does metabolic alkalosis cause respiratory depression?

Metabolic acidosis causes hyperventilation, but not all patients with metabolic alkalosis hypoventilate. It is possible to predict the PCO_2 for a given degree of metabolic alkalosis based on the empiric formula:

Expected $PCO_2 = 20 + 0.7 * [HCO_3^-] \pm 1.5$

❒❒ What characteristic lab findings are associated with primary adrenal insufficiency?

Hyperkalemia, hyponatremia, hypoglycemia, azotemia (if volume depletion is present) and a mild metabolic acidosis.

❒❒ How should acute adrenal insufficiency be treated?

Administration of hydrocortisone IV and crystalloid fluids containing dextrose.

❒❒ What are the main causes of death during an adrenal crisis?

Circulatory collapse and hyperkalemia induced arrhythmias.

❒❒ What is thyrotoxicosis? What causes it?

A hypermetabolic state occurring secondary to excess circulating thyroid hormone. Thyrotoxicosis is caused by thyroid hormone overdose, thyroid hyperfunction or thyroid inflammation.

❒❒ What are the hallmark clinical features of myxedema coma?

Hypothermia and coma.

❒❒ What is the most important initial step in treating DKA?

Volume replacement.

❒❒ What are the neurologic signs and symptoms associated with hypoglycemia?

Hypoglycemia may produce behavioral and neurologic dysfunction. Neurologic manifestations include paresthesias, cranial nerve palsies, transient hemiplegia, diplopia, decerebrate posturing and clonus.

❒❒ What laboratory findings occur in diabetic ketoacidosis?

Elevated beta-hydroxybutyrate, acetoacetate, acetone and glucose. Ketonuria and glucosuria are present. Serum bicarbonate levels, PCO_2 and pH are decreased. Potassium levels may be elevated but will fall when the acidosis is corrected.

❒❒ What is the basic treatment for DKA?

Administer fluids. Start with 0.9% normal saline, switch to 0.5 normal saline, include potassium (after the patient begins to urinate and if not hyperkalemic). Give insulin, 0.1 units/kg bolus followed by 5 to 10 units/hour. Add glucose to the IV fluid when the glucose level falls below 250 mg/dl and give the patient a phosphate supplement when the level drops below 1.0 mg/dL. The need for phosphate repletion in the ED (in the first 6-12 hours) is highly unlikely. Religiously monitor glucose, electrolytes (including anion gap), ketones, volume status and the patient's symptoms.

❒❒ A 42 year-old female presents with a history of palpitations, sweating, diplopia, blurred vision and weakness. The husband states she has been confused, most notably before breakfast. What is the probable diagnosis?

Islet cell tumor of the pancreas, which can result from fasting hypoglycemia.

❒❒ What are the key features of non-ketotic hyperosmolar coma?

Hyperosmolality, hyperglycemia and dehydration. Blood sugar levels are > 800 mg/dl, serum osmolality is > 350 mOsm/kg and serum ketones are negative.

❒❒ What is the treatment for non-ketotic hyperosmolar coma?

This is treated much like DKA with the caveat that the patient requires less insulin. It is important to initiate IV normal saline before giving insulin. Some suggest that an IV insulin bolus is not necessary in this condition.

❒❒ What pathognomonic findings and confirmatory lab tests are diagnostic of thyroid storm?

None. Diagnosis and thyroid storm is based on a clinical impression.

❒❒ What is the most common precipitant of thyroid storm?

Infection.

❒❒ What signs and symptoms are helpful for diagnosing thyroid storm?

Eye signs of Graves' disease, a history of hyperthyroidism, widened pulse pressure, hypertension, a palpable goiter, tachycardia, fever, diaphoresis, increased CNS activity, emotional lability, heart failure and coma.

❒❒ T/F: Elderly patients may manifest thyrotoxicity with a decrease in CNS activity.

True.

❒❒ What are some diagnostic findings of thyroid storm?

Tachycardia, CNS dysfunction, cardiovascular dysfunction, GI system dysfunction and a temperature > 37.8 °C (100° F).

❒❒ What are the hemodynamic changes seen with thyroid storm?

Tachycardia, increased cardiac output and decreased systemic vascular resistance (SVR).

❒❒ What are the ophthalmologic signs in hyperthyroidism?

Exophthalmos, lid lag, lid retraction and periorbital swelling.

❒❒ What are the associated laboratory findings in hyperthyroidism?

Hypercalcemia, hypokalemia, hyperglycemia, anemia, leukocytosis with a left shift, hyperbilirubinemia and increased alkaline phosphatase.

❒❒ What is the initial treatment of thyroid storm?

Intravenous fluids, acetaminophen, propranolol, propylthiouracil (PTU) and iodine.

❒❒ What are the CNS manifestations of myxedema?

Depression, memory loss, ataxia, frank psychosis and coma.

❒❒ What are the common causes of hypothyroidism?

Cessation of thyroid medication, autoimmune thyroid disease, decreased TSH, radioactive and surgical ablation and iodine deficiency/excess.

❒❒ What is the first thyroid function test abnormality seen in hypothyroidism?

TSH elevation (usually associated with a low T4).

❒❒ A 45 year-old female presents with a two year history of diffuse, tender thyroid enlargement, lethargy and a 20 pound weight gain. What is the most likely diagnosis?

Hashimoto's thyroiditis.

❒❒ What is the appropriate treatment for the above patient?

Thyroid replacement therapy.

❒❒ What is the mechanism of action of propylthiouracil (PTU)?

PTU interferes with the incorporation of iodine into the tyrosine residues of thyroglobulin. It also inhibits the peripheral conversion of T4 to T3.

❒❒ What are the signs/symptoms of hyperthyroidism?

Anxiety, weight loss, heat intolerance, gastrointestinal disturbances, fever, arrhythmias, muscle weakness and tremors.

❒❒ What is the differential diagnosis of thyrotoxicosis?

Sepsis, pheochromocytoma, cocaine/amphetamine overdose, neuroleptic malignant syndrome and malignant hyperthermia.

❒❒ What is the most common cause of chronic primary adrenal insufficiency (Addison's Disease)?

Autoimmune disease.

❒❒ What are the most common (non-medication) causes of acute secondary adrenal insufficiency?

Sheehan's Syndrome (postpartum pituitary necrosis), bleeding into a pituitary macroadenoma and head trauma.

❑❑ **What diseases produce a slow insidious progression to primary adrenal insufficiency?**

Autoimmune diseases, tuberculosis, systemic fungal infections, CMV, Kaposi's sarcoma, metastatic carcinoma and lymphoma.

❑❑ **In a critical care setting, refractoriness to what type of medication suggests adrenal insufficiency?**

Catecholamines/vasopressors.

❑❑ **T/F: Orthostatic hypotension and electrolyte abnormalities are more common in primary adrenal insufficiency than secondary.**

True.

❑❑ **What are the most specific signs of primary adrenal insufficiency?**

Hyperpigmentation of the skin and mucosal membranes.

❑❑ **What therapy should be instituted in the interval until the results of an ACTH stimulation test is known in a critically ill patient?**

Empiric stress dose steroids should be given to treat a critically ill patient with adrenal insufficiency. Therapy can begin before the ACTH stimulation test using dexamethasone, as this will not interfere with cortisol assays.

❑❑ **What is the emergent steroid replacement in adrenal insufficiency?**

Hydrocortisone 100 mg intravenously every 8 hours.

❑❑ **What patients should receive fluorocortisone?**

Those with primary adrenal insufficiency.

❑❑ **What is the characteristic hemodynamic pattern of adrenal insufficiency?**

Decreased systemic vascular resistance and to a lessor degree, decreased cardiac contractility.

❑❑ **What drugs can impair cortisol synthesis in the critically ill patient?**

Ketoconazole, etomidate and aminoglutethimide.

❑❑ **T/F: Corticosteroids are effective in the treatment of septic shock.**

False.

❑❑ **A 45 year-old male develops hypotension, lethargy, a hemoglobin of 12 gm/dL and a blood glucose of 34 mg/dl 24 hours after colectomy. His history is significant for a renal transplant 3 years ago. What is the most likely diagnosis?**

Addisonian crisis.

❑❑ **Where does aldosterone exert its primary effect?**

On the distal tubules and collecting ducts of the kidney, leading to an increase in the absorption of sodium from the urine in exchange for potassium, thereby aiding in water retention and restoring intravascular volume.

❑❑ **What are the metabolic effects of catecholamines seen during periods of stress?**

Increased glycogenolysis, gluconeogenesis, lipolysis and ketogenesis and inhibition of insulin use in peripheral tissues.

❑❑ **What stimuli cause release of ADH (vasopressin)?**

Plasma osmolality greater than 285 mOsm/L, decreased circulating blood volume, catecholamines, the renin-angiotensin system and opiates.

❑❑ **What are the classic electrolyte findings of hyperaldosteronism?**

Hypernatremia and hypokalemia.

❑❑ **What are the clinical manifestations of adrenal insufficiency?**

Fatigue, lethargy, anorexia, weight loss, depression, dizziness, orthostatic hypotension, nausea, vomiting, diarrhea, hyponatremia, hyperkalemia, hypoglycemia, normochromic/normocytic anemia, lymphocytosis and eosinophilia.

❑❑ **What symptoms should increase the suspicion of adrenal insufficiency in critically ill patients?**

Unexplained circulatory instability, fever without cause, hypoglycemia, hyponatremia, hyperkalemia, eosinophilia, unexplained mental status changes and disparity between the anticipated severity of disease and the actual state of the patient.

❑❑ **What is the syndrome of inappropriate antidiuretic hormone (SIADH)?**

Hypersecretion of vasopressin.

❑❑ **What tumor most commonly causes ectopic ACTH secretion?**

Small cell carcinoma of the lung.

❑❑ **What medications are likely to lead to acute hyperkalemia in a diabetic patient?**

NSAIDs, ACE inhibitors, beta-blockers, potassium sparing diuretics and salt substitutes (these are usually potassium salts).

❑❑ **What key complication is seen in diabetic patients on peritoneal dialysis?**

Peritonitis.

❑❑ **What are the major causes of sudden mortality in diabetic patients on dialysis?**

Vascular events including cardiac ischemia and stroke.

❑❑ **What are common causes of abdominal pain, nausea and vomiting in a diabetic patient?**

Diabetic gastroparesis, gallbladder disease, pancreatitis and ischemic bowel.

❑❑ **What is a necrotizing perineal infection in a diabetic male?**

Fournier's gangrene which can spread very rapidly.

❑❑ **What necrotizing ear infection is seen in patients with DKA?**

Necrotizing otitis externa (NEO).

❒❒ **Are thyroid function tests necessary prior to the initiation of treatment for thyroid storm?**

No, this is a life threatening process and therapy should be initiated based upon the clinical findings and not waiting for results of thyroid testing.

❒❒ **Differentiate between non-ketotic hyperosmolar coma and DKA.**

In non-ketotic hyperosmolar coma, glucose is very high, often > 800. The serum osmolality is also very high, with average about 380. Nitroprusside test is negative.
In DKA, glucose is more often in the range of 600. The serum osmolality is approximately 350. Nitroprusside test is weakly positive and becomes more positive with treatment for DKA.

❒❒ **What focal signs may be present in a patient with non-ketotic hyperosmolar coma?**

These patients may have hemisensory deficits or hemiparesis. 10 to 15% of these patients have a seizure.

❒❒ **What ECG finding would you expect in myxedema coma?**

Bradycardia.

❒❒ **What is the major mineralocorticoid?**

Aldosterone. Aldosterone is regulated by the renin angiotensin system. Aldosterone increases sodium reabsorption and increased potassium excretion.

❒❒ **What key lab findings are expected in SIADH?**

Serum sodium is low and urine sodium is high.

❒❒ **What are the symptoms of thyrotoxicosis?**

Symptoms include weight loss, palpitations, dyspnea, edema, chest pain, nervousness, weakness, tremor, psychosis, diarrhea, abdominal pain, myalgias and disorientation.

Signs include fever, tachycardia, wide pulse pressure, CHF, shock, thyromegaly, tremor, weakness, liver tenderness, jaundice, stare and hyperkinesis. Mental status changes include somnolence, obtundation, coma or psychosis. Pretibial myxedema may be found.

❒❒ **What type of alcohol ingestion is associated with hypocalcemia?**

Ethylene glycol.

❒❒ **What type of alcohol ingestion is associated with hemorrhagic pancreatitis?**

Methanol.

❒❒ **What type of lung cancer is commonly associated with hypercalcemia?**

Squamous cell carcinoma. The production of parathormone related peptide could produce hypercalcemia even without bony metastases.

❒❒ **What non-neoplastic pulmonary disease is often associated with hypercalcemia and hypercalciuria?**

Sarcoidosis.

❑❑ What type of lung tumors can cause excessive ACTH production and Cushing's syndrome?

Small cell carcinoma and carcinoid tumor.

PEDI PEARLS

"Somebody BOUNCED me. I was just thinking by the side of the river -
...when I received a loud BOUNCE."
Eeyore

❒❒ What is the normal pulse rate of a newborn?

120 - 160 bpm.

❒❒ External chest compressions should be initiated for a newborn with assisted ventilation who has a heart rate less than _____ beats per minute.

50 bpm.

❒❒ Outline the Apgar scoring system.

Index	0 points	1 point	2 points
Pulse	Ø	< 100	> 100
Resp. effort	Ø	Weak cry	Strong cry
Color	Cyanotic	Extremities cyanotic	Pink
Tone	Flaccid	Weak tone	Strong
Response	Ø	Motion	Cry

❒❒ A normal appearing term neonate presents with tachypnea and cyanosis. Likely pathology?

Congenital cardiac pathology.
CHF can be presenting symptomatology for VSD, severe aortic coarctation or transposition of the great vessels. The "hyperoxia" test may help differentiate cardiac etiology - Place the infant in 100% O_2, the PaO_2 will increase less than 20 mmHg with R→L shunting of cardiac decrease.

❒❒ Stridor in the neonate is usually caused by congenital anomalies. Is infection also a common cause of neonatal stridor?

No.

❒❒ What is the <u>most common</u> cause of neonatal stridor?

Laryngotracheomalacia.

❒❒ Define apnea.

No respiration for > 20 s.

❒❒ Does apnea always indicate a serious problem and require admission?

True apnea represents serious pathology and always merits immediate appropriate intervention and admission.

❑❑ **Physiologic jaundice occurs at about 2-4 d. How high may the bilirubin level be expected to climb?**

5-6 mg/dL.

❑❑ **A neonate presents with a history of poor feeding, vomiting, respiratory distress, has abdominal distention and is found to have hyperbilirubinemia. What is the likely cause of this complex?**

This neonate is septic!

❑❑ **Name some causes of jaundice occurring at age less than 1 d.**

Sepsis, congenital infections, ABO/Rh incompatibility.

❑❑ **Jaundice due to breast feeding occurs after 7 d and can reach very high levels over weeks; how high?**

Levels of bilirubin near 25 mg/dl can be reached.

❑❑ **A cyanotic infant's SaO_2 & PaO_2 do not increase with oxygen therapy. What cause does this suggest?**

Intracardiac (R→L) shunting, not pulmonary disease.

❑❑ **Do not skip to the answer to this question, make a real attempt to answer it - Name 8 clinical presentations of pediatric heart disease.**

1. Cyanosis
2. CHF
3. Pathologic murmur
4. Cardiogenic shock
5. HTN
6. Tachyarrhythmias
7. Abnormal pulses
8. Syncope

❑❑ **Tetralogy of Fallot (TOF) consists of VSD, an "overriding" aorta, pulmonary stenosis and right ventricular hypertrophy. What type of intracardiac shunting occurs?**

Right-to-left shunting whose severity is related to the degree of pulmonary stenosis.

❑❑ **Describe the murmurs of TOF.**

1. Holosystolic murmur of VSD - 3rd ICS @ LSB.
2. Crescendo-decrescendo murmur of pulmonary stenosis - 2nd ICS @ LSB.

N.B. - If you can differentiate these two murmurs in a sick cyanotic infant in a busy ED, go directly to Pediatric Cardiology, Pass Go, and collect $200!

❑❑ **Describe the three aspects of acute treatment of TOF.**

Positioning -	Place in knee-chest position. Keep patient unstimulated (i.e., upright on lap in parent's arms).
Oxygenation -	Deliver high FiO_2.
Pharmacologic -	Morphine 0.1 mg/kg.

❒❒ SVT in adults usually occurs with a ventricular rate of about 150 - 200. What is the range of ventricular rates in children?

220 - 360 bpm.

❒❒ What is the dose of adenosine given to a pediatric patient with SVT?

0.1 mg/kg.

❒❒ Verapamil should not be used to treat infants of less than what age?

Do not use verapamil in infants less than two years of age (can lead to asystole).

❒❒ If cardioversion is necessary to treat an infant with unstable SVT, what is the appropriate energy to use?

0.25 - 1 J/kg.

❒❒ Differentiate sepsis from bacteremia.

Bacteremia is the symptom of fever with a positive blood culture; sepsis is bacteremia with focal findings identified.

❒❒ What are the two most common organisms causing bacteremia?

S. pneumoniae and *H. influenzae*.

❒❒ What are the two most common organisms causing sepsis in the neonate?

Group B streptococcus and *E. coli.*

❒❒ What are the three most common organisms causing sepsis after the newborn period?

H. influenzae, N. meningitidis and *S. pneumoniae*.

❒❒ There is much controversy surrounding the question of when to check a WBC in a pediatric patient with suspected bacteremia and if results of this test should be used to decide whether or not to draw a blood culture or decide to initiate treatment with antibiotics. What is the current recommendation of when to draw a WBC for suspected bacteremia?

Draw a WBC for patients 3 mo to 2 year-old with temperature ≥ 39.4° C (102.9° F) and no clear source.
Draw a WBC for patients 3 mo to 2 year-old who appear toxic with fever < 39.4° C.

❒❒ What is the current recommendation, from the same source, of what level of WBC and absolute polymorphonuclear cell count should then lead to drawing blood for culture?

WBC ≥ 15,000/mm^3 or absolute polymorphonuclear cell count > 9,000/mm^3 should lead to drawing blood for culture.

N.B. Answers to these two questions are controversial.

❒❒ A septic pediatric patient is in shock. An initial bolus of normal saline at 20 mL/kg has been given. Urine output should be maintained at what level by delivery of appropriate fluid?

1 mL/kg/h.

❒❒ What is the appropriate dose of diazepam to be administered to a seizing pediatric patient with suspected meningitis?

0.3 mg/kg. Load with phenytoin or phenobarbital after termination of seizure activity.

❒❒ Many authors believe in giving methylprednisolone to pediatric patients with meningitis to decrease sequelae, especially deafness. What is the appropriate dose of methylprednisolone in meningitis?

30 mg/kg.

❒❒ What are the two <u>most common</u> organisms causing meningitis in the first month of life?

Group B streptococci and *E. coli.*

❒❒ Describe antibiotic selection to treat meningitis in patients aged < 1 mo.

Use ampicillin plus an aminoglycoside*.

❒❒ What is the most common organism causing meningitis after the second mo of life?

H. influenzae.

❒❒ Describe antibiotic selection to treat meningitis in patients aged > 1 mo.

Ampicillin and chloramphenicol*.
This change in antibiotic choice is due to the increasing rate of *H. influenzae* as the causative organism during the second mo of life and the resistance of some of these organisms.

*N.B. Many physicians currently feel there is a role for third-generation cephalosporins in treatment of meningitis; e.g., ampicillin + cefotaxime (or ceftriaxone).

❒❒ What percentage of children with asthma are likely to have symptoms that persist into adulthood?

50%.

❒❒ What is the <u>most common</u> cause of bronchiolitis?

RSV.

❒❒ What is the most common organism causing epiglottitis?

H. influenzae.

❒❒ What is the usual age range for presentation of retropharyngeal abscess?

6 months - 3 years.

❒❒ Surprisingly, extrinsic asthma is the <u>most common</u> form in children. Does extrinsic asthma involve IgE production?

Yes, extrinsic asthma involves IgE production in response to allergens.

❒❒ Current recommendations include obtaining a CXR on all pediatric patients with first presentation of symptoms of reactive airway disease or asthma who are less than one year of age. Name some of the etiologies of these symptoms that may be discovered by CXR.

Foreign body aspiration, bronchiolitis, parenchymal pulmonary disease and heart disease.

❒❒ What is the common age range for bronchiolitis?

Though it may occur in patients up to age 2 years, bronchiolitis commonly occurs between ages 2 - 6 months.

❑❑ Sympathomimetic agents are used to treat asthma. What enzyme is activated by these agents?

Adenyl cyclase.

❑❑ What reaction is catalyzed by adenyl cyclase?

Adenyl cyclase catalyzes ATP to cyclic AMP.

❑❑ What effect does increased levels of cyclic AMP have on bronchial smooth muscle and on the release of chemical mediators (histamine, proteases, platelet activation factor and chemotactic factors) from airway mast cells?

Smooth muscle relaxation and decreased release of mediators.

Recall that the effects of cyclic AMP are opposed by cyclic GMP - this provides another treatment approach by *decreasing* levels of cyclic GMP which is achieved via anticholinergic (antimuscarinic) agents such as ipratropium bromide.

❑❑ As discussed above, stimulation of ß-adrenergic receptors increases cyclic AMP availability and results in smooth muscle relaxation. Which flavor of ß-adrenergic receptors primarily control bronchiolar and arterial smooth muscle tone?

$ß_2$-adrenergic receptors.

❑❑ What is the current understanding of the mechanism of action of the methylxanthines?

The mechanism of action of these agents is not known.

❑❑ Pediatric patients presenting with severe asthma may be treated with "high-dose" albuterol. What dose of nebulized albuterol is considered "high-dose," and how frequently may it be given?

0.15 mg/kg (0.03 mL/kg of 0.5%) per dose to a maximum of 5 mg may be provided every 20 min up to six times.

❑❑ How may albuterol dosing be changed if the patient has not responded to the above 6 doses?

Consider switching to continuous delivery of albuterol nebulized at 0.5 mg/kg/h up to a rate of 15 mg/h. Monitor heart rate.

❑❑ What makes albuterol the usual agent of choice?

Of nebulized ß-adrenergic agonists it has the longest duration of action and the greatest degree of $ß_2$-adrenergic selectivity.

❑❑ Terbutaline is given SQ for asthma in what dose?

0.01 mL/kg (of 1 mg/mL) up to 0.25 mL (0.25 mg) which may be repeated once in 20 minutes.

❑❑ Is theophylline of use in the emergency management of severe asthma in pediatric patients?

No. It has not been shown to cause further bronchodilatation in patients fully treated with ß-adrenergic agents. Theophylline does have a role in inpatient management of asthma and may be started in the ED.

❑❑ If corticosteroids are given, how should prednisone be dosed?

1 - 2 mg/kg/d in two divided doses; no tapering is necessary if duration of therapy is 5 days or less.

❒❒ **What effect can acidosis have on treatment with ß-adrenergic agonists?**

Decreased efficacy.

❒❒ **What is the appropriate parenteral dose of methylprednisolone (Solu-Medrol) to give a pediatric patient with status asthmaticus?**

1 - 2 mg/kg every 6 hours.

❒❒ **If mechanical ventilation is required for such a patient, what is an appropriate setting for initial tidal volume?**

10 mL/kg.

❒❒ **Parents of a child who has suffered a febrile seizure often want to know what the risk of a recurrence is. What is it?**

Risk of recurrence is the chance that the same thing will happen again.
About 35%.

❒❒ **Is LP usually an appropriate component of the evaluation of a first febrile seizure?**

Yes. Many clinicians prefer LP in this situation only if a prolonged postictal period or clinical symptoms such as lethargy are present.

❒❒ **Treatment of febrile seizures is primarily directed at gradual cooling and treatment for the source of the fever. If anticonvulsant therapy is begun, which medication is best?**

Phenobarbital.

❒❒ **Phenobarbital is also the drug of choice in neonatal seizures. Its half-life in children over one mo of age is about 65 h. The half-life is even longer in newborns up to one week of age. How long is it in this age group?**

100 hours.

❒❒ **Neonatal seizures have a broad range of presentations. What are the two frequent causes of myoclonic seizures?**

Metabolic disorders and hypoxia.

❒❒ **The initial treatment of neonatal seizures is directed initially at reversible causes; insure adequate oxygenation, provide pyridoxine (B_6), glucose, calcium and magnesium. Following these measures, pharmacologic intervention can be considered. Outline this treatment.**

Phenobarbital load, 10 - 15 mg/kg IV.
Phenytoin load, 10 - 15 mg/kg IV.
Diazepam, 0.2 mg/kg IV, may repeat.
Lorazepam, 0.05 mg/kg IV, may repeat.
Clonazepam, 0.1 mg/kg NG.

❒❒ **Infantile spasms are usually first noted in children of about 6 months of age. Is it true that these patients have a high rate of developmental disorders, and if so, what percentage of patients have such disorders?**

Yes, it is true; 85%.

❑❑ **Are infantile spasms a form of seizures?**

Yes.

❑❑ **Infantile spasms represent a significant disorder and require aggressive evaluation and management. In addition to anticonvulsants, what hormone plays a role in management of infantile spasms?**

Adrenocorticotropic hormone.

❑❑ **Febrile seizures occur relatively commonly; about what percentage of children will experience such a seizure?**

3.5%; about 35% of these patients will experience a recurrence.

❑❑ **Phenobarbital is probably the most efficacious drug used to treat febrile seizures. Should all patients with a febrile seizure receive phenobarbital as prophylaxis against future similar seizures?**

Probably not, though its use may be warranted in patients who are particularly ill, who have had repeated febrile seizures or who have underlying neurologic disease.

❑❑ **Posttraumatic seizures that occur immediately are associated with a very low rate of subsequent epilepsy. About what are the rates of subsequent epilepsy in patients suffering early (within 1 wk) and late (after 1 wk) posttraumatic seizures?**

Early ≈ 25%.
Late ≈ 70%.

❑❑ **For how long must a continuous seizure last to be defined as status epilepticus?**

30 minutes.

❑❑ **You appropriately elect to administer diazepam to a patient in "status" at a loading dose of 0.3 mg/kg and a rate of 1 mg/min. This dose should be repeated prn up to a total of how many mg/kg?**

2.6 mg/kg maximum dose of diazepam.

❑❑ **The Valium given above does not break the seizure and phenytoin is appropriately selected as the next agent. Dose and rate of administration?**

Phenytoin load 15 mg/kg at 25 mg/min (cf. adults ≈ 17 mg/kg @ 50 mg/min!).

❑❑ **Your patient is** still **seizing!@#! What is the dose of phenobarbital to load?**

10 - 15 mg/kg.

❑❑ **The seizure has stopped! What three alternative treatments remained?**

Paraldehyde, lidocaine and general anesthesia.

❑❑ **Hepatic failure is associated with which anticonvulsant?**

Valproic acid.

❑❑ **What antibiotic can cause carbamazepine to accumulate quickly?**

Erythromycin.

❒❒ Bronchopulmonary dysplasia (BPD) is commonly caused by hyaline membrane disease, prematurity and/or mechanical ventilation. BPD is treated with O_2, hydration and time. Describe the clinical features of BPD.

Tachypnea, reactive airways, hypoxia, and hypercarbia, on occasion with pulmonary edema and cor pulmonale.

❒❒ Patients with BPD may have chronic hypercarbia; does administering O_2 blunt respiratory drive in such patients?

No.

❒❒ A youngster presents with signs and symptoms that suggest a pneumonia. She describes chest pain that is pleuritic. Is such pain more commonly associated with viral or with bacterial pneumonia?

Bacterial.
Strep. pneumoniae in particular is the most common cause in this age group, and is often associated with pleuritic pain and a pleural effusion.

❒❒ The spectrum of likely etiology of a pneumonia changes with patient age. What are likely agents causing pneumonia in neonates?

Bacterial -
Group B *streptococci* (Lancefield group B, mostly *S. agalactiae*).
Listeria monocytogenes.
Enteric Gram negative bacilli.
Chlamydia.
Viral -
Rubella.
CMV.
Herpes.

❒❒ A neonate presents at 2 wk of age febrile with tachypnea and a history of poor feeding. Your suspicion of a pneumonia is confirmed by a CXR revealing diffuse homogenous infiltrates. You correctly presume a bacterial origin, likely with group B Strep., given the young age and fever (Chlamydia **usually presents between about 4 - 10 wk and afebrile, RSV presents between 1 - 6 mo). Though group B Strep. is always susceptible to penicillin G, you are aware that some strains require higher doses of penicillin G and that other less common causes still need to be considered, such as** Listeria monocytogenes **and Gram negative enteric bacteria. Thus you wish to add a second agent to this patient's treatment, one that is synergistic with penicillin G and will help cover these pathogens. Treat with:**

Penicillin G and gentamicin.

❒❒ Causes of pneumonia in patients aged 1 month to 5 years?

Bacterial - *Streptococcus pneumonia* and *Hemophilus influenzae*.
Viral - RSV, parainfluenza, adenovirus. RSV occurs primarily in patients less than 6 months of age.

❒❒ Hemophilus influenzae **is the second most common cause of pediatric pneumonia; what percentage of cases of** H. influenzae **occur in patients of less than 1 year of age?**

50%, half of remaining cases occur between ages 1 - 2 years.
H. influenzae pneumonia is common primarily in young infants.

❑❑ Causes of pneumonia in patients greater than 6 year-old?

Strep. pneumonia, *Mycoplasma pneumoniae* and influenza virus.

❑❑ Mycoplasma pneumoniae **is the second most common cause of pneumonia in children greater than 6 years old. Contrast pneumonia due to Mycoplasma with that due to** Strep. pneumoniae**.**

Characteristic	S. pneumoniae	M. pneumoniae
Prodrome	Little	Mild fever, malaise, cough, HA.
Onset	Rapid	Gradual
URI sx	Tachypnea, cough, occasional pleuritic pain.	Little
Associated findings	High fever.	Exanthem, arthritis, GI complaints, neurologic complications.
Pleural effusion	Occasional	Rare
Lab	Leukocytosis	WBC normal or sl. elevation.
Tx	Penicillin	Erythromycin

❑❑ What are the three stages of pertussis?

Catarrhal stage - rhinorrhea, cough, conjunctivitis.
Paroxysmal stage - after 1 week of above, paroxysms of continuous coughing. Lasts up to 6 weeks.
Convalescent stage - Coughing decreases. (NSS).

Dangerous pneumonias are usually superinfections; treat patient and household contacts with erythromycin (provide broader coverage if pneumonia present), immunize household contacts who are less than 7 y. old.

❑❑ SIDS is the <u>most common</u> cause of death of infants between 1 mo and 1 year of age (incidence 2 per 1000 = 10,000/y). What are the four risk factors that increase an infant's risk of SIDS?

Prematurity with low birth weight.
Previous episode of apnea or apparent life threatening event (ALTE).
Mother is a substance abuser.
Sibling of infant who died of SIDS.

❑❑ SIDS has a bimodal distribution. At what ages do the peaks occur?

2.5 & 4 months.

❑❑ What is the <u>most common</u> cause of neonatal conjunctivitis?

A trick question, as chemical conjunctivitis due to silver nitrate is most common. Chlamydia trachomatis is the <u>most common</u> clinically significant cause in the first 14 days with a usual incubation period of at least 5 days. Gonococcal conjunctivitis has a shorter incubation and may present as soon as 2 days.

❑❑ What is the name of the condition of fluid collected in the middle ear that is usually painless, is without sign of infection and that may result in a hearing deficit?

Serous otitis media, aka otitis media with effusion (OME). An underused diagnosis.

❑❑ Which type of agent is the most common cause of acute otitis media (AOM), found in about 70% of cases, bacteria or viruses?

Bacteria, most commonly *S. pneumoniae* and *H. influenzae*.

❑❑ **How useful is the light reflex in evaluation of suspected AOM?**

It is useless. Loss of TM mobility is the most valuable sign.

❑❑ **Describe the use of topical steroids, midazolam, antihistamines or decongestants in the management of AOM.**

All these agents are of no use in AOM. Antihistamines may decrease Kleenex® use.

❑❑ **What solution is appropriate treatment of otitis externa?**

Acetic acid ear drops. Treat for ≥ 7 days.

❑❑ **Among pediatric emergency patients, what is the <u>most common</u> skin infection?**

Impetigo.
Impetigo is a bacterial infection of the dermis, most commonly caused by group A ß-hemolytic streptococcus; it comes in two flavors - impetigo contagiosa and the bullous form.

❑❑ **What is the recommended treatment for impetigo?**

Erythromycin, 50 mg/kg/d.
Some authors recommend penicillin.
Dicloxacillin and cephalexin in the same dose as erythromycin and topical mupirocin may also be used.

❑❑ **Impetigo is the most common skin infection affecting children presenting to the emergency department. Honey-colored serous fluid from ruptured vesicles and similarly colored crusts are typical. Erysipelas (St. Anthony's fire) is another pediatric exanthem that represents a primary bacterial infection. What organism causes this uncommon cellulitis that is usually characterized by pain at the affected site, malaise and fever?**

Erysipelas is also caused by group A, ß-hemolytic streptococci.
Penicillin or, in penicillin allergic patients, erythromycin usually cause rapid improvement.
Recurrences are common and can lead to irreversible lymphedema (termed elephantiasis nostras).

❑❑ **"Strawberry tongue" is a physical finding associated with what systemic bacterial infection also caused primarily by group A, ß-hemolytic streptococci?**

Scarlet fever. Also seek characteristic Pastia's lines found in the antecubital area.
Recall the scarlet rash that spares the perioral area usually has onset 1 - 2 d after high fever, sore throat, headache and occasional vomiting and abdominal pain.
Mucocutaneous lymph node syndrome (Kawasaki disease), a disorder of unclear etiology, may also present with this finding.

❑❑ **Speaking of rashes...Dermacentor andersoni is a vector for** Rickettsia rickettsii **which cause Rocky Mountain spotted fever. The rash of RMSF usually begins on the wrists and ankles and spreads centripetally. What is the underlying pathologic lesion that causes the serious sequelae of this disease, as well as the hemorrhagic rash?**

Vasculitis 2° to rickettsial invasion of endothelial cells in small blood vessels, including arterioles.

❑❑ **Cellulitis in childhood is <u>most commonly</u> caused by** S. aureus. **The** least common **causative organism is responsible for most of the dangerous forms of this disease - striking younger children in more dangerous locations (e.g.. periorbital cellulitis), causing fever and bacteremia. What is the** least common **cause (overall) of pediatric cellulitis?**

H. influenzae.

❒❒ **A pediatric patient presents with cellulitis. As this patient does not have a violaceous lesion, nor a fever, nor a markedly elevated WBC,** *H. influenzae* **is not considered likely and discharge is planned. What antibiotic selection is appropriate in such a case?**

Dicloxacillin or cephalexin.

❒❒ *H. influenzae* **is the most common cause of periorbital cellulitis. What is the most common cause of** *orbital* **cellulitis?**

S. aureus.

❒❒ **Group A ß-hemolytic streptococcus is the most common cause of pharyngitis in older children. About what percentage of such patients with pharyngitis will have GABHS?**

≈ 50 %.

❒❒ **T/F: GABHS is a** frequent **cause of pharyngitis in patients less than 3 year of age.**

False.

❒❒ **We all know that the streptococcal antigen sampling tests for pharyngitis have a high false-negative rate (sensitivity variable, generally > 50%). What is the false-negative rate for a single throat culture?**

≈ 10 %.

❒❒ **For how long should a school-age child receive antibiotic treatment for GABHS before being allowed to return to school?**

1 day.

❒❒ **Rheumatic fever is preventable if antibiotic therapy is begun prior to how many days after the start of GABHS?**

9 days.

❒❒ **Poststreptococcal glomerulonephritis is preventable if antibiotic therapy is begun prior to how many days after the start of GABHS?**

TRICK QUESTION! Poststreptococcal glomerulonephritis is not an infectious complication of GABHS and is not preventable with antibiotic therapy.

❒❒ **What is the maximum dose of lidocaine for infiltration, a.) without epi and b.) with epi?**

a) 5 mg/kg without epinephrine.
b) 7 mg/kg with epinephrine.

❒❒ **Midazolam (Versed) may be given IV, IM, PO, PR and intranasally. The usual IV or IM dose is 0.15 mg/kg. What is a usual PR dose?**

0.25 mg/kg.

❒❒ **A child presents in DKA. On average, how dehydrated is this patient likely to be (give answer in mL/kg)?**

≈ 125 mL/kg average fluid volume deficit.

❑❑ You are managing a child in DKA. After initial 20 mL/kg bolus with 0.9% NS and careful fluid replacement with 0.45% NS for maintenance and replacement you are considering switching to D_5 0.45% NS. At about what glucose level should this change in fluid selection occur?

250 mg/dl.

❑❑ What is the dose of insulin to be used for low-dose continuous infusion therapy?

0.1 unit/kg/h of regular insulin.

❑❑ Insulin is usually mixed in NS at 1 unit/5 mL NS. How much of this fluid should be run through the tubing to saturate binding sites in the plastic?

50 mL = 10 units!

❑❑ A child known to have IDDM presents unconscious. What is the correct amount of $D_{50}W$ (expressed in mL/kg) to administer to this patient?

0.5 mL/kg.

❑❑ You have given the dose of medication from the previous question with no real improvement after 5 minutes. Now what should you do?

Try to sit tight, clinical response to glucose often takes 10 minutes. Use the time to think of other causes in this patient's d/dx, including sepsis, meningitis, metabolic abnormalities, poisoning, head injury, postictal state.

❑❑ Is intestinal intussusception associated with GI bleeding?

Yes, though the classic history of sudden onset of severe pain that often is relieved as quickly as it arose and is recurrent is more sensitive. The currant jelly stool associated with this disorder is present in about half of cases.

❑❑ About how old is the average patient presenting with intussusception?

One year, +/- 6 months.

❑❑ Pyloric stenosis usually presents at about what age?

5 weeks.

❑❑ What is the eponym for congenital aganglionic megacolon (the disease in which a portion of the distal colon lacks ganglion cells impairing the normal inhibitory innervation in the myenteric plexus impairing coordinated relaxation which can in turn cause clinical symptoms of obstruction, and that presents 85% of the time <u>after</u> the newborn period)?

Hirschsprung's disease.

❑❑ Acute enterocolitis with development of "toxic" megacolon is the life-threatening complication of Hirschsprung's disease. Between what range of ages does this complication most frequently present?

2 - 3 months.

❑❑ What signs and symptoms are associated with increased probability of a bacterial pathogen causing diarrhea?

Fever, acute onset of multiple diarrhea stools/day and blood in the stool.

❒❒ **T/F: Antibiotic therapy for gastroenteritis is limited in utility to children with high or prolonged fevers, those with inflammatory cells present in stool, those with protracted diarrhea and infants of less than 6 mo of age.**

True.

❒❒ **Among infants less than 3 mo of age, are UTI's more common in males or in females?**

Males.

❒❒ **Dysuria among female pediatric patients; more common cause - vulvovaginitis or UTI?**

Vulvovaginitis.
Maternally acquired - Candida, Trichomonas, condyloma.
Prepubertal –
  No cause determined (most common).
  Enterobius vermicularis, characterized by nocturnal pruritus.
  Candida, associated with antibiotics, IDDM.
  Foreign body.
  STDs - suggests sexual contact.

❒❒ **About what percentage of injuries in children less than 5 year of age seen in the ED are due to child abuse?**

10%.

❒❒ **Of abused children seen in the ED, about what percentage will be killed by future abuse?**

5%.

❒❒ **What is the most concerning aspect of the definition of Reye's syndrome provided by the CDC?**

Two of the criteria required may be determined at autopsy. Mortality is about 25% or less overall and varies with age of patient and clinical stage. The underlying abnormality is one of mitochondrial morphology and function, affecting primarily brain and liver.

❒❒ **Signs and symptoms of Reye's syndrome:**

Patient age usually between ages 6 - 11 y with prior viral illness, possible use of ASA, followed by intractable vomiting. Patient may present irritable, combative, or lethargic, and may c/o right upper quadrant tenderness. Seizures may occur, check for papilledema. Lab findings would include hypoglycemia, and an elevated ammonia level greater than 20 times normal. Bilirubin level is NORMAL.

❒❒ **Describe stage I and stage II of Reye's syndrome.**

Stage I - Vomiting, lethargy and liver dysfunction.
Stage II - Disorientation, combativeness, delirium, hyperventilation, increased deep tendon reflexes, liver dysfunction, hyperexcitable, tachypnea, fever, tachycardia, sweating and pupillary dilatation.

❒❒ **Treatment of stages I and II?**

Supportive.

❐❐ Describe Stages III, IV, and V of Reye's syndrome.

Stage III - coma, decorticate rigidity, increased respiratory rate, mortality rate of 50%.
Stage IV - coma, decerebrate posturing, no ocular reflexes, loss of corneal reflexes, and liver damage.
Stage V - loss of DTRs, seizures, flaccid, respiratory arrest, 95% mortality.

❐❐ Treatment for advanced stages of Reye's syndrome?

Manage ICP - elevate HOB, paralyze, intubate and hyperventilate, furosemide, mannitol, dexamethasone, pentobarbital coma. Also consider hypertonic glucose and bowel sterilization.

NEURON PEARLS

"Examinations are formidable even to the best prepared, for the greatest fool may ask more than the wisest man can answer."
Unknown

❑❑ **As you walk into the room, your patient gives you a BIG smile. What CN is intact?**

7th.

❑❑ **How can upper motor neuron (UMN) lesions of CN VII (facial nerve) be distinguished from peripheral lesions?**

UMN - Unilateral weakness of the lower half of the face.
Peripheral - Involve entire half of the face.

❑❑ **A 35 year-old woman with a history of flu like symptoms (URI) one wk ago now presents with vertigo, nausea, and vomiting. No auditory impairment or focal deficits are noted. What is the most likely cause of her problem?**

Labyrinthitis or vestibular neuronitis.

❑❑ **A patient presents with facial droop on the left and weakness of the right leg. What is the most likely site of the lesion?**

Brainstem (for you neuro fans, specifically the left pons).

❑❑ **During a routine Romberg exam a patient is asked to stand with his eyes open. He falls to the left. Diagnosis?**

Cerebellar dysfunction. An unsteady, broad-based gait suggests cerebellar problems. If the patient only falls with their eyes closed, the problem is with sensation, usually as a result of abnormality in position sense, most commonly posterior column dysfunction.

❑❑ **A 30 year-old presents with progressively severe intermittent vertigo for six months and progressive unilateral hearing loss for 3 months. Diagnosis?**

Cerebellopontine angle tumor. Confirm diagnosis with MRI scan.

❑❑ **Describe the key signs and symptoms of classic, common, cluster, ophthalmoplegic, and hemiplegic migraine headache.**

Classic -	Prodrome lasts up to 60 min. Most common symptom is visual disturbance, such as homonymous hemianopsia, scintillating scotoma, and photophobia. Lips, face, and hand tingling as well as aphasia and extremity weakness may occur. Nausea and vomiting may also occur.
Common -	Most common. Slow evolving headache over hours to days. A positive family history as well as two of the following: nausea or vomiting, throbbing quality, photophobia, unilateral pain, and increase with menses. Distinguishing feature from "Classic" migraine is the lack of visual symptoms.
Cluster -	Mostly males. Intense unilateral ocular or retroocular pain which lasts less than 2 hours

and occurs several times a day for weeks or months. Symptoms include lacrimation, facial flushing, rhinorrhea, sweating, and conjunctival injection. Often awakes patient from sleep.

Ophthalmoplegic - Most commonly seen in young adults. Patient has an outwardly deviated, dilated eye, with ptosis. The 3rd > 6th > 4th nerves are typically involved.

Hemiplegic - Unilateral motor and sensory symptoms, mild hemiparesis to hemiplegia.

❑❑ Treatment of a cluster headache?

100% O_2 and 5-10% cocaine solution, 4% lidocaine in the ipsilateral nostril, and a short course of steroids.

❑❑ A 29 year-old drunken male presents after having his head pounded into the concrete by his wife. The patient had a brief episode of LOC, but was then ambulatory and alert. Now he appears drowsy and just threw up on you. Diagnosis?

Epidural hematoma.

❑❑ A 25 year-old presents with a history of being knocked unconscious for 10 seconds while playing touch football one week ago. Since then he has felt malaise, intermittent vertigo, nausea, vomiting, blurred vision, and a headache. Neuro exam and CT are normal. Diagnosis?

Post-traumatic vertigo. Expect recovery to normal over 2 to 6 wk.

❑❑ A 64 year-old presents with a bilateral "burning" headache. She describes jabs of pain which are worse at night. Treatment?

Temporal arteritis is treated with long-term steroids. Treatment should begin immediately, do not wait for biopsy confirmation. ESR over 50 mm/h is highly suggestive.

❑❑ A 53 year-old female presents with unilateral right sided sudden-onset lancinating pain in the distribution of the second and third branches of the fifth cranial nerve. Treatment?

Carbamazepine treats trigeminal neuralgia. An MRI to rule out a brainstem process (tumor) is indicated.

❑❑ A 28 year-old woman raised in Minnesota complains of weakness and tingling in the right arm and leg for 2 days. She reports an episode of right eye pain and blurred vision which resolved over one mo that occurred 2 years ago. She also recalls a two wk episode of intermittent blurred vision one year ago. Diagnosis?

Presumptive MS. Confirm with MRI and CSF (oligoclonal bands).

❑❑ What artery is most commonly associated with epidural hematomas?

Middle meningeal artery.

❑❑ Which way do the eyes look with a major hemispheric abnormality (CVA or tumor)?

Toward the lesion.

❑❑ Which way do the eyes look with a brainstem abnormality?

Away from the lesion.

❑❑ A 50 year-old female presents with acute vertigo, nausea, and vomiting. She reports similar episodes over the last 20 years, sometimes but not always associated with hearing change and/or hearing loss and tinnitus. She has permanent right > left sensorineural hearing loss. Diagnosis?

Ménière's Disease.

❑❑ What is the most common cause of a subarachnoid hemorrhage?

Saccular aneurysm.

❑❑ For the following clinical presentations identify if each is most consistent with peripheral or central vertigo.

1. Intense spinning, nausea, hearing loss, diaphoresis.
2. Swaying or impulsion, worse with movement, tinnitus, acute onset.
3. Unidirectional nystagmus inhibited by ocular fixation, fatigable.
4. Mild vertigo, diplopia, and ataxia.
5. Multidirectional nystagmus not inhibited by ocular fixation, non-fatigable.

1,2, and 3 - Peripheral.
4 and 5 - Central.

❑❑ The Nylen-Bárány maneuver is performed as follows: the patient is rapidly brought from the sitting to supine position and the head is turned 45°. Match the findings with peripheral and central vertigo:

1. Nystagmus is multidirectional, non-fatiguing, has no latent period, and lasts over a minute.
2. Vertigo increased. Nystagmus is unidirectional, fatiguing, latent period is 2-20s, with duration less than a minute.

1 - Central.
2 - Peripheral.

❑❑ A 42 year-old air traffic controller presents with attacks of vertigo whenever he scans the skies for landing airplanes. Symptoms last about a minute. He is worried sick. What do you tell him about his disease?

The patient has benign positional vertigo. Attacks usually subside in a few weeks.

❑❑ A 50 year-old female presents with hearing loss over the last 6 months. She now presents at 2 A.M. with vertigo which has progressively become worse over the last 2 months. On exam, she is mildly ataxic. Diagnosis?

8th nerve lesion, possibly an acoustic schwannoma or meningioma.

❑❑ Dangerous diagnosis of a purpuric, petechial rash?

Think meningococcemia. Other causes include *Hemophilus influenzae*, *Streptococcus pneumoniae*, and *Staphylococcus aureus*.

❑❑ On LP, opening pressure is markedly elevated. What should be done?

Close 3-way stopcock, remove only a small amount of fluid from manometer, abort LP and initiate measures to decrease intracranial pressure.

❑❑ A patient presents with acute meningitis; when should antibiotics be initiated?

Immediately. Do not wait. Patients should receive a CT prior to LP only if papilledema or focal deficit is present.

❑❑ What is the most common presenting symptom of MS?

Optic neuritis (about 25%).

❐❐ A patient with MS presents with a fever. The nurse asks "should I give the patient Tylenol?" What is your response?

YES! Lowering temperature is important in MS patients as small increases in temperature can worsen existing signs and symptoms.

❐❐ What rhythm disturbance would make phenytoin relatively contraindicated?

Second or third degree heart block. If the patient is in status, you may have no choice.

❐❐ What three bacterial illnesses present with peripheral neurologic findings?

Botulism, tetanus, and diphtheria.

❐❐ What are the components of the mental status examination?

Attention, memory, orientation, language, calculation, visuospatial skills, praxis, gnosis, frontal (executive) function, mood and affect, thought processes and ideation.

❐❐ What types of memory are impaired earliest in Alzheimer's disease?

Episodic, explicit, declarative and short-term memory.

❐❐ Define apraxia and its etiology.

Apraxia is the inability to perform a complex motor task to command which cannot be attributed to deficits in attention, language, cooperation, strength, sensation or coordination. The task may be accomplished spontaneously. Apraxia usually results from a lesion in dominant hemisphere association areas. Apraxia may be described by the body part (oral apraxia) or task involved (gait apraxia).

❐❐ How does one test praxis?

Ask the patient to perform tasks such as blowing out a match or combing hair and observe the performance to command alone (hardest), by imitation of the examiner, or with use of the real object (easiest). Transitive (involving a tool or object), distal limb gestures, e.g., pounding a hammer, are also more difficult than intransitive, proximal gestures, e.g., taking a bow.

❐❐ What is agnosia?

Agnosia is the inability to recognize complex sensory stimuli despite preservation of elemental perception. More specific terms are used to denote the precise impairment.

❐❐ How can one determine if hearing loss is due to a middle ear problem?

Rinne: Check if conducted sound is heard better than air transmitted sound. If so, there is a problem with the middle ear.

❐❐ What are the main eye findings in multiple sclerosis?

Bilateral internuclear ophthalmoplegia (the eyes face straight ahead at rest, but on deviation, the adducted eye has weak movement).

❐❐ A patient presents complaining of a sudden onset of severe vertigo which doesn't change with position, and which is associated with horizontal nystagmus. You find yourself having to repeat a lot of questions. What is the most likely diagnosis?

Labyrinthitis.

❒❒ If the above patient had a history of chronic problems with middle ear infections, what would be your concern?

Acute suppurative labyrinthitis which is also associated with severe hearing loss.

❒❒ A patient presents complaining of sudden onset of severe vertigo, which doesn't change with position, and is associated with horizontal nystagmus, but the patient can hear you well. What is the most likely diagnosis?

Vestibular neuronitis.

❒❒ A patient presents with profound muscular weakness, and some respiratory difficulty. After adequately caring for the airway, you learn from the family that the patient has a history of myasthenia gravis, and is under treatment. What do you do for the patient?

A Tensilon test, to differentiate over treatment with cholinergics from under treatment. 1 to 2 mg of edrophonium (an AchE blocker) IV will transiently worsen the weakness of a cholinergic crisis and will transiently improve the weakness of a myasthenic crisis.

❒❒ A patient presents to the emergency department complaining of weakness that has been going on for some time now. He reports to you that he has had weakness primarily of his proximal arms and legs, and reports that he most notices it when he first starts a given activity. What should you be concerned about?

Eaton-Lambert syndrome.

❒❒ You have just gotten an ESR of 95 back on a 60 year-old patient with a throbbing unilateral headache who also is complaining of some generalized fatigue and some visual problems. What do you do now?

Get an emergent surgical consult for a temporal artery biopsy. You should also start steroids. The most likely diagnosis is temporal arteritis

❒❒ What is the most likely diagnosis for a patient with progressive dementia, ataxia, and incontinence?

Normal pressure hydrocephalus.

❒❒ What is the most likely cause of pinpoint pupils if metabolic and pharmacologic causes are excluded?

Pontine hemorrhage.

❒❒ When you perform cold calorics on a patient and his eyes slowly deviate toward the irrigated ear, but there is no rapid return phase, what does this mean?

The patient is comatose. The rapid phase is only present in awake patients. Neither phase will be present in brainstem injured patients.

❒❒ Define atopognosia, astereognosis, agraphesthesia and autopagnosia.

Atopognosia: inability to localize touch
Astereognosis: inability to identify an object by manipulation or palpation
Agraphesthesia: inability to identify a number or letter traced on the hand
Autopagnosia: inability to identify body parts (e.g., finger agnosia)

❒❒ What terms describe disordered perception of one's body?

Hemi-neglect (hemiasomatognosia): unawareness of half of one's body

Macro- or microsomatognosia: perception that a body part is unusually large or small
Autoscopy: seeing one's double, an "out of body" experience

❒❒ **What is the difference between dysarthria and aphasia?**

Dysarthria is a disorder of speech (a motor function); aphasia is a disorder of language (a higher cortical function).

❒❒ **Which types of aphasia have spared repetition?**

The transcortical aphasias (motor, sensory, and mixed) and anomic aphasia.

❒❒ **What components of language are used to characterize aphasias?**

Fluency, repetition, comprehension, naming, reading and writing comprise the language examination. The first three are used in characterizing aphasias as follows:

Aphasia	Fluency	Repetition	Comprehension
Broca's	impaired	impaired	intact
Wernicke's	intact	impaired	impaired
Conduction	intact	impaired	intact
Global	impaired	impaired	impaired
Transcortical motor	impaired	intact	intact
Transcortical sensory	intact	intact	impaired
Transcortical mixed	impaired	intact	impaired
Anomic	intact	intact	intact

❒❒ **What is anomic aphasia?**

Inability to name object.

❒❒ **Are reading and writing impaired in anomic aphasia?**

No, except for anomia with writing. Anomic aphasia is poorly localized within the dominant hemisphere.

❒❒ **Where is the lesion that results in a conduction aphasia?**

In the arcuate fasciculus, which connects Wernicke's to Broca's area.

❒❒ **What types of paraphasic errors are most common in Broca's aphasia?**

Literal (phonemic), such as "ladder" for "letter." Semantic (verbal) paraphasias (e.g., "table" for "chair" are more common in Wernicke's aphasia. Paralexic errors may also be of two types, phonemic or semantic.

❒❒ **How is delirium distinguished from dementia?**

In contrast to dementia, delirium is characterized by rapid onset, fluctuations in alertness and level of consciousness and reversibility over hours to days with correction of the underlying toxic or metabolic disturbance. Delirium may also be accompanied by asterixis, tremulousness and a diffusely slow EEG.

❒❒ **How is depression ("pseudodementia") distinguished from dementia?**

In depression, onset of symptoms is usually more acute, progression more rapid, self-report of mental impairment more common, and affect is depressed. Memory impairment is more inconsistent over time, and psychometric testing produces variable and effort-related results. There may be a history of psychiatric illness, recent life stressor, and somatic disturbances (anorexia and insomnia).

❑❑ The post-concussive syndrome includes what symptoms?

Headaches, dizziness, impaired memory and concentration, irritability and depression.

❑❑ What is the Wernicke-Korsakoff syndrome?

Chronic, severe impairment in anterograde memory (Korsakoff's syndrome) with acute confusion, ataxia, ophthalmoplegia, and nystagmus (Wernicke's encephalopathy). This syndrome results from lesions of the dorsomedial nuclei of the thalamus and mamillary bodies.

❑❑ How should Wernicke's encephalopathy be treated?

Immediate intravenous thiamine replacement.

❑❑ The NINDS t-PA study demonstrated the effectiveness of t-PA in the treatment of acute ischemic stroke. What was the time window for treatment?

The maximum allowed time from onset of symptoms to treatment is 3 hours.

❑❑ What laboratory studies are required prior to the administration of t-PA?

Noncontrast head CT, CBC, platelet count and glucose. PT and PTT are also required if the patient has a suspected or known coagulopathy or recently received warfarin or heparin.

❑❑ A 63-year-old previously healthy man awakens at 6 AM with weakness of the left arm and leg and difficulty walking. He arrives at the hospital at 7 AM and a CT scan is immediately performed, the results of which are normal. What dose of t-PA should he receive?

None. It must be assumed that the stroke onset was the time the patient was last known to be normal, i.e., when he went to sleep. Thrombolysis is contraindicated beyond 3 hours.

❑❑ What blood pressure parameters must be met for an acute stroke patient to receive thrombolytic treatment?

The SBP must be no greater than 185 mmHg and the DBP no greater than 110 mmHg. Hypertension increases the risk of hemorrhagic conversion.

❑❑ What was the risk of symptomatic intracerebral hemorrhage in patients who received t-PA in the NINDS study?

Six percent. The risk of fatal intracerebral hemorrhage was 3 percent.

❑❑ What effect does t-PA have on 3-month mortality?

The 3-month mortality of patients receiving t-PA was 17%, compared to 21% for conventional treatment.

❑❑ What is the single most important modifiable risk factor for stroke?

Hypertension.

❑❑ When is maximum cerebrospinal fluid xanthochromia observed after subarachnoid hemorrhage?

48 hours.

❑❑ What ocular sign is most frequently observed in extracranial carotid dissection?

Horner's syndrome.

❑❑ Name two risk factors for stroke.

Modifiable: Hypertension, diabetes, cholesterolemia, cigarette smoking, OSA
Non modifiable: Age > 65, family history (genetic)

❑❑ What are other risks of ischemic stroke?

Vasculitis, temporal arteritis, PAF, and cardiomyopathy.

❑❑ What are common causes of stroke in young people?

1. Vasculitis (SLE, rheumatoid)
2. Hypercoagulable states
3. Patent foramen ovale
4. Moyamoya
5. Fibromuscular dysplasia

❑❑ What is the initial workup of stroke?

CT without contrast, carotid ultrasound, 2-D echo; labs: glucose, ESR, fasting lipids, RPR.

❑❑ What should be added in young people?

Angiogram, antithrombin III, prot C, prot S, double contrast transesophageal echo, antiphospholipid antibody.

❑❑ After successful resuscitation from cardiac arrest, computed tomography of an elderly patient shows unilateral watershed infarct. What is the etiology?

After circulatory arrest, the cerebral cortex is commonly affected bilaterally but may occur unilaterally if there is carotid stenosis on one side.

❑❑ A comatose patient following a cerebrovascular accident presents with generalized repetitive movement of the limbs not affected by stimuli. What is the diagnosis?

Seizure. Seizures following a stroke can be generalized or focal, and present with only eyelid twitching or several clonic jerking of the limbs. Focal seizures indicate a focal cortical lesion but may also occur in hypoglycemia, hyperosmolarity, and in some drug intoxications (e.g., with aminophylline and tricyclic antidepressants).

❑❑ What is the implication of doll's eyes in a comatose patient?

When the cortical influences are depressed with an intact brain stem, doll's eyes (oculocephalic response) can be present in patients. Doll's eyes indicate the integrity of proprioceptive fibers from the neck structures, the vestibular nuclei, and the nuclei of the third, fourth and sixth cranial nerves. Unilateral lesions of the brain stem eliminate the doll's eyes response to the side of the lesion. In the event of absent doll's eyes in a comatose patient, performance of the ice-water caloric test (oculovestibular response) is a necessary requisite. In some cases, the doll's eyes response may be absent initially since the ice-water caloric response is produced by a stronger stimulus.

❑❑ A patient presents with eyes closed, is unresponsive to painful stimuli, and has flaccid muscle tone. What is the diagnosis?

Coma. Individuals in coma have no physiological response to external stimuli. They are without speech and do not respond to noxious stimuli.

❑❑ A patient presents with eyes closed but is aroused by deep, painful stimuli. What is the diagnosis?

Stupor. Stupor is a condition of deep sleep or behaviorally similar unresponsiveness from which the subject can be aroused only by vigorous and repeated stimuli. As soon as the stimulus ceases, stuporous subjects lapse back into the unresponsive state.

❒❒ A patient presents with acute agitation, fear, irritability and hallucinations. What is this state of consciousness?

Delirium. Delirium is acute in onset and can present with mental fluctuations between agitation and lethargy. In addition, the motor signs of tremor, myoclonus and asterixis may be present. The behavior of such patients commonly places them completely out of contact with the environment. Delirium is commonly found in hypoxic injury, sepsis, uremic encephalopathy and drug intoxication.

❒❒ A previously healthy 65-year-old individual presents with gradual loss of memory. What is the diagnosis?

Dementia. Dementia is the loss of intellectual abilities previously attained (memory, judgment, abstract thought and higher cortical functions) severe enough to interfere with social and/or occupational functioning. Dementia is commonly found in Alzheimer's disease, Pick's disease, AIDS and multiple cerebral infarctions (multi-infarct dementia).

❒❒ Following cardiac arrest, a patient presents with eyes open, no response to the environment and preserved sleep/wake cycles. What is the diagnosis?

Vegetative state. The vegetative state implies a subacute or chronic condition that sometimes emerges after severe brain injury. The condition comprises a return of wakefulness accompanied by an apparent total lack of cognitive function. Individuals in the vegetative state demonstrate eye opening spontaneously in response to verbal stimuli, sleep/wake cycles, maintenance of vital signs (blood pressure, heart rate and respirations). Patients do not display discrete localizing motor response and offer no comprehensible words or follow any verbal commands.

❒❒ A patient acutely develops contralateral hemiparesis with oculomotor palsy. What is the diagnosis?

Weber syndrome. Central midbrain infarction, usually due to occlusion of interpeduncular branches of the basilar artery, that disrupts the cerebral peduncle and the oculomotor nerve nuclei on one side of midbrain.

❒❒ What is the thalamic syndrome of Dejerine-Roussy?

The thalamic syndrome of Dejerine-Roussy is a result of thalamic infarction due to occlusion of the thalamo-geniculate branches. There is severe sensory loss, both deep and cutaneous, of the opposite side of the body. In some instances there is a dissociation of sensory loss with pain and thermal sensation affected more than touch, vibration and position. After an interval, sensation begins to return and the patient may then become afflicted with pain in the affected parts. Thus, the thalamic syndrome of Dejerine-Roussy is a late complication of thalamic infarct.

❒❒ A patient presents with a severe temporal headache and stiffness of the proximal muscles of the limbs. What is the diagnosis?

Temporal arteritis with polymyalgia rheumatica. Serum sedimentation rate can be markedly elevated in these patients. Some patients respond to high dose oral steroids, but patients who develop amaurosis fugax require treatment with intravenous steroids.

❒❒ A patient presents with fluent speech but poor comprehension. What is the diagnosis?

Wernicke's aphasia. The lesion involves the temporal auditory association area and/or the disconnection from the angular gyrus and the primary auditory cortex. Wernicke's aphasia is a fluent aphasia that implies maintenance of normal sentence length and intonation, but speech that is devoid of meaning.

❑❑ A patient presents with intact comprehension and writing skills but is unable to speak fluently. What is the diagnosis?

Broca's (motor) aphasia. Patients with Broca's aphasia have telegraphic speech. Their word-strings rarely exceed three or four words in length. They generally lack the short, functionally important words that indicate syntactic structure (e.g. as if, and, but, by, for). They have a deficit in the organization of speech output and aspects of grammar.

❑❑ A patient presents with sudden onset of severe headache with nuchal rigidity. What is the most important investigation?

Non-contrast computed tomography. Good quality non-contrast high resolution computed tomography will detect subarachnoid hemorrhage in >95% of cases if scanned within 48 hours of subarachnoid hemorrhage.

❑❑ What other additional information can be obtained from computed tomography in patients with subarachnoid hemorrhage?

1. Ventricular size (hydrocephalus occurs acutely in 21% of patients with subarachnoid hemorrhage)
2. Associated increased intracranial pressure which may need emergent management
3. Infarct
4. Amount of blood in cisterns (important predictor for the development of vasospasm)
5. In the event of multiple aneurysms, computed tomography may identify which aneurysm bled
6. Computed tomography can predict aneurysm location in 70% of cases

❑❑ An elderly, hypertensive woman presents with sudden headache, vomiting and inability to walk. The patient has loss of coordination in the right extremities and paralysis of upward and right gaze. She is alert with no motor and sensory deficit and pupils are normal and reactive. What is the diagnosis?

Cerebellar hemorrhage. The onset is sudden without loss of consciousness, within minutes patient is unable to walk or stand. Headache, dizziness and vomiting occur in most of the patients. There is often paresis of gaze to the affected side (cranial nerve VI palsy). Loss of upward gaze is sign of compression on the tectal plate. Intact motor strength and sensation is characteristic. Rapid diagnosis is crucial such as with magnetic resonance imaging since surgical decompression can lead to complete recovery.

❑❑ A middle-aged woman presents with a generalized seizure. There is a three-day history of headache, fever and lethargy but no history of prior seizures. Plantar response on the right is extensor, and cranial computed tomography is normal. What is the diagnosis?

Herpes encephalitis. Initially, patients may present with febrile illness followed by headaches and malaise that soon progress to seizures, alteration of consciousness, personality change and focal deficits. Cranial computed tomography is unremarkable for a mass lesion. Cerebral spinal fluid reveals pleocytosis and a raised immunoglobulin. Brain biopsy can confirm the diagnosis.

❑❑ A 30-year-old man presents with acute, severe headache and nuchal rigidity. Cranial computed tomography is negative. What is the next investigation?

Lumbar puncture. When subarachnoid hemorrhage is suspected in patients with unremarkable cranial computed tomography, a lumbar puncture is a requisite to examine for blood in the cerebral spinal fluid. The cerebral spinal fluid should be examined with the first and last collection tubes and for evidence of xanthochromia.

❑❑ A 50-year-old female presents with paroxysmal lancinating right-sided facial pain precipitated by exposure to gusts of cold wind and brushing the teeth. The pain persists for less than a minute. What is the diagnosis?

Trigeminal neuralgia. The majority of cases with trigeminal neuralgia (tic douloureux) are due to microvascular compression in the in the root entry zone where the trigeminal nerve enters the pons. Most often a loop of the superior cerebellar artery is responsible.

❒❒ What are the types and treatment of trigeminal neuralgia?

The pain of tic douloureux affects the face within the trigeminal distribution of the ophthalmic (first), the maxillary (second) and the mandibular (third) divisions of the trigeminal nerve. The second or third divisions of the trigeminal nerve are involved more often than the first. The medical treatment can consist of carbamazepine with approximately 70% of patients obtaining relief. Alternative drugs include phenytoin and baclofen. Surgical treatment may be an option for microvascular decompression or rhizotomy.

❒❒ In addition to microvascular compression of the trigeminal nerve, what are additional causes of trigeminal neuralgia?

Tumors are the cause in 5-8% of cases (e.g. schwannomas, meningiomas or epidermoid tumors in the cerebellopontine angle). Multiple sclerosis is the cause in 3% of cases. Cranial computed tomography or magnetic resonance imaging can diagnose tumors. If multiple sclerosis is suspected, evoked potentials, cerebral spinal fluid analysis and magnetic resonance imaging are helpful in making the diagnosis.

❒❒ An elderly alert male is distressed because of his severe disorientation to time and space. His recent memory is impaired, but remote memory is intact. He had one similar spell before that persisted for two hours. What is the diagnosis?

Transient global amnesia. These patients suffer from a severe but isolated deficit in retrograde memory that gradually resolves. Most attacks affect middle aged or elderly persons and reflect temporary vascular insufficiency affecting the hippocampal memory area or the subsequent thalamic connections. Most attacks neither leave residual limitations nor carry a strong risk of recurrence.

❒❒ What is the differential diagnosis of transient global amnesia?

Transient global amnesia may be a result of vascular transient ischemic attacks, temporal lobe seizures or drug therapy.

❒❒ A 60-year-old ex-boxer presents with slowness of thinking, gross memory loss (remote and recent), broad-based shuffling gait, incontinence and bilateral upper motor neuron dysfunction. What further investigations are necessary?

Cranial computed tomography or magnetic resonance imaging. The patient is suffering from hydrocephalic dementia. Brain imaging may reveal dilated ventricles and effaced hemispheric sulci. The condition is caused by chronic interference with the cerebral spinal fluid (CSF) absorption pathways over the surface of the hemispheres. Ultimate causes include acute or chronic inflammatory meningitis, subarachnoid hemorrhage and traumatic head injury. CSF pressure is normal in most cases.

❒❒ A 65-year-old, hypertensive male presents with gross memory loss. Cranial magnetic resonance imaging reveals multiple high signal intensity areas reflecting past infarctions. What is the diagnosis?

Multi-infarct dementia. This condition occurs as a result of successive large and small strokes, affecting the cerebral hemispheres and their deep subcortical nuclei. Hypertension, diabetes mellitus, or hyperlipidemia most often underlies the vascular changes. The usual clinical picture is of successive cumulative episodes of focal neurologic worsening, resulting in a disheveled appearance accompanied by aphasia, focal neurologic deficits, and progressive amnesia.

❒❒ What are the toxic side effects of phenytoin?

Toxic symptoms that are related to blood levels of the drug include nystagmus, ataxia and blurred vision. Other side effects not related to blood levels of the drug include skin eruptions, teratogenesis, hepatitis, blood dyscrasias and lupus. Hypertrichosis, gingival hyperplasia and coarsening of facial features may trouble patients but rarely require withdrawal of medication.

❒❒ An elderly man during a hot summer day following an alcoholic binge develops confusion, fever of 42° C and anhydrosis. What is the diagnosis?

Heat stroke. The risk factors for heat stroke include a lack of acclimatization, increased age, alcoholic excess and, especially, the ingestion of anticholinergic or antipsychotic drugs. The disorder results when high ambient temperatures and humidity combine to generate heat and prevent its loss while at the same time, age, neurologic disease or drugs impair central autonomic mechanisms. Clinical signs include hyperpyrexia greater than 41° C, hot, dry skin, increasing prostration, confusion, stupor and, finally, coma accompanied by signs of brain stem dysfunction. Treatment is aimed at bringing core temperature below 39° C in an ice tub bath and meeting systemic problems.

❒❒ An adolescent boy presents with unilateral severe headache associated with malaise, vomiting and photophobia that persists for three hours. Prior to his headache, he experienced hemiparesis, which disappeared with the onset of headache. What is the diagnosis?

Classic migraine. In classic migraine, brief (up to 30 minutes) neurologic dysfunction precedes or less often, accompanies headache. The neurologic symptoms are usually visual, consist of bright flashing lights beginning in the center of visual half-field and radiate toward the periphery. In addition, unilateral paresthesias (hand and perioral), aphasia, hemiparesis and hemisensory defects can occur.

❒❒ An adolescent boy presents with unilateral severe headache associated with malaise, vomiting and photophobia that persists for four hours. During his headache, he developed hemisensory loss, which is now persisting. What is the diagnosis?

Complicated migraine. In migraine, if the neurologic dysfunction continues into or outlasts the duration of the headache, the disorder is called complicated migraine. In rare instances, such as in this case, a neurologic disorder may be permanent with the subsequent vasoconstriction resulting in cerebral infarction.

❒❒ An adolescent boy presents with recurrent attacks of unilateral paresthesias in the hand for 15 minutes, which occur approximately 1-2 times per month. Evidence of headache or loss of consciousness is not evident. What is the diagnosis?

Migraine equivalent. The clinical presentation of recurrent attacks of neurologic dysfunction that mimic the migraine alone but do not culminate in headache is known as a migraine equivalent, which is sometimes confused with transient ischemic attack or a focal seizure.

❒❒ A 35-year-old male presents with a severe unilateral headache that persists for 20 minutes associated with chemosis and rhinorrhea. What is the diagnosis?

Cluster headache. Cluster headaches are short-lived (15-180 minutes) attacks of extremely severe, unilateral orbital or supraorbital headache that occur in clusters, often occurring several times daily and lasting several weeks. These headaches are most common in males and may disappear for months or years before recurring. This headache is associated with conjunctival injection, lacrimation, nasal congestion, rhinorrhea, forehead and facial sweating, miosis, ptosis and eyelid edema. Frequency of attacks varies from 1 every other day to 8 per day.

❒❒ A 5-year-old boy presents with focal motor epilepsy and Port wine nevus in the right fronto-temporal region. What is the diagnosis?

Sturge-Weber disease. This condition is defined as a port wine-colored capillary hemangioma accompanied by a similar vascular malformation of the underlying meninges and cerebral cortex. The cause is unknown. Diagnosis is made by observing the disfiguring stain involving the sensory dermatomal distribution of the first, second, and third division of trigeminal nerve. General or focal motor seizures may occur with or without associated mental retardation and require antiepileptic medication.

❒❒ A 15-year-old high school student succumbs to stupor six hours following a hit with a baseball to his left temporal region. What is the diagnosis?

Epidural hematoma. Bony breaks across the groove of the middle meningeal artery in the temporal bone can lacerate the artery, leading to epidural hematoma. Typically, such clots enlarge progressively to produce signs of neurologic worsening beginning from a few hours to as much as 3 days following initial injury. Unilateral headache followed by restlessness, agitation, or greater obtundation is characteristic. Such hematomas can be fatal unless surgically treated. If cranial computed tomography is not available, skull radiographs are useful.

❒❒ A 50-year-old hypertensive female presents with sudden headache followed by acute onset coma with irregular breathing and pinpoint pupils. What is the diagnosis?

Pontine hemorrhage. The onset usually is cataclysmic with sudden headache followed by coma shortly and accompanied by irregular breathing, pinpoint pupils, bilateral conjugate gaze paralysis or ocular bobbing, tetraparesis and, often, decerebrate or decorticate rigidity. Most patients die, and those who survive usually are left quadriplegic.

❒❒ A 25-year-old female presents with headache and bilateral papilledema. Cranial computed tomography is unremarkable. Lumber puncture reveals low protein (<15 mg/dl) with a cerebral spinal fluid (CSF) pressure of 320 mm. What is the diagnosis?

Pseudotumor cerebri. This disorder is characterized by increased intracranial pressure in the absence of tumor or obvious obstruction of CSF pathways. Pseudotumor cerebri can follow head trauma, middle ear disease, internal jugular vein ligation, oral contraceptive use, pregnancy, polycythemia vera and any condition that suggest possible cerebral venous occlusion. The disorder has also been reported in patients with steroid therapy or steroid withdrawal, Addison's disease or hypoparathyroidism. It is also seen with ingestion of drugs such as vitamin A, nalidixic acid and tetracycline.

The disorder usually affects young (20-30-year-old), obese females. It is characterized by headache, papilledema and, at times, visual changes (sudden momentary, usually bilateral visual loss). It has benign prognosis. The diagnosis is established by the presence of elevated intracranial pressure in a patient without a mass occupying. The CSF pressure is usually above 300 mm and its composition is normal, although some patients may have a relatively low protein (<15 mg/dl).

❒❒ What is the treatment of pseudotumor cerebri?

Treatment is symptomatic. Repeated lumber punctures sometimes relieve the headache. Only if there is evidence of progressive visual loss, therapeutic intervention is mandatory. In that instance, the best treatment appears to be lumbo-peritoneal cerebral spinal fluid shunt.

❒❒ A comatose patient with presents with nuchal rigidity. Following a lumber puncture that is positive for blood in the cerebral spinal fluid with elevated pressure, the patient develops respiratory arrest. What is the diagnosis?

Tonsillar herniation. In patients with raised intracranial pressure (supra- or infra-tentorial lesions), lumber puncture precipitates tonsillar herniation. Cerebellar tonsils cone through the foramen magnum, compressing the medulla and result in respiratory arrest.

❒❒ Following a motor vehicle accident, a 17-year-old patient presents with coma, right side decerebrate posture, left-side decorticate posture and anisocoria. What is the diagnosis?

Left hemispheric expanding mass lesion. This is the feature of Kernohan's phenomenon, usually due to expanding epidural hematoma leading to uncal herniation. The impaired consciousness results from compression of the reticular activating system in the rostral brain stem. The left-side dilated pupil is secondary to the compression of left third nerve. The right side hemiplegia (decerebrate) is secondary to compression of the left cerebral peduncle which carries fibers to the right side. The herniating uncus is compressing the left third cranial nerve and cerebral peduncle. Left-side hemiplegia (decorticate) is a result of compression of the right cerebral peduncle along the tentorial notch.

❐❐ A patient omits the left half of a clock when asked to sketch a clock. What is the diagnosis?

Hemispatial neglect secondary to a nondominant parietal lobe lesion, such as a middle cerebral artery infarct. Patients with right parietal (nondominant) lesions have a profound disturbance of visuospatial skills, i.e. they omit the left half of the figure which they attempt to copy it. They are unable to interpret maps, provide directions or describe the floor plan of their house.

❐❐ Following a successful resuscitation from cardiac arrest, a 65-year-old man presents with paraplegia, pain and temperature sensation loss at T6 and below, but intact vibratory and position sense. What is the diagnosis?

Spinal cord ischemia. The midthoracic anterior spinal segments (the territory of anterior spinal artery) has tenuous vascular supply, possessing only the radicular artery at T4 to T5 and the artery of Adamkiewicz at T9 to T12. This region is known as the watershed zone and is more susceptible to vascular insults, especially during systemic hypotension.

❐❐ A patient notes that when he looks at the trunk lock of a car in front of him he cannot see either of the tail lights of the vehicle. What do you suspect?

Chiasmal field defect (optic chiasm mass with bitemporal hemianopsia).

❐❐ What is the most sensitive ancillary test for multiple sclerosis (MS):

MRI (greater than 95%).

❐❐ What is the most common visual deficit in MS?

Unilateral optic neuritis (ON).

❐❐ What is ON?

Inflammation of the optic nerve leading to demyelination. The disc may initially appear normal if the process is retrobulbar.

❐❐ What is the most common urinary bladder dysfunction in MS?

Urgency from contraction of the detrusor muscle (spastic bladder).

❐❐ Which gastrointestinal disturbance is commonly observed in MS?

Constipation.

❐❐ Describe Lhermitte's sign.

Descending electric shock upon flexion of the neck.

❐❐ What are the most common presenting complaints in MS?

Fatigue, sensory and/or motor symptoms, visual complaints, and ataxia.

❐❐ Rapid correction of chronic hyponatremia will cause which neurologic disorder?

Rapid correction of serum sodium level (> 0.5 mEq/L) may cause central pontine myelinolysis.

❑❑ **What are the clinical features of myxedema coma?**

Non-pitting edema, hypothermia, bradycardia, dry skin and brittle hair.

❑❑ **What are the neurological causes of diabetes insipidus?**

Lesions of the hypothalamus or pituitary such as postoperative state, head trauma, sarcoid, lymphoma, craniopharyngioma, pituitary adenoma and metastatic tumors.

❑❑ **What are the clinical features of epidural abscess?**

Spinal tenderness, fever, radicular pain, myelopathy, elevated CSF protein and CSF pleocytosis.

❑❑ **What is the treatment of epidural abscess?**

Immediate laminectomy, drainage of the abscess and antibiotic therapy. A delay in treatment may result in permanent myelopathy.

❑❑ **What are the causes of subdural empyema?**

Sinusitis, meningitis, head trauma, otitis and osteomyelitis.

❑❑ **What are the complications that occur following subarachnoid hemorrhage?**

Vasospasm, recurrent hemorrhage, hydrocephalus, seizures, cardiac arrhythmias, hypertension, neurogenic pulmonary edema, stress ulcers and SIADH.

❑❑ **What is the drug treatment for convulsive status epilepticus?**

Lorazepam (0.1 mg/kg) administered at 2 mg/minute, followed by intravenous fosphenytoin (18 mg of phenytoin equivalent/kg).

❑❑ **What are the clinical features of spinal cord compression from metastatic cancer?**

Localized spinal tenderness, radicular pain, sensory level, paraparesis or quadriparesis, bowel-bladder incontinence, brisk deep tendon reflexes, upgoing plantar reflexes and spasticity.

❑❑ **What is the treatment for acute spinal cord compression from metastatic cancer?**

High dose corticosteroids and radiation therapy. Surgical therapy is used in place of radiation therapy when the primary cancer type is unknown, when the tumor is radioresistant, spinal instability makes surgery necessary or when the patient has received the maximum radiation dose to the involved area.

❑❑ **What are the medical complications in Guillain-Barré syndrome?**

Respiratory failure, dysautonomia, deep vein thrombosis, pulmonary embolus, SIADH, respiratory and urinary tract infections.

❑❑ **What is myasthenic crisis?**

Myasthenic crisis occurs in a person with myasthenia gravis when the person has significant impairment in respiratory function. A person with myasthenic crisis may require emergency intubation and assisted ventilation.

❑❑ **What is the treatment for neuroleptic induced acute dystonic reaction?**

Diphenhydramine (25-50 mg IV).

❑❑ **What are the features of neuroleptic malignant syndrome?**

Altered mental status, fever, rigidity, irregular pulse, irregular blood pressure, tachycardia, diaphoresis and elevated CPK.

❑❑ **What is the treatment for neuroleptic malignant syndrome?**

Immediate withdrawal of the neuroleptic drug. Sinemet, bromocriptine or dantrolene may be used as needed.

❑❑ **What is the treatment for hepatic coma?**

Treat precipitating causes such as GI bleeding, alkalosis, hypokalemia, narcotics, sedatives, and infection. Treatment may include: reduced dietary protein, lactulose, oral neomycin and flumazenil.

❑❑ **What are the features of botulism infection?**

A history of recent ingestion of home canned or prepared foods, followed by sudden onset of diplopia, dysphagia, muscle weakness, dry mouth, fixed dilated pupils and respiratory paralysis.

❑❑ **What is the medical treatment of confirmed botulism?**

Botulism antitoxin.

❑❑ **What are the features of hypertensive encephalopathy?**

The features are diastolic blood pressure usually over 130 Torr, papilledema and impaired mental status.

❑❑ **What are the features of giant cell arteritis (temporal arteritis)?**

Age > 50 years, visual loss, unilateral headache, tender nodular temporal artery, pain and stiffness of shoulders and pelvic girdle area, malaise, fever, weight loss, jaw claudication, anemia, elevated sedimentation rate and a temporal artery biopsy showing giant cell arteritis.

❑❑ **What is the treatment for giant cell arteritis?**

Prednisone (60 mg/day) is started immediately prior to biopsy to prevent blindness.

❑❑ **What are the clinical features of a cerebellar hemorrhage?**

The symptoms may begin with headache, vomiting and inability to stand or walk. Other symptoms may include vertigo, diplopia, ataxia, gaze palsies, peripheral facial palsy, altered mental status and coma.

❑❑ **What is the treatment for cerebellar hemorrhage?**

Immediate surgical evacuation is performed for patients with rapid progression of symptoms, patients with hydrocephalus and patients with large (> 3 cm diameter) hematomas. The remaining patients are carefully followed.

❑❑ **What are the earliest clinical features of uncal herniation?**

Uncal herniation begins with a unilateral enlarged pupil and a sluggish pupillary light reaction.

❑❑ **What intravenous injection must every patient with coma of unknown cause receive?**

Glucose and thiamine.

❑❑ **How is a subarachnoid hemorrhage diagnosed?**

CT scan may show blood in the suprasellar cistern, interhemispheric fissure, sylvian fissure, or surface of the brain. If the CT scan is normal, a spinal tap may show xanthochromia.

❒❒ What is the Cushing reflex?

This brainstem mediated reflex is a elevation in blood pressure and reduction in pulse that follows an increase in intracranial pressure.

❒❒ What is the Glasgow coma scale?

This scale measures eye, verbal and motor responses that occur spontaneously, in response to voice, and in response to painful stimuli. The scale ranges from 0 - 15; higher scores indicate a more normal level of functioning.

❒❒ What are the criteria for diagnosis of brain death?

The criteria are: (1) coma is present from a known cause, (2) reversible causes of coma such as hypothermia (temperature < 32 degrees Celsius) or drug intoxication have been excluded, (3) there is no clinical evidence of brain or brainstem function.

❒❒ What are typical features of tension-type headache?

Diffuse and bilateral location, mild to moderate intensity, pressure or tightening quality and no aggravation upon physical activity.

❒❒ What are typical features of migraine headaches?

Unilateral headache (60% of cases), pulsating quality, moderate to severe intensity, nausea and/or vomiting, photophobia and phonophobia and aggravation by routine physical activity.

❒❒ What are typical features of cluster headache?

Periodic attacks of sharp, severe, unilateral head pain, referred to the orbital or periorbital regions, associated with at least one autonomic symptom (miosis, rhinorrhea, ptosis, conjunctival hyperemia).

❒❒ Which features are important in eliciting a headache history?

Attack onset, duration, frequency, and timing. Pain location, severity, and quality. Associated symptoms, aggravating and ameliorating factors. Past medical, social, and family history.

❒❒ Which elements are considered "alarms" in the evaluation of headache disorders?

Onset of headache after the age of 50 years, sudden onset of headache, accelerating pattern of headaches, new-onset headache in a patient with cancer or HIV, headache with systemic illness (fever, stiff neck, rash), focal neurological symptoms or signs of disease, headache aggravated by Valsalva maneuver.

❒❒ Which type of acute headache is highly responsive to oxygen?

Cluster headache (100% oxygen at 7-10 l/min for 15 min).

❒❒ Which drugs are effective in the acute attack of cluster headache?

Sumatriptan 6 mg SC, Dihydroergotamine (DHE) 1.0 mg IV or IM, Intranasal lidocaine.

❒❒ What is the cardinal feature of post-lumbar puncture headache?

Pain aggravated by upright position and relieved by recumbency.

❒❒ **What are the signs and symptoms of giant cell arteritis?**

Headache, fatigue, myalgia, arthralgia, jaw claudication, associated with tenderness, induration and diminished or absent pulse of the temporal artery.

❒❒ **Which is the most consistent laboratory abnormality in giant cell arteritis?**

Elevation of Westergren ESR. Generally, well above 50 mm/h.

❒❒ **What is the main risk factor to suffer post-herpetic neuralgia following Herpes Zoster infection?**

Age. The older the patient the higher the risk.

❒❒ **What are the four cardinal signs of Parkinson's disease?**

Tremor, bradykinesia/akinesia, rigidity, postural instability/gait problems.

❒❒ **A 23-year-old college student presents to your neurology clinic with a history of acute onset of rigidity, bilateral and symmetric resting tremor, akinesia and inability to walk. What do you suspect and what history should you try to elicit?**

His history is suspicious for MPTP (1-methyl-4-phenyl-1, 2,3,6-tetrahydropyridine) induced parkinsonism. Ask the patient about illicit drug use, particularly exposure to "designer drugs" synthesized to substitute for heroin. MPTP was a contaminant found in such drugs in the late 1970s and early 1980s.

❒❒ **What are the side effects of dopaminergic therapy?**

Nausea, vomiting, orthostatic hypotension, constipation, dyskinesias and hallucinations.

❒❒ **What medications are contraindicated for patients with parkinsonism?**

Neuroleptics and related agents - phenothiazine (e.g., prochlorperazine (Compazine)), butyrophenones (e.g., haloperidol), thioxanthenes, benzamide (e.g., metoclopramide-Reglan), dihydroindolone (Mobane), dibenzoxazepine (Loxitane)

❒❒ **An elderly woman with a history of diabetes presents with complaints of repetitive grimacing and lip smacking. She is taking glyburide, hormone supplements and metoclopramide. Her examination is remarkable for mild peripheral neuropathy and repetitive mouth movements. She can suppress the mouth movements for brief periods of time. What do you suspect?**

She is likely suffering from tardive dyskinesia due to her taking metoclopramide.

❒❒ **What is benign positional vertigo (BPV)?**

Recurrent episodes of vertigo triggered by postural changes.

❒❒ **What is the most common cause of benign positional vertigo?**

The majority of cases have no known precipitating cause. When a cause can be identified, it is either head trauma or a previous viral syndrome.

❒❒ **How does one diagnose benign positional vertigo?**

Fatigable vertical/torsional nystagmus on head hanging positional testing (Dix and Hallpike maneuver), in the context of a normal neurological examination is consistent with benign positional vertigo.

❒❒ **How is Dix-Hallpike maneuver performed?**

In the sitting position, the head is turned 45 degrees to one side and the patient is rapidly taken from the sitting to the supine position. The final position is one in which the head hangs off the edge of the exam table.

❐❐ How does one distinguish recurrent positional vertigo of central origin from that of peripheral origin?

Positional vertigo of central origin is non-fatiguing and usually purely vertical.

❐❐ What is thought to be the cause of benign positional vertigo?

Free floating otoconia (calcium carbonate crystals) in the semicircular canal are thought to coalesce into a relatively larger mass which will suddenly displace the cupula with sudden movement of the head, resulting in vertiginous symptoms.

❐❐ What are the most common signs and symptoms of spinal cord compression?

Back pain, weakness, autonomic dysfunction, sensory loss and ataxia.

❐❐ How does Adie's pupil react?

Unilateral dilated pupil usually in a middle-aged female with diminished deep tendon reflexes (mainly knee jerk and ankle reflex) results from damage to the ciliary ganglion. This pupil may show denervation supersensitivity and will constrict to a very dilute pilocarpine 0.125% strength. A normal pupil will not constrict to such dilute pilocarpine. On slit lamp examination this pupil may show segmental constriction. Chronic Adie's pupil can become a miotic nonreactive pupil. Adie's pupil can be bilateral.

❐❐ Enumerate some causes of Horner's syndrome.

1. Brain stem and cerebral CVA, basal meningitis, cervical cord lesion, Wallenberg syndrome, trauma, sarcoidosis can cause central first order preganglionic Horner's syndrome.
2. Trauma, head and neck tumor, cervical rib, tuberculosis and lymphadenopathy can cause second order pre-ganglionic Horner's syndrome.
3. Cavernous sinus lesions, Internal carotid artery disease, CAE (carotid artery end-arterectomy), and orbital trauma can cause third order or post-ganglionic Horner's syndrome.

❐❐ What are the CSF characteristics of tuberculous meningitis?

Lymphocytic pleocytosis, very high protein (several hundred to a thousand mg/dl) and very low glucose.

❐❐ Radial deviation on wrist extension is indicative of a lesion of which nerve?

Posterior interosseous nerve.

❐❐ What is the predominant root innervation of the tibialis posterior muscle?

L5 ventral root via the tibial nerve.

❐❐ What is the most sensitive test for carpal tunnel syndrome?

Comparing conduction latencies in a short segment of the median versus ulnar nerves across the carpal tunnel. This is done by stimulating the median and ulnar mixed nerves in the palm while recording over the wrist.

❐❐ A 39-year-old patient presents to the emergency department with weakness and fatigue. She is diagnosed with a bacterial infection and given gentamicin. Shortly after, the patient develops respiratory distress and requires intubation. What is her likely diagnosis and why did this occur?

Signs of weakness and fatigue, although non specific, are compatible with the diagnosis of myasthenia gravis. Impaired transmission at the neuromuscular junction, as found in myasthenia gravis, can be exacerbated by aminoglycoside antibiotics due to their actions as non-depolarizing neuromuscular blocking agents.

❒❒ A 16-year-old patient presents with recent onset (48 hours) of progressive weakness with numbness. Her reflexes are absent. She complains of back pain and numbness. What are the likely underlying pathophysiology and preferred treatment?

Acute, progressive motor and sensory symptoms along with hypoactive deep tendon reflexes are compatible with the diagnosis of Guillain-Barré syndrome. This acquired *demyelinating* neuropathy can be life threatening and requires prompt attention. Frequent monitoring of her vital signs (especially respiratory) is required. Plasmapheresis or intravenous gamma-globulin are both accepted first-line treatments.

❒❒ Following a motor vehicle accident, a patient presents with inability to extend the left arm or wrist. Despite an apparent traumatic injury to the radial nerve, fibrillation potentials are not seen when the weak muscles are examined in the emergency department soon after the accident. If the nerve was apparently crushed in the accident, why would fibrillation potentials not be present?

Fibrillation potentials occur following denervation which results in an enhanced excitability of the muscle membrane to spontaneous release of acetylcholine. This process usually does not begin for seven to ten days following acute injury.

❒❒ What structures are commonly affected in carbon monoxide intoxication?

Bilateral necrosis of globus pallidus.

❒❒ How does rabies spread to the brain?

An RNA virus that spreads to the brain along the nerves from the inoculation site.

❒❒ What is the most common cause of epidural hematoma?

Laceration of the middle meningeal artery by a skull fracture.

❒❒ What causes subdural hematoma?

Tearing of the bridging veins.

❒❒ What are symptoms and signs of neuroleptic malignant syndrome?

Fever, muscle rigidity, myoglobinuria and elevation of CPK, autonomic instability with labile pulse and blood pressure.

❒❒ What is the treatment for neuroleptic malignant syndrome?

Dopamine agonist treatment (bromocriptine) and supportive measures (cooling, sedation with benzodiazepines, some would advocate dantrolene).

❒❒ A myasthenic crisis is characterized by weakness, which can also be present in overmedication with anticholinesterases. What might differentiate the two?

Cramping, diarrhea and fasciculations tend to occur in anticholinesterase excess. Alternatively, edrophonium (Tensilon) can be administered. If dramatic improvement is observed, then it is likely that the weakness is due to myasthenic crisis. If no improvement or worsening occurs, the effect is short-lived with this short-acting agent.

❑❑ Which antibiotics may exacerbate myasthenia gravis?

Aminoglycoside.

❑❑ What is an important feature to keep in mind when initiating corticosteroid therapy in a patient with myasthenia gravis?

Initiation of steroid therapy is often associated with initial worsening of weakness.

❑❑ What therapy should be used for a patient with hemophilia A who suffers a traumatic brain injury?

Cryoprecipitate: Cryoprecipitate has an increased concentration of factor VIII complex than does fresh frozen plasma.

❑❑ Do "hangman's fractures" usually lead to quadriplegia?

No: While there is often some dislocation, these laminar C2 fractures are usually without significant distraction or displacement of C2 on C3.

❑❑ Laceration of which artery is the most common cause for epidural hematoma?

The middle meningeal artery: This usually occurs in association with skull fracture.

❑❑ What is the most common pathology of acute subdural hematoma?

Disruption of bridging or cortical surface veins: Other causes include cortical contusion or laceration.

❑❑ Is an intracranial pressure > 40 mmHg always fatal?

No: This is exemplified by patients with pseudotumor cerebri who may have little or no significant neurological dysfunction.

❑❑ What are pontine pupils?

Pinpoint, but reactive, pupils secondary to injury of the sympathetic fibers descending through the tegmentum, either from intrinsic pontine tegmental injury or from cerebellar or other posterior fossa mass effect causing compression of the tegmentum: Similar pupillary findings can be seen after narcotic administration.

❑❑ A patient complains of difficulty walking not associated with numbness or pain. Examination is remarkable for loss of position sense and vibration in the toes, bilateral leg spasticity and Babinski's signs. What diagnoses should be considered?

This is a posterior column and corticospinal tract syndrome. Subacute combined degeneration of the spinal cord from vitamin B12 deficiency, myelopathy from HIV infection, and posterior cord compression need to be considered. Cervical spondylosis and cervical disc protrusion are surgical lesions to be considered. Mass lesions, such as metastatic tumors, should be considered.

❑❑ This patient also has electric shock-like sensations extending down the back and sometimes the arms. What is this symptom called?

Lhermitte's phenomenon. The symptom is usually associated with multiple sclerosis but may occur with any compressive lesion of the cervical spinal cord or with radiation myelopathy or chronic meningeal inflammation.

❑❑ A patient has spasticity of all extremities, hyperreflexia, and bilateral Babinski's signs. Examination reveals fasciculations of the tongue only. What diagnoses do you consider?

ALS is certainly a consideration. The examination is consistent with a lesion at the base of the skull and a MRI of the head with particular attention to the cranio-cervical junction should be performed. Correctable lesions such as tumors (meningiomas, clivus chordomas, metastases), atlantoaxial subluxation, syringobulbia and Chiari malformations should be considered.

❐❐ **What are the manifestations of a spinal epidural abscess?**

Fever, back pain, leukocytosis and an elevated erythrocyte sedimentation rate.

❐❐ **What cosmetic side effects are seen with valproate?**

Excessive weight gain, hair loss and dose-related hand tremor may be seen.

❐❐ **What hypersensitivity reactions are seen with valproate?**

Severe valproate hepatotoxicity and acute hemorrhagic pancreatitis may develop.

❐❐ **Which antipsychotic agents lower seizure threshold?**

Chlorpromazine is one of the worst offenders. Clozapine also carries a high risk of seizures.

❐❐ **What is status epilepticus?**

Status epilepticus is defined as more than 30 minutes of continuous seizure activity or operationally as two or more sequential seizures without recovery of consciousness between seizures.

❐❐ **What is the drug of choice for status epilepticus?**

Benzodiazepines are recommended initially due to their efficacy and rapid onset of action. Lorazepam and diazepam are similar in efficacy, though lorazepam has a longer duration of action.

❐❐ **Permanent brain injury can occur after seizures of what duration?**

Approximately one hour.

❐❐ **What is the most commonly used medication in refractory generalized convulsive status epilepticus?**

Pentobarbital is used when combinations of benzodiazepines, phenytoin, and phenobarbital fail to control status. Pentobarbital is titrated to seizure control or burst-suppression on EEG.

❐❐ A 13-year-old is hit by a car. What is the diagnosis? What cranial nerve deficit in the more distant future might be considered possible?

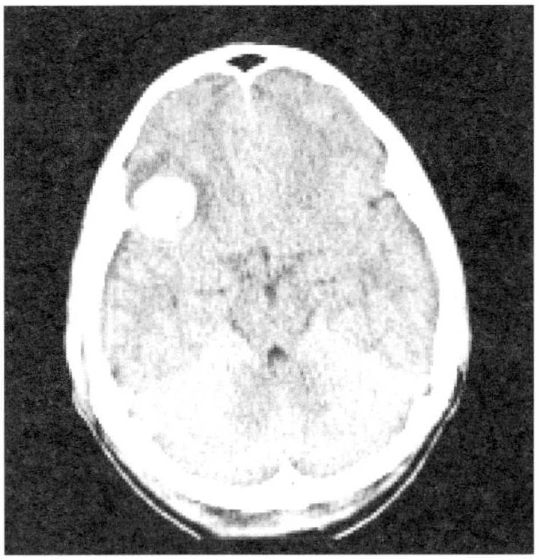

Fig. A

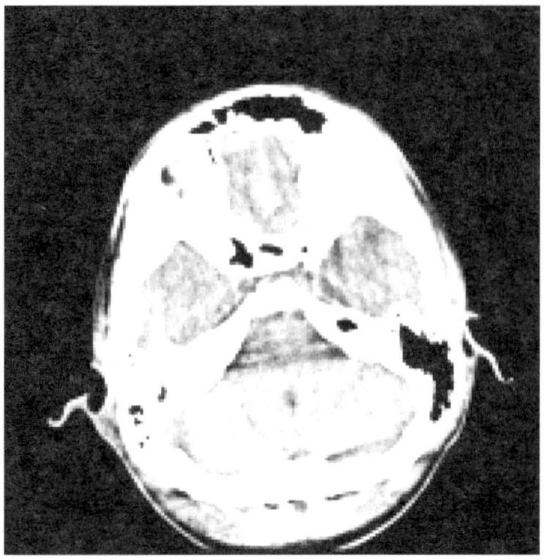

Fig. B

In the right frontal lobe posteriorly a 3 cm acute intracerebral hematoma is identified with mild surrounding edema (Fig. A). Note the blood in the subfrontal region indicating trauma in this location (Fig. B). The cribriform plate has a rough surface and can damage the subfrontal region and particularly the cranial nerve I (olfactory nerve) resulting in decreased smell or anosmia.

❐❐ A 21-year-old fell from a horse. The patient is unconscious and has decerebrate posturing. What is the diagnosis?

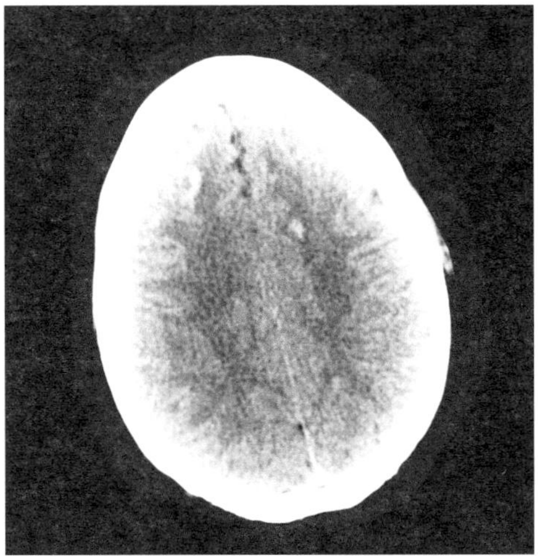

Petechial acute hemorrhages at the gray/white junction in a patient with diffuse axonal injury caused by shearing at the junction of axons and cell bodies from rotational forces.

❒❒ A 66-year-old presents with new onset left ptosis. What is the diagnosis?

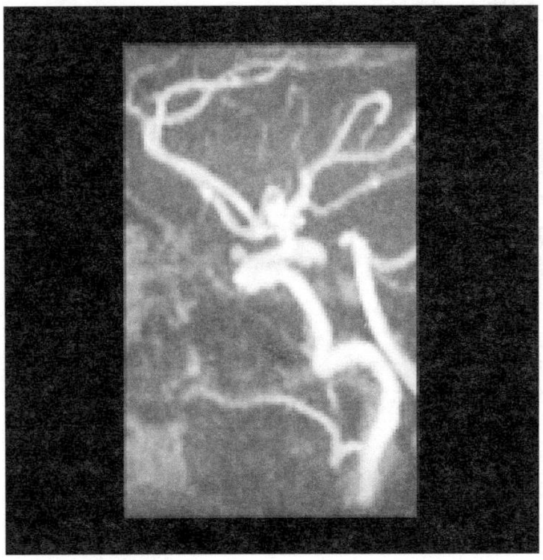

MR angiography demonstrates a large left posterior communicating artery aneurysm. Did you also note the left ophthalmic artery origin aneurysm? Not shown is a right posterior communicating artery aneurysm incidentally noted.

❒❒ A 36-year-old presents with altered mental status and history of a fall with severe headache. What is the diagnosis after viewing only the CT? (Fig. A)

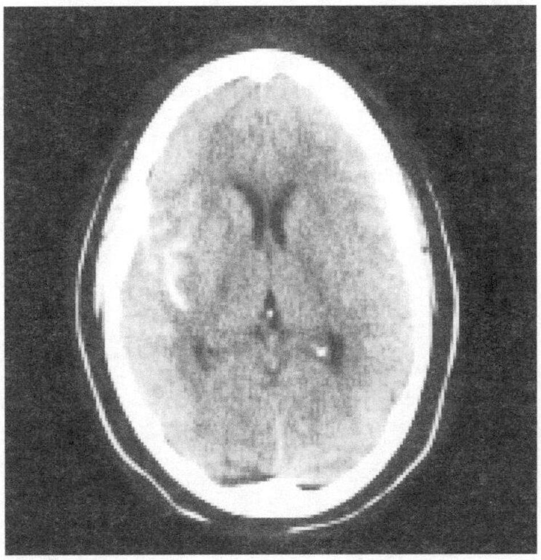

Fig. A

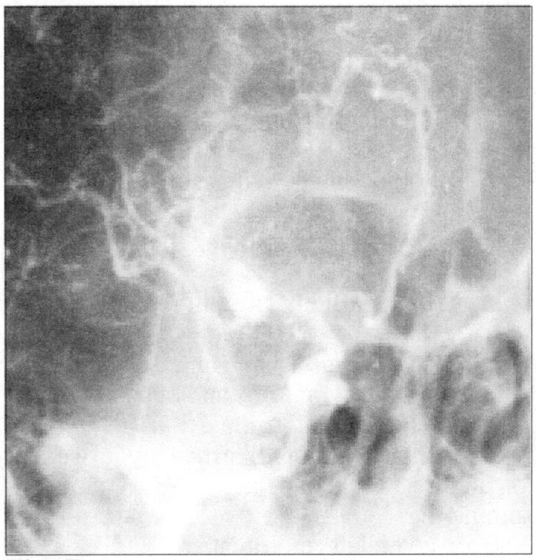

Fig. B

Acute right-sided subarachnoid hemorrhage confined mostly to the sylvian fissure. The differential diagnosis is between trauma and ruptured intracerebral aneurysm. In this patient, a large right middle cerebral artery trifurcation aneurysm is confirmed by contrast angiography. (Fig. B)

TOX PEARLS

"Prepare for the difficult while it is still easy.
Deal with the big while it is still small.
Difficult undertakings have always started with what is easy,
And great undertakings have always started with what is small....
He who takes things too easily will surely encounter much difficultly.
For this reason even the sage regards things as difficult,
And therefore he encounters no difficulty."

Tao-te Ching, 63; Lao Tzu

❑❑ A patient presents in shock, lethargic, bordering on comatose, with vomiting, hematemesis and diarrhea? What could cause this?

Iron, stage III. Check an abdominal x-ray for concretions.

❑❑ What iron level is toxic?

Moderate OD is considered with serum level 350 µg/dl, measured 4 h after ingestion.
Alternatively, try to determine the amount of <u>elemental</u> iron ingested, 20-40 mg elemental iron/kg is toxic.
Treat symptomatic patients without waiting for lab test results.

❑❑ Discuss the 4 stages of iron toxicity.

I (h) .... Abdominal pain, vomiting, diarrhea, possible GI bleeding and 2° lethargy and metabolic acidosis. Due to direct corrosive effect of iron.

II (3-12 h) .... Resolution of GI symptoms, physician falsely reassured.

III (>12 h) .... Iron makes it into cells, blocks oxidative phosphorylation, catalyzes formation of free radicals. Cellular and organ disruption ensue with edema and venous pooling. Hepatic dysfunction, renal and cardiac failure can occur. Stage III occurs earlier in severe poisoning.

IV (days-wk) .. Small bowel and gastric outlet obstruction.

(N.B: Some sources prefer to break this up into 5 stages.)

❑❑ What is the treatment of iron ingestion?

If patient has Ø symptoms for 6 h and is completely normal on exam, go home.
If patient has minimal symptoms and appears fine and has iron level close to maximum normal level (150 µg/dl) measured 4 h after ingestion, go home.
Cathartics for patients without diarrhea (controversial).
Hydration and treat GI hemorrhage.
Deferoxamine if:
- Moderate or severely symptomatic,
- Serum iron level > TIBC,
- Serum iron level > 350 µg/dl.

Deferoxamine is a specific agent for iron and will not chelate other metals.
Give 15 µg/kg/h IV x 8 h for serum iron > 500 µg/dl or 90 mg/kg IM q 8 h for serum iron < 500 µg/dl.

❑❑ What are the symptoms and signs of cyanide overdose?

Dryness and burning in the throat, air hunger, and hyperventilation. If not removed from the toxic environment loss of consciousness, seizures, bradycardia and apnea occur prior to asystole.

❒❒ What is the treatment for cyanide overdose?

Oxygen, CPR prn.
Amyl nitrite perle inhaled.
Sodium nitrite 10 mL of 3% solution in an adult which is 300 mg, or 0.2 - 0.33 mL/kg in a child.
Sodium thiosulfate - give 5 times the volume of sodium nitrite; 12.5 mg in an adult which is 50 mL of a 25% solution or 1.0 - 1.5 mL/kg in a child.

❒❒ Interesting treatment! The mechanism of action of nitrites is not completely clear, though formation of methemoglobin is probably important. Methemoglobin rapidly combines with cyanide to form cyanomethemoglobin. O.K., so now you've stripped the cyanide off it's binding to cytochrome A_3, but how is the cyanomethemoglobin handled?

The intrinsic enzyme rhodanase catalyzes the transport of cyanide from cyanomethemoglobin to sulfur forming thiocyanate. This reaction is limited by sulfur availability. Sodium thiosulfate is given to act as a sulfur donor. Thiocyanate is excreted by the kidney.

❒❒ What order are the kinetics of elimination of ASA overdose?

Zero-order elimination with hepatic enzymatic clearance saturated and renal clearance becoming important.

❒❒ What is the mechanism of ASA leading to respiratory alkalosis?

Direct stimulation of brainstem respiratory centers.
When even greater levels of ASA are present, respiratory depression can occur.

❒❒ By what mechanism does ASA lead to a metabolic acidosis?

ASA uncouples oxidative phosphorylation.
ASA enhances lipolysis leading to ketoacid production.

❒❒ We all remember to think of ASA poisoning when a patient presents with mental status changes associated with respiratory alkalosis and metabolic acidosis. Many of us may recall that salicylate toxicity may be associated with elevated, normal, or decreased glucose levels. By what mechanisms are hyper-glycemia and hypoglycemia caused?

Hyperglycemia is caused by salicylate induced mobilization of glycogen.
Hypoglycemia is caused by salicylate inhibition of gluconeogenesis.

❒❒ Is ARDS more likely to be a complication of acute or chronic ASA poisoning?

Chronic.

❒❒ ARDS is <u>not</u> a common complication of acute ASA OD. However, with acute ingestion, does ARDS occur more often in adults or children?

Adults.

❒❒ What is the "magic number" for the dose of non-enteric coated ASA which must be exceeded to cause toxicity (mg/kg)?

150 mg/kg.

❑❑ **What is the "magic number" for the dose of enteric coated ASA which must be exceeded to require admission for observation and serial salicylate levels?**

150 mg/kg.

❑❑ **Metabolic acidosis favors formation of what form of salicylate, ionized or un-ionized?**

UN-IONIZED.
This is a KEY point because:
a) It is the reason to therapeutically produce an alkaline urine which then makes more of the free salicylate ionized, not reabsorbed by tubules, and excreted.
b) It is the reason for the large changes in amount of free drug able to diffuse into tissue. Small decreases in pH result in decreased protein binding and more salicylate in the un-ionized form able to diffuse into tissue thereby increasing its volume of distribution. [Thus, always treat the patient and not the level - serum levels can decrease as salicylate moves into tissue!!].

❑❑ **Under what circumstances is use of A.D. Done's nomogram O.K.?**

Only when the patient has an acute, single ingestion of non-enteric coated ASA without recent prior use.

❑❑ **Can a patient who is symptomatic with mental status changes from chronic salicylate poisoning have a level in the therapeutic range?**

Yes! Interestingly, patients taking acetazolamide are at particular risk for chronic salicylate poisoning because the carbonic anhydrase inhibitor results in acidified plasma (leading to increased V_d) and more alkalotic CSF, thereby encouraging salicylate concentration in the CNS.

❑❑ **Is hemodialysis used to treat salicylate toxicity?**

Yes, in severe poisoning (coma, ARDS, cardiac toxicity, serum level > 100 mg/dL), and for patients who are unresponsive to maximal therapy.

❑❑ **What is the "magic number" for the minimum ingestion of acetaminophen (N-acetyl-para-aminophenol, APAP) necessary to cause hepatic toxicity in an adult?**

7.5 gm.

❑❑ **In a child?**

140 mg/kg.

❑❑ **Let's review some aspects of hepatic anatomy and metabolism of APAP in the next few questions to help recall particulars of acetaminophen's toxicity.**

O.K.

❑❑ **What region of liver lobules contains the greatest amount of P_{450} related mixed-function oxidases (P_{450}MFO)?**

The centrilobular regions, accounting for primarily centrilobular necrosis.

❑❑ **How is APAP usually metabolized under non-overdose conditions?**

Most APAP metabolism is by glucuronidation.
Some APAP metabolism is by conjugation with sulfate. This percentage increases with decreasing age.
4% or less is transformed into an extremely toxic intermediary compound by P_{450}MFO's. This toxic metabolite is likely immediately conjugated with glutathione and harmlessly excreted in the urine.

❑❑ How does N-acetylcysteine (NAC, Mucomyst) work?

Precise mechanism is still unknown. We know that NAC enters cells and is metabolized to cysteine which serves as a glutathione precursor.

❑❑ Summarize, in the simplest possible outline, the 4 stages of APAP toxicity.

I - Primarily N, V; first d.
II- N, V decrease, abdominal pain begins, LFT's increase; 1-2 d.
III- N, V recur, LFT's peak; 3-4 d.
IV- get better or die; 4 d - 2 wk.

❑❑ Which measures of hepatic function are better indicators of prognosis, liver enzyme levels or bilirubin level and prothrombin time?

Bilirubin level and prothrombin time.

❑❑ Clonidine is a centrally acting presynaptic a_2-adrenergic agonist that results in decreased central sympathetic outflow. While its primary use is to treat hypertension, it has additional emergency utility in blunting withdrawal symptoms from opiates and EtOH. Clonidine overdose closely resembles OD with what other class of drugs?

Opiates.

❑❑ Can clonidine ever cause hypertension?

Yes; high serum levels can result in direct peripheral α–adrenergic stimulation. Such hypertension usually yields to ensuing hypotension.

❑❑ Toxicity from clonidine (Catapres) usually occurs within what time period?

4 hours.

❑❑ What agent may be useful as an "antidote" for clonidine OD.

Naloxone.

❑❑ Name a few substances that have anticholinergic properties.

Antihistamines, cyclic antidepressants, phenothiazines, atropine, amanita sp., Jimson weed.

❑❑ Sure, patients who suffer anticholinergic toxicity have mental status changes, mydriasis, urinary retention, cardiogenic pulmonary edema, dry skin, tachycardia and decreased salivation, but what is the <u>most common</u> ECG abnormality?

Sinus tachycardia. Other, dangerous, arrhythmias include conduction problems and V-Tach.

❑❑ What is "cornpicker's pupil?"

Mydriasis from contact of Jimson weed with the eye. Jimson weed contains atropine, scopolamine and hyoscyamine. It is a common plant and is available through health food stores.

❑❑ Intermediate-chain aliphatic hydrocarbons are responsible for most of the exposures to hydrocarbons. What is the <u>most common</u> complication from these liquids?

Chemical pneumonitis caused by direct injury to pulmonary parenchyma after aspiration.

❑❑ Which hydrocarbons carry the greatest risk of aspiration?

Those with low viscosity, less than 60 SSU.
(We'll return to the SSU in the random question section.)

❑❑ **Aromatic hydrocarbons, such as toluene present in glue, may be sniffed. Resulting effects most closely resemble those of what other class of compounds?**

Effects are similar to those of inhalational anesthetic agents: initial excitatory response gives way to CNS depression.

❑❑ **Can solvent abusers be scared to death?**

Yes. Halogenated hydrocarbons can "sensitize" myocardium to catecholamines, thus exertion or fright can lead to fatal arrhythmias.

❑❑ **What is the relationship between toluene and A MUDPILE CAT?**

Toluene is the "T"!

❑❑ **Is charcoal useful in hydrocarbon ingestions?**

No.

❑❑ **Is gastric emptying useful in hydrocarbon ingestions?**

Yes and no.
Yes for the following:

- Halogenated hydrocarbons - Carbon tetrachloride, other solvents and dry-cleaning agents.
- Aromatic hydrocarbons - Toluene, benzene, xylene.

❑❑ **For what period of time should an asymptomatic patient with hydrocarbon ingestion be observed prior to discharge?**

6 hours.

❑❑ **Sure, digitalis increases myocardial inotropy by inhibiting Na^+-K^+-ATPase, thereby allowing intracellular Na^+ to increase providing more substrate for the Na^+-Ca^{2+} membrane exchange that leads to increased intracellular (sarcoplasmic) Ca^{2+} concentration, but does it also increase vagal tone and slow conduction through the AV node?**

Yes.

❑❑ **Serum potassium can soar to very high levels with acute digitalis toxicity; is this also true for chronic digitalis poisoning?**

No, not really.

❑❑ **T/F- A patient with acute digitalis OD presents with frequent multifocal PVC's, peaked T-waves and a K^+ of 6.2 mEq/l; correct treatment is to first administer $CaCl_2$ as this is the fastest acting agent for reducing hyperkalemia.**

No, no, this is a trick question! Yes, $CaCl_2$ is the fastest acting agent for decreasing hyperkalemia, but you don't want to give any more Ca^+ to a patient with digitalis-induced cardiac toxicity. Digitalis toxicity promotes increases in intracellular Ca^+ concentration.

❑❑ **Phenytoin has an appropriate role in the treatment of digitalis-induced arrhythmias. For which arrhythmias is consideration of use of phenytoin appropriate?**

Digitalis-induced ventricular arrhythmias.

❑❑ Signs and symptoms of phenytoin toxicity?

Seizure, heart blocks, bradyarrhythmias, hypotension, coma. All dangerous cardiovascular complications of phenytoin OD result from parenteral administration; high levels after PO doses do not cause such signs in a stable patient.

❑❑ Treatment of phenytoin overdose?

Systemic support, charcoal, atropine for bradyarrhythmias, and phenobarbital 20 mg/kg IV for seizures.

❑❑ At what serum level of phenytoin do nystagmus, ataxia, and lethargy generally occur?

Nystagmus -	20 µg/mL.
Ataxia -	30 µg/mL.
Lethargy -	40 µg/mL.

❑❑ What rhythm and ECG findings are expected with phenytoin toxicity?

Bradycardia, AV block, ventricular tachycardia, VF, and asystole. ECG findings might include increased PR interval and a wide QRS.

❑❑ What is the treatment of phenytoin toxicity?

Charcoal. Seizures are treated with benzodiazepine or phenobarbital. Extravasation may be limb threatening, consult an orthopedic or plastic surgeon. Hemodialysis and hemoperfusion are not helpful.

❑❑ How many vials of digoxin-specific Fab should be administered to a patient in critical condition from digitalis toxicity in whom neither the ingested dose nor the serum level is known?

10 vials = 400 mg Fab.

❑❑ Is orally administered activated charcoal useful in treating digitalis toxicity?

Right again.

❑❑ ß-adrenergic antagonists have 3 main effects on the heart - name them.

Negative chronotropy.
Negative inotropy.
Decrease AV nodal conduction velocity.

❑❑ T/F: ß-adrenergic antagonists can cause mental status changes and seizures.

True.

❑❑ What is the agent of choice to counteract the effects of ß-adrenergic antagonists, and how does it work?

Glucagon should be given in boluses of 3 - 5 mg q 5 min until response is obtained or 10 -15 mg has been administered. It has rapid onset and a short-lived effect (≈ 15 min); therefore, administer a continuous infusion at the same number of mg/hr as the number of mg initially provided in boluses to obtain a response. The initial dose is 50 - 150 µg/kg in children. Glucagon works by increasing intracellular cAMP by direct glucagon (non-adrenergic) receptors, bypassing ß-adrenergic receptors.

❑❑ Activated charcoal for ß-adrenergic antagonist toxicity?

Sure.

❑❑ Calcium channel blocking agents (CCB's) come in several flavors and all have the potential to be lethal. Which CCB has the most depressing effect on sinus nodal activity and AV nodal conduction?

Verapamil.

❑❑ Which CCB causes the greatest degree of systemic vasodilation?

Nifedipine.

❑❑ Describe the dosing of calcium for CCB OD.

$CaCl_2$ 10 - 20 mL of 10% solution.
$CaCl_2$ 10 - 30 mg/kg for children.
Calcium gluconate 0.2-0.5 mL/kg/dose up to 10 mL/dose.

❑❑ What is the <u>most common</u> cause of acute heavy metal poisoning?

a) Twisted Sister
b) Metallica
c) Arsenic

❑❑ Arsenic is initially housed in RBC's, WBC's and bound to serum proteins. From there it is distributed to major organs, bone, hair and nails. What is the primary mechanism of toxicity of arsenic?

It blocks the conversion of a cofactor necessary for oxidative phosphorylation (Krebs cycle).
Arsenic also substitutes for phosphate, disrupting high-energy phosphates.

❑❑ What is the resultant pathology of arsenic intoxication?

N, V, D, cerebral edema, cerebral hemorrhage, arrhythmias, encephalopathy associated with mental status changes, and seizures, pulmonary edema, ARF, rhabdomyolysis.

❑❑ T/F- Chronic arsenic poisoning tends to present less dramatically with constitutional symptoms and peripheral neuropathy.

True.

❑❑ Charcoal probably doesn't absorb arsenic much. What chelating agents are appropriate?

Play BAL with a DMSAl named MAG!

This means that Mercury, Arsenic and Gold (MAG) can be chelated with BAL and with DMSA. D-Penicillamine can also be used.

❑❑ Arsine is a gaseous form of arsenic; is chelation also used to treat arsine?

No.

❑❑ What are the effects of arsine poisoning?

Binds to hemoglobin; causes anemia with jaundice, ARF. Manage with transfusions and dialysis for ARF.

❑❑ Which two antidepressants tend to cause less problems when taken in large quantities?

Trazodone (Desyrel) and fluoxetine (Prozac).

❒❒ Describe the signs and symptoms of cyclic overdose.

Anticholinergic toxicity. CNS depression. Cardiac depression of contractility and conduction. The earliest signs of toxicity tend to be lethargy, slurred speech, and tachycardia. Other signs include myoclonic jerks, seizures, and coma.

❒❒ A patient with a history of CA overdose is found by paramedics awake and alert. Prognosis?

25% of patients who die from cyclic overdose are awake and alert at the scene. Treat with O_2, IV, monitor, multiple doses of 50 to 100 grams of activated charcoal q 2 h and alkaline diuresis. The drug has a high tissue binding, thus once absorbed, it is poorly removed.

❒❒ Is degree of toxicity in CA overdose closely related to QRS duration?

NO! QRS > 100 ms has a specificity of 75 percent and a sensitivity of 60% for serious complications. A normal ECG will not rule out serious overdose!

❒❒ What electrolytes should be followed closely in a CA overdose?

Potassium increases toxic effects. Sodium antagonizes CAs.

❒❒ How should seizures be treated in a patient with cyclic overdose?

Most patients do not need treatment as seizures tend to be brief. Diazepam, 5-10 mg IV has been used but its efficacy is questionable. Phenytoin is used to treat conduction defects and seizures, it will not treat myoclonic jerks. Alkalinize with IV sodium bicarbonate 1-5 mEq/kg.

❒❒ What agent should be used as part of the intubation protocol in a cyclic overdose patient.

A nondepolarizing agent, such as vecuronium. Succinylcholine (the depolarizing agent) has potent vagal effects and should be avoided.

❒❒ How should cardiac complications of cyclic overdose be treated?

Alkalinize the blood to a pH of 7.5. Either hyperventilate the patient or administer sodium bicarb IV 1-5 mEq/kg over several minutes. For hypotension, epinephrine, norepinephrine, and phenylephrine may be tried. Dobutamine is contraindicated. Any drug that prolongs the QRS or QT interval is also contraindicated.

❒❒ Which IV fluid should be used in a patient with cyclic overdose?

Isotonic saline (0.9% NS).

❒❒ For how long should an asymptomatic CA overdose patient be monitored?

6 hours.

❒❒ A schizophrenic patient presents to the ED with muscular rigidity, confusion, and a high temperature. Diagnosis and treatment?

Neuroleptic malignant syndrome. Treat with supportive care, IV diazepam for skeletal muscle relaxation, and cooling measures. Dantrolene and bromocriptine are also effective. Consider paralysis with a non-depolarizing agent.

❒❒ What lithium level is considered toxic?

2.0 mEq/l.

❒❒ **Signs and symptoms of lithium toxicity?**

Confusion, lethargy, tremor, and muscle jerking are early signs. GI symptoms are frequent. Stupor, seizures, and coma occur in severe toxicity. Bradycardia, conduction defects, and ST-T wave changes may occur. Hypotension secondary to volume depletion may also occur.

❒❒ **Treatment of lithium toxicity?**

Gastric lavage, IV NS, alkalinize the urine, and supportive care. **Charcoal does not bind lithium**. Hemodialysis is effective and should be used if urine output decreases or renal failure is present, severe, signs of severe poisoning develop, or for deteriorating clinical condition.

❒❒ **Clinical signs and symptoms of barbiturate overdose?**

Emotional lability, lethargy, impaired thinking, slurred speech, decreased coordination, and nystagmus. Hypotension, hypothermia, vasodilation, shock, and skin bullae may also occur.

❒❒ **Treatment of barbiturate overdose?**

Systemic support, gastric lavage, charcoal q 6 h, and diuresis. Alkalinization of the urine for long-acting barbiturates.

❒❒ **A narcotic addict presents to the ED with bone and joint pain. Two causes that should be considered are __________ and __________.**

Osteomyelitis and septic arthritis. *Pseudomonas aeruginosa* and *Serratia marcescens*. In a patient with back pain, think of osteomyelitis.

❒❒ **What is the most frequent neurologic complication of narcotic abuse?**

Non-traumatic mononeuropathy (painless weakness occurring 2 to 3 h post injection). Other CNS complications include traumatic mononeuritis, seizures, subarachnoid hemorrhage, and spinal epidural abscess (Staphylococcus aureus is the most common).

❒❒ **What are the common causes of bacterial pneumonia in narcotic addicts?**

Streptococcus pneumoniae, Haemophilus, Staphylococcus aureus, and *Klebsiella.*

❒❒ **How is pulmonary edema associated with heroin use treated?**

Naloxone and ventilatory support. Diuretics, digitalis, and rotating tourniquets are not effective.

❒❒ **What valve is most commonly infected in narcotic IV drug abusers?**

Tricuspid valve, usually with *Staphylococcus aureus*.

❒❒ **What is the treatment of narcotic overdose?**

Naloxone, 0.4 to 2.0 mg in an adult, and 0.01 mg/kg in a child. Naloxone's duration of action is about 1 h.

❒❒ **What signs and symptoms are expected with cocaine overdose?**

Tachycardia, hyperthermia, hypertension, seizures, and agitation may occur. Extremely high doses cause depressant effects, bradycardia, hypotension, and coma.

❒❒ **A cocaine addict presents with chest pain. The ECG is normal. What are the odds they will have abnormal CPK and CPK-MB isoenzymes?**

19%.

❒❒ Treatment of cocaine overdose?

Sedation with benzodiazepine to control hypertension and tachycardia; nitroprusside to treat resistant hypertension. Phentolamine (a peripheral alpha blocker) may also be used to control hypertension. Most physicians do not have clinical experience using this agent. Fortunately, most patients respond to initial Tx with adequate doses of benzodiazepine. The only indication for use of a beta blocker (labetalol) in cocaine poisoning is the setting of serious resistant tachyarrhythmias that don't respond to sedation.

❒❒ What is the treatment of amphetamine overdose?

Gastric lavage, charcoal, diazepam for seizures, haloperidol for hyperactivity, and nitroprusside for hypertension.

❒❒ What type of nystagmus is expected with PCP overdose?

Vertical, horizontal, and rotary. Vertical nystagmus is not common with other conditions/ingestions. The most common findings of PCP overdose are hypertension, tachycardia, and nystagmus.

❒❒ What are the two most common complications of PCP intoxication?

Hyperpyrexia and rhabdomyolysis with myoglobinuria. Urine acidification as a treatment to promote renal excretion was abandoned more than a decade ago. It can increase complications related to myoglobinuria..

❒❒ What type of necrosis does lye produce?

Base ⇒ Liquefaction necrosis. Lye is the most common cause of severe caustic injuries. Esophageal stricture is a complication of lye ingestion.
Acids ⇒ Coagulation necrosis. Pyloric stricture is a complication of acid ingestion.

❒❒ Principle signs and symptoms of NSAID toxicity?

Nephrotoxicity, tinnitus, headache, GI intolerance, platelet dysfunction, and peripheral edema. Toxic ingestions most commonly cause drowsiness and GI upset. Seizures can occur.

❒❒ What respiratory complication can occur in children who ingest NSAIDS?

Apnea. NSAIDs can cause toxic respiratory symptoms ranging from rhinitis to bronchospasm.

❒❒ What effect do NSAIDs have on lithium?

They can increase the serum lithium concentration.

❒❒ Should charcoal be given for an NSAID overdose?

Yes.

❒❒ For how long should an asymptomatic patient with NSAID overdose be observed in the ED?

4 to 6 hours.

❒❒ Treatment for benzodiazepine overdose?

First, protect the airway and provide assisted ventilation (endotracheal intubation) as needed. Next, gastric lavage and charcoal. Hemodialysis, hemoperfusion, and forced diuresis have not been found to be effective. The use of flumazenil for benzodiazepine overdose is very risky. Patients with chronic benzodiazepine use or concomitant cyclic antidepressant use may develop intractable seizures after single dose of flumazenil.

❐❐ Treatment of mercury salt ingestion?

Egg whites or milk to bind the mercury, lavage, and charcoal. BAL and D-penicillamine for chelation therapy. DMSA can be used for mercury.
PLAY BAL!

❐❐ What is the most common cause of chronic heavy metal poisoning?

Lead.

❐❐ A patient presents with neurologic dysfunction and abdominal complaints. Lab studies reveal a hemolytic anemia. Diagnosis?

Lead toxicity. Diagnosis is confirmed by finding an elevated PbB level. If indication of PB are found on abdominal x-ray, initiate whole-bowel irrigation with Golytely. Chelate with BAL followed by EDTA. Oral chelating agents , D-penicillamine and DMSA, may also be considered.

❐❐ What is the serotonin syndrome like?

Agitation, anxiety, restlessness, tachycardia, hypertension, diaphoresis, shivering, tremor, diarrhea, myoclonus (especially of the lower extremities).

❐❐ How is serotonin syndrome treated?

Of course, stop the serotonin agonists, and otherwise treat the patient supportively. Admit patients with symptoms for more than 6 hours. A detailed medication history is imperative, many drugs in combination can induce serotonin syndrome.

❐❐ What is the difference between carbamates and organophosphates?

Carbamates produce similar symptoms as organophosphates. The bonds in carbamate toxicity are reversible. Organophosphates cross the blood brain barrier; carbamates don't.

❐❐ A patient presents with miotic pupils, muscle fasciculations, diaphoresis and diffuse oral and bronchial secretions. The patient has an odor of garlic on his breath. What is the most likely diagnosis?

Organophosphate poisoning.

❐❐ What ECG changes may be associated with organophosphate poisoning?

Prolongation of the QT interval and ST and T wave abnormalities.

❐❐ What is the key laboratory finding in the diagnosis of organophosphate poisoning?

Decreased red blood cell (true) cholinesterase activity. The serum cholinesterase level (pseudocholinesterase) is more sensitive but less specific. RBC cholinesterase is regenerated slowly and can take months to approach normal levels.

❐❐ Treatment of organophosphate poisoning?

First and foremost, support airway and breathing with endotracheal intubation using a high FiO_2. Next, decontamination, charcoal, atropine and pralidoxime. Atropine should be administered in a large enough doses to produce multiple clinical signs of atropinization and not just mydriasis.

❐❐ What is the toxic metabolic end product in methanol poisoning?

Formic acid.

❐❐ What methanol level mandates dialysis?

25 mg/dL.

❐❐ What cofactors should be administered to a patient with ethylene glycol poisoning?

Thiamine and pyridoxine. These cofactors will aid in transforming glyoxylic acid to nontoxic metabolites.

❐❐ What are the three clinical phases of ethylene glycol poisoning?

Stage I:	Neurological symptomatology (inebriation)
Stage II:	Metabolic acidosis and cardiovascular instability
Stage III:	Renal failure

❐❐ When should dialysis be initiated for ethylene glycol poisoning?

For a serum level > 25 mg/dL, renal insufficiency or severe metabolic acidosis. Don't forget that fomepizole (Antizol) has been shown to be highly antidotal Tx for the treatment of EG poisoning.

❐❐ What may occur with too large a dose of naloxone in a chronic heroin user?

It may precipitate acute withdrawal.

❐❐ A patient is administered a topical Cetacaine spray prior to endoscopy. The patient then complains of dyspnea and is noted to be cyanotic. What is the antidote?

Methylene blue. Methemoglobinemia developed secondary to the local anesthetic.

❐❐ A 32 year-old female complains of vomiting and diarrhea which developed eight hours after ingesting an unknown type of mushroom. Is the mushroom potentially a hepatotoxin?

Yes. Hepatotoxic cyclopeptide containing mushrooms induce a delayed onset of gastrointestinal symptomatology, generally occurring 6 hours after ingestion.

❐❐ Can solvent abusers be "scared to death"?

Yes. Halogenated hydrocarbons can "sensitize" myocardium to catecholamines. Exertion or fright can lead to fatal arrhythmias. Epinephrine is contraindicated.

❐❐ Is charcoal useful for hydrocarbon ingestion?

No.

❐❐ T/F: Serum potassium tends to increase with digitalis intoxication.

True.

❐❐ What are the signs and symptoms of phenytoin toxicity?

Seizure, heart blocks, bradyarrhythmias, hypotension and coma.

❐❐ In life threatening theophylline overdose, what is definitive management?

Charcoal hemoperfusion.

❑❑ What are the typical CNS findings in mild lithium toxicity?

Rigidity, tremor and hyperreflexia.

❑❑ What are the typical CNS findings in severe lithium toxicity?

Seizures, coma and myoclonic jerking.

❑❑ What is the primary system affected by lithium toxicity?

Central nervous system.

❑❑ T/F: Hydration status has little effect on lithium toxicity.

False. Patients with lithium toxicity and dehydration require aggressive rehydration to establish euvolemia and normal urine output, while avoiding fluid overload. In addition, any drug or circumstance that promotes sodium loss can augment the toxic effects of lithium.

❑❑ What constitutes definitive therapy for moderate to severe lithium toxicity?

Hemodialysis.

❑❑ What are the indications for hemodialysis in lithium toxicity?

Serum lithium level above 4.0 mEq/l, renal failure and severe clinical symptoms.

❑❑ You are treating a 25 year-old South American man who was resuscitated in an international airport terminal. His initial rhythm was ventricular fibrillation. Presently he is tachycardic and hypotensive. What drug toxicity and specific treatment modality should be strongly considered?

Cocaine smugglers may swallow packets of cocaine ("body packers") and develop significant toxicity if only one packet rupture, including arrhythmias, hyperthermia and intractable seizures. In fact, rupture of only one packet is very likely to be lethal. Whole bowel irrigation can be employed to eliminate drug packets from the GI tract.

❑❑ What major pathophysiologic mechanisms underlie cocaine's toxic effects on the cardiovascular system?

1) Potentiates the actions of the sympathetic nervous system by blocking presynaptic reuptake of dopamine and norepinephrine. This results in increased inotropy, tachycardia and hypertension.
2) Induces coronary artery spasm, with possible increased focal effects in atherosclerotic areas.
3) Induces platelet activation and aggregation, which may help to induce thrombus formation.

❑❑ What arrhythmia is pathognomonic for digoxin toxicity?

Bidirectional ventricular tachycardia. It is characterized by a regular (beat-to-beat) alteration of two QRS complexes. The site of origin may be junctional or ventricular.

❑❑ What happens to the digoxin level immediately after the administration of digoxin Fab fragments?

Total serum digoxin levels rise, sometimes more than tenfold, secondary to displacement of drug from tissue and extracellular compartments into plasma where it binds to the Fab fragments. When there is concern of a possible rebound phenomenon (Fab-digoxin complex dissociation in patients with renal failure and delayed drug excretion), free plasma levels should be measured.

❐❐ A 13 year-old boy is brought into the emergency department with what you believe to be a cholinesterase inhibitor poisoning. After initial stabilization what study can you obtain to definitively establish the diagnosis?

Plasma and red blood cell cholinesterase levels.

❐❐ What drugs should be avoided in G-6-PD deficiency?

ASA, phenacetin, primaquine, quinine, quinacrine, nitrofurantoin, sulfamethoxazole, sulfacetamide and methylene blue. These are all oxidants which may cause an hemolytic reaction in a patient with G-6-PD deficiency.

ID PEARLS

"Nobody will fly for a thousand years!"
Wilbur Wright, 1901, in a fit of despair.

❒❒ **Describe the pathophysiologic features of HIV:**

HIV attacks the T4 helper cells. HIV genetic material consists of single-stranded RNA. HIV has been found in saliva, urine, cerebrospinal fluid, tears, alveolar fluid, synovial fluid, breast milk, and amniotic fluid.

❒❒ **How quickly do patients infected with HIV become symptomatic?**

5-10% develop symptoms within three years of seroconversion. Predictive characteristics include low T4 count, and hematocrit less than 40. Mean incubation time is about 8 years for adults and 2 years for children less than 5.

❒❒ **Name the most common causes of fever in HIV infected patients:**

HIV-related fever, Mycobacterium avium-intracellular, CMV, non-Hodgkin's and Hodgkin's lymphoma. Common cause of fever (e.g., those which produce fever in otherwise healthy patients) should not be ignored.

❒❒ **An HIV positive patient presents with a history of weight loss, diarrhea, fever, anorexia, and malaise. They are also dyspneic. Lab studies reveal abnormal LFTs and anemia. Diagnosis?**

Mycobacterium avium-intracellular. Lab confirmation is made by acid-fast stain of body fluids or by blood culture.

❒❒ **What is the second most common complication (presentation) of AIDS?**

Kaposi's sarcoma. PCP is the most common.

❒❒ **What is the most common cause of focal encephalitis in AIDS patients?**

Toxoplasmosis. Symptoms include focal neurologic deficits, headache, fever, altered mental status, and seizures. Ring enhancing-lesions are seen on CT. The initial scan is often negative; delayed CT or MRI may be necessary.

❒❒ **The differential diagnosis of ring-enhancing lesions in AIDS patients is:**

Lymphoma, cerebral tuberculosis, fungal infection, CMV, Kaposi's sarcoma, toxoplasmosis, and hemorrhage.

❒❒ **What are the signs and symptoms of CNS cryptococcal infection in an AIDS patient?**

Headache, depression, lightheadedness, seizures, and cranial nerve palsies. Diagnosis is made by India ink prep, fungal culture, or by cryptococcal antigen in the CSF.

❒❒ **Presentation of an AIDS patient with tuberculous meningitis:**

Fever, meningismus, headache, seizures, focal neurologic deficits, and altered mental status.

❑❑ On physical exam, what is the most common eye finding in AIDS patients?

Cotton-wool spots thought to be associated with PCP. These may be hard to differentiate from fluffy-white, often perivascular retinal lesions that are associated with CMV.

❑❑ An AIDS patient presents with complaints of decreased visual acuity, photophobia, redness, and eye pain. Diagnosis?

Retinitis or malignant invasion of the periorbital tissue or eye.

❑❑ What is the most common cause of retinitis in AIDS patients?

Cytomegalovirus.
Findings include photophobia, redness, scotoma, pain, or change in visual acuity. On exam, findings include fluffy white retinal lesions.

❑❑ Most common opportunistic infection (presentation) in AIDS patients?

PCP. Symptoms may include non-productive cough and dyspnea. Chest x-ray may show diffuse interstitial infiltrates or uncommonly, it may be negative. Gallium scanning is more sensitive but results in false positives. Initial treatment includes TMP-SMX. Pentamidine is an alternative.

❑❑ How is Candida of the esophagus diagnosed in the ED?

Air-contrast barium swallow will show ulcerations with plaques. In contrast, herpes esophagitis will produce punched-out ulcerations with no plaques.

❑❑ What is the most common gastrointestinal complaint in AIDS patients?

Diarrhea. Hepatomegaly and hepatitis are also common. Jaundice is an uncommon finding.

❑❑ A patient is infected with Treponema pallidum, what is the treatment?

Syphilis is treated with benzathine penicillin G, 2.4 million units IM or tetracycline 500 mg qid po for 15 d or erythromycin 500 mg qid po for 15 d.

❑❑ Describe lesions associated with lymphogranuloma venereum:

LV caused by Chlamydia presents as painless skin lesions with lymphadenopathy. Lesions may be papular, nodular or herpetiform vesicles. Sinus formation involving the vagina and rectum are common in women with chronic untreated disease.

❑❑ What is the cause of chancroid? Describe the lesions?

Haemophilus ducreyi. Presents with one or more painful necrotic lesions. Suppurating inguinal lymphadenopathy may also be present.

❑❑ What is the cause of granuloma inguinale; describe the lesions?

Calymmatobacterium granulomatis. Typically begins with small papular, nodular, or vesicular lesions that develop slowly into ulcerative or granulomatous lesions. Lesions are PAINLESS and are located on mucous membranes of the genital, inguinal, and anal areas.

❑❑ What are the two major types of tetanus infection?

1). Localized wherein the toxin is not absorbed but does act locally to cause muscle spasm.
2). Generalized, the more common presentation, wherein the toxin is absorbed and the patient presents with the classic symptoms.

❑❑ What is the incubation period in tetanus?

Hours to over one month. The shorter the incubation the more severe the disease. Most patients in the U.S. who get the disease are over 50.

❑❑ What is the most common presentation of tetanus?

"Generalized tetanus" with pain and stiffness in the trunk and jaw muscles. Trismus develops and results in risus sardonicus (sardonic smile). The three other presentations include cephalic tetanus, localized tetanus, and neonatal tetanus.

❑❑ What cranial nerve is most commonly involved in cephalic tetanus?

Cephalic tetanus usually occurs after injuries to the head and typically involves the 7th cranial nerve.

❑❑ Outline tetanus treatment.

1. Respiratory -	Succinylcholine for immediate intubation if required.
2. Immunotherapy -	Human tetanus immune globulin will neutralize circulating tetanospasmin and toxin in the wound (it will not neutralize toxin fixed in the nervous system). Dose TIG 500 units. Tetanus toxoid, 0.5 mL IM at 1 and 6 wk and 6 mo.
3. Antibiotics -	*Clostridium tetani* is sensitive to metronidazole, cephalosporins, erythromycin, and penicillin. Metronidazole is the drug of choice.
4. Muscle Relaxants -	Diazepam or dantrolene.
5. Neuromuscular blockade -	Pancuronium bromide, 2 mg plus sedation.
6. Autonomic dysfunction -	Labetalol 0.25-1.0 mg/min IV or magnesium sulfate 70 mg/kg IV load then 1-4 g/h continuous infusion is used to treat autonomic dysfunction. MS, 5-30 mg IV infusion q 2-8 h. Clonidine, 300 µg q 8 h per NG.

NOTE: FATAL CARDIOVASCULAR COMPLICATIONS HAVE OCCURRED IN PATIENTS TREATED WITH ß-ADRENERGIC BLOCKING AGENTS ALONE. ADRENERGIC BLOCKING AGENTS USED TO TREAT AUTONOMIC DYSFUNCTION MAY PRECIPITATE MYOCARDIAL DEPRESSION.

❑❑ What is the most common tapeworm in the U.S.?

Hymenolepis nana.

❑❑ A patient presents with fever, dyspnea, cough, hemoptysis and eosinophilia. Diagnosis?

Ascaris lumbricoides. This helminth is a roundworm. Serologic tests: ELISA, bentonite flocculation, and indirect hemagglutination. Treat with pyrantel pamoate (pyrimidine pamoate) or mebendazole. Obstruction of the intestine may require surgery.

❑❑ How is hookworm infection acquired?

In areas where "human fertilizer" is used and people don't wear shoes.
Patients present with chronic anemia, cough, low-grade fever, diarrhea, abdominal pain, weakness, weight loss, eosinophilia and guaiac positive stools. Diagnosis is made by finding ova in the stool. Treatment is mebendazole or pyrantel pamoate [This is not a zebra - SHP].

❑❑ What are the signs and symptoms of Trichuris trichiura?

This hookworm lives in the cecum. Complaints include anorexia, abdominal pain especially RUQ, insomnia, fever, diarrhea, flatulence, weight loss, pruritus, eosinophilia, and microcytic hypochromic anemia.
Diagnosis is made by ova in the stool. Mebendazole is the treatment.

❑❑ A patient presents with a history of attending a walrus, bear, and pork roast. He now has N/V/D/F, urticaria, myalgia, splinter hemorrhages, muscle spasm, headache, and a stiff neck. What physical finding will clinch the diagnosis?

Periorbital edema is pathognomonic of infection with *Trichinella spiralis*.
Patients may have acute myocarditis, nonsuppurative meningitis, catarrhal enteritis, or bronchopneumonia.
Lab studies may reveal leukocytosis, eosinophilia, ECG changes, and elevated CPK.
Diagnosis is confirmed with latex agglutination, skin test, or complement fixation or bentonite flocculation test.
Stool exam is not helpful after the initial GI phase in confirming the diagnosis.

❑❑ Explain the pathophysiology of rabies:

Infection occurs within the myocytes for the first 48 to 96 h. It then spreads across the motor endplate, ascends and replicates along peripheral nervous axoplasm into the dorsal root ganglia, the spinal cord, and CNS. From the gray matter, the virus spreads by peripheral nerves to tissues and organ systems.

❑❑ What is the characteristic histologic finding in rabies?

Eosinophilic intracellular lesions found within cerebral neurons called **Negri** bodies are the site of CNS viral replication. They are found in 75% of rabies cases; although pathognomonic for rabies, their absence does not rule out rabies.

❑❑ What are the signs and symptoms of rabies?

Initial - fever, headache, malaise, anorexia, sore throat, nausea, cough, and pain or paresthesias at the bite site.

CNS stage - agitation, restlessness, altered mental status, painful bulbar and peripheral muscular spasms, bulbar or focal motor paresis, and opisthotonos. Similar to Landry-Guillain-Barré syndrome, 20% develop ascending, symmetric flaccid and areflexic paralysis. Hypersensitivity to water (even sayings, "water") and sensory stimuli (light, touch, and noise) may occur.

Progressive stage - lucid and confused intervals with hyperpyrexia, lacrimation, salivation, and mydriasis may occur along with brainstem dysfunction, hyperreflexia and extensor plantar response.

Final stage - coma, convulsions, and apnea, followed by death at days 4 to 7 in the untreated patient.

❑❑ What is the diagnostic procedure of choice in rabies?

Fluorescent antibody testing (FAT).

❑❑ How is rabies treated?

RIG 20 IU/kg, half at wound site and half in the DELTOID muscle. HDCV 1-mL doses IM on days 0,3,7,14, and 28 also in the opposite DELTOID muscle.

❑❑ What is the <u>second</u> <u>most</u> <u>common</u> tick borne disease?

Rocky Mountain spotted fever.
Causative agent - *Rickettsia rickettsii.*
Vector - Female Ixodid ticks, *Dermacentor andersonii* (wood tick) and *D. variabilis* (American dog tick).

❑❑ A patient presents with fever up to 40° C followed by a rash which is erythematous, macular, and blanching. The rash progresses to deep red, dusky, papular and becomes petechial. The patient also complains of a headache, vomiting, myalgias, and cough. Where did the rash begin?

RMSF rash typically begins on the flexor surfaces of the ankles and wrists and spread centripetally and centrifugally.

❑❑ **How do you diagnose RMSF?**

Immunofluorescent antibody staining of skin biopsy or serologic fluorescent antibody titer. The Weil-Felix reaction and complement fixation tests are no longer recommended.

❑❑ **Tests of confirmation for RMSF?**

Tetracycline or chloramphenicol. Antibiotic therapy should not be withheld pending serologic confirmation.

❑❑ **What is the most deadly form of malaria?**

Plasmodium falciparum.

❑❑ **What is the vector for malaria?**

The female anopheline mosquito.

❑❑ **What lab findings would you expect in a patient with malaria?**

Normochromic normocytic anemia, normal or depressed leukocyte count, thrombocytopenia, an elevated sed rate, abnormal kidney and LFTs, hyponatremia, hypoglycemia, and false-positive VDRL.

❑❑ **How is the definitive diagnosis of malaria established?**

Visualization of parasites on Giemsa-stained blood smears. In early infection, especially with *P. falciparum*, parasitized erythrocytes may be sequestered and be undetectable.

❑❑ **How is** P. falciparum **diagnosed on blood smear?**

1. Small ring forms with double chromatin knobs within the erythrocyte.
2. Multiple rings infected within red blood cells.
3. Rare trophozoites and schizonts on smear.
4. Pathognomonic crescent-shaped gametocytes.
5. Parasitemia exceeding 4%.

❑❑ **What is the drug of choice for treating** P. vivax, ovale, **and** malariae?

Chloroquine.

❑❑ **How is uncomplicated chloroquine-resistant** P. falciparum **treated?**

Quinine + pyrimethamine-sulfadoxine + doxycycline or mefloquine.

❑❑ **How is complicated chloroquine-resistant** P. falciparum **treated?**

Quinidine gluconate IV + doxycycline IV.

❑❑ **What complication of quinine and quinidine therapy should be considered?**

Insulin release which may result in hypoglycemia.

❑❑ **What are the adverse effects of chloroquine?**

N/V/D/F, pruritus, headache, dizziness, rash, and hypotension.

❑❑ **What type of parasitic infection commonly presents with a papular pruritic rash?**

Schistosomiasis.

❒❒ What type of parasite infections do not typically result in eosinophilia?

Protozoa infections such as amebas, Giardia, Trypanosoma, and Babesia.

❒❒ What is the most common intestinal parasite in the U.S.?

Giardia. Cysts are obtained from contaminated water or passed by hand-to-mouth transmission.
Symptoms include explosive foul smelling diarrhea, abdominal distention, fever, fatigue, and weight loss. Cysts reside in the duodenum and upper jejunum.
Treatment is quinacrine.

❒❒ How is Chagas disease transmitted?

The blood-sucking Reduviid (kissing) bug, blood transfusion, or breast feeding. A nodule or chagoma develops at the site of the bite. Symptoms include fever, headache, conjunctivitis, anorexia, and myocarditis. CHF and ventricular aneurysms can occur. The myenteric plexus is involved and may result in megacolon. Lab findings include anemia, leukocytosis, elevated sed rate, and ECG changes (PR interval, heart block, T-wave changes, and arrhythmias).

❒❒ What two diseases does the deer tick, Ixodes dammini **transmit?**

Lyme disease and Babesiosis.

❒❒ How do patients present with Babesia infection?

Intermittent fever, splenomegaly, jaundice, and hemolysis. The disease may be fatal in patients without spleens. Standard treatment is with clindamycin and quinine. Newer agents are also used. Long-term or repeat therapy is not unusual.

❒❒ What is the most frequently transmitted tick-borne disease?

Lyme disease.
Causative agent - spirochete *Borrelia burgdorferi.*
Vector - *Ixodes dammini* (deer tick) also *I. pacificus*, *Amblyomma americanum*, and *Dermacentor variabilis.*

❒❒ When are patients most likely to acquire Lyme disease?

Late spring and late summer, peaks in July.

❒❒ How is Lyme disease diagnosed?

Immunofluorescent and immunoabsorbent assays diagnose the antibodies to the spirochete.
Treatment includes doxycycline or tetracycline, amoxicillin, IV penicillin V in pregnant patients, or erythromycin.

❒❒ What type of paralysis does tick paralysis cause?

Ascending paralysis. The venom which causes paralysis is probably a neurotoxin which causes a conduction block at the peripheral motor nerve branches. This prevents acetylcholine release at the neuromuscular junction. 43 species of ticks are implicated as causative agents.

❒❒ What is the most common sign of tularemia?

Lymphadenopathy, usually cervical in children and inguinal in adults. It is caused by *Francisella tularensis* and is transmitted by the vectors *Dermacentor variabilis* and *A. americanum*.

❒❒ What two tick born diseases are transmitted by the tick vector I. dammini? **FEEL the Force, Luke...**

Lyme disease and babesiosis.

❒❒ A patient presents with sudden-onset of fever, lethargy, headache, myalgias, anorexia, nausea and vomiting. They describe the headache as retro-orbital and are extremely photophobic. They have been on a camping trip in Wyoming. What tick borne disease might cause these symptoms?

Colorado tick fever is caused by a virus of the genus Orbivirus of the family Reoviridae. The vector is the tick *D. andersoni*. The disease is self-limited and treatment is supportive.

❒❒ A patient presents to the emergency department with proximal and bulbar muscle weakness, pupils are fixed and dilated. What is the most likely diagnosis?

Botulism.

❒❒ What are the symptoms of Toxic shock syndrome?

1). Fever >39.2. 2). Rash-diffuse and macular. 3). Desquamation. 4). Involvement of 3 or more organ systems. 5). Hypotension. 6). Negative blood and CSF cultures.

❒❒ What infection presents like Toxic shock syndrome, and what are the major differences?

Group A Strep sepsis. The infection site in GASS is usually obvious unlike Toxic shock, and the cultures are usually positive for the Strep organism.

❒❒ What causes cutaneous larva migrans?

Classically caused by a dog or cat hookworm after walking barefoot on a contaminated soil or beach. The organism meanders under the skin producing the classic skin lesion.

❒❒ What patients require more than a three day course of antibiotics for a UTI?

Diabetics, those with symptoms for more than 7 days, those with a history of recent UTI, those that use a diaphragm, patients over age 65, and pregnant patients.

❒❒ What is the treatment for asymptomatic bacteriuria?

These patients require a 10 day course of antibiotics.

❒❒ What causes Typhoid fever?

The ingestion of large numbers of Salmonella typhi.

❒❒ What is the presentation of Typhoid fever?

Fever with a relative bradycardia, headache, and abdominal pain initially, then after approximately 1 week, a rose spot rash starts, and the patient will develop abdominal distension, hepatomegaly, and watery diarrhea.

❒❒ What are the prognostic bad signs in meningococcal infection?

Petechial rash starting less than 12 hours before presentation, shock, absence of meningitis, low WBC count and erythrocyte sedimentation rate, purpura (the worst of all), and age <1 or >10.

❒❒ Who gets mumps orchitis?

Only post-pubescent males.

❑❑ Where does Babesiosis occur?

Primarily in the islands off of the Northeastern U.S.

❑❑ Contrast pneumonia due to Mycoplasma with pneumonia due to pneumococcus.

	S. pneumoniae	M. pneumoniae
Prodrome	Uncommon	Mild fever, malaise, cough, headache
Onset	Rapid	Gradual
Severe respiratory symptoms	Tachypnea, cough, occasionally pleuritic pain	Uncommon
Associated findings	High fever	Exanthem, arthritis, GI complaints, neurologic complications
Pleural effusion	Occasionally	Rarely
Lab	Leukocytosis	WBC normal or slight elevation
Treatment	Penicillin	Erythromycin

❑❑ Describe the skin lesions associated with a *Pseudomonas aeruginosa* infection.

Pale, erythematous lesions, 1 cm in size, with an ulcerated necrotic center.

❑❑ A 56 year-old smoker with COPD presents with chills, fever, green sputum and extreme shortness of breath. CXR shows a right lower lobe pneumonia. What is expected from the sputum culture?

Haemophilus influenza. This organism is generally found in COPD patients who develop pneumonia and bronchitis. The two other common organisms in COPD patients are *Streptococcus pneumoniae* and *Moraxella catarrhalis.*

❑❑ A 67 year-old alcoholic was found in an alley, covered in his own vomit and beer. Upon examination, he is shaking, has a fever of 103.5° F and is coughing up currant jelly sputum. What is the most likely diagnosis?

Pneumonia induced by *Klebsiella pneumoniae*. This is a likely etiology in alcoholics, the elderly, the very young and immunocompromised patients. Other gram-negative bacteria, such as *E. coli* and other Enterobacteriaceae, may cause pneumonia in alcoholics.

❑❑ A 23 year-old male presents with a dry cough, malaise, fever and a sore throat that developed in the past two weeks. What is the most likely diagnosis?

Mycoplasma pneumonia. This condition usually has a slow onset and occurs in the young. Treat the patient with erythromycin, azithromycin or clarithromycin.

❑❑ What are the extrapulmonary manifestations of mycoplasma?

Erythema multiforme, pericarditis, GI and CNS disease.

❑❑ What common type of community acquired pneumonia is typically spread by aspiration of microdroplets from common water supplies?

Legionnaire's disease.

❑❑ What is the most common etiologic agent of atypical pneumonia?

Mycoplasma pneumoniae.

❒❒ **What is considered to be the second most common cause of atypical pneumonia?**

Chlamydia pneumoniae.

❒❒ **What is the most important risk factor for Moraxella catarrhalis pneumonia?**

Chronic obstructive lung disease.

❒❒ **What category of bacteria is most important in hospital acquired pneumonia?**

Gram negative bacilli and *Staphylococcus aureus.*

❒❒ **What is the treatment of choice for Legionella pneumonia?**

Erythromycin +/- rifampin.

❒❒ **What is the leading identifiable cause of acute community acquired pneumonia in adults?**

Streptococcus pneumoniae.

❒❒ **What is the most common cause of community acquired pneumonia among alcoholic patients?**

Streptococcus pneumoniae.

❒❒ **Which other bacteria are seen with increased frequency as causes of pneumonia among alcoholic patients?**

Klebsiella pneumoniae and *Hemophilus influenzae.*

❒❒ **What pulmonary fungal infection grows in soil, is endemic to the Mississippi River basin and rarely results in symptoms?**

Histoplasmosis.

❒❒ **What fungus is endemic to the deserts of the southwestern United States, produces a granulomatous tissue reaction and can cause the triad of pneumonitis, erythema nodosum and arthralgias known as "valley fever"?**

Coccidioidomycosis.

❒❒ **What is the most frequently transmitted tick borne disease?**

Lyme disease. The causative agent is the spirochete *Borrelia burgdorferi.*

❒❒ **What is the most common cause of cellulitis?**

Streptococcus pyogenes. Staphylococcus aureus can also cause cellulitis, though it is generally less severe and more often associated with an open wound.

❒❒ **What is the most common cause of cutaneous abscesses?**

Staphylococcus aureus.

❒❒ **What degree of leukocytosis is considered a risk factor for poor outcome among patients with bacterial pneumonia?**

Greater than 30,000 cells/mm^3.

❑❑ What degree of leukopenia is considered a risk factor for poor outcome among patients with bacterial pneumonia?

Less than 4000 cells/mm^3.

❑❑ What bacteria are associated with pneumonia following influenza?

Streptococcus pneumoniae, Staphylococcus aureus and *Hemophilus influenzae.*

❑❑ What category of bacteria is most important in community acquired aspiration pneumonia?

Anaerobic.

❑❑ What is the antibiotic of choice for patients with community acquired aspiration pneumonia?

Clindamycin.

❑❑ What antibiotic has been consistently effective against penicillin resistant Streptococcus pneumoniae?

Vancomycin.

❑❑ Of the following organisms, which is commonly spread by person-to-person contact: Legionella pneumoniae **or** Mycoplasma pneumoniae?

Mycoplasma pneumoniae.

❑❑ Is single antibiotic therapy typically effective in the treatment of Klebsiella pneumonia?

Yes.

❑❑ What is the most common cause of community acquired bacterial pneumonia among patients infected with HIV?

Streptococcus pneumoniae.

❑❑ What are the CSF findings in viral meningitis?

Lymphocytic pleocytosis, normal (or slightly elevated) protein and normal glucose.

❑❑ What are the CSF characteristics of tuberculous meningitis?

Lymphocytic pleocytosis, high protein and low glucose.

❑❑ What is the management of herpes simplex encephalitis?

Early treatment with acyclovir, anticonvulsants for seizures and general supportive care.

❑❑ Clinically, how can you distinguish orbital cellulitis from periorbital cellulitis?

Extraocular muscle dysfunction, decreased pupillary reflexes, decreased visual acuity and change in globe position are seen only in orbital cellulitis.

❑❑ What CSF protein and WBC findings occur in Guillain-Barré?

An increase in cerebrospinal fluid protein without a corresponding increase in cerebrospinal fluid white cells.

❑❑ **What is the most common infectious disease problem in patients with lupus that are not on steroid therapy?**

Urinary tract infections and urosepsis.

❑❑ **What rapid diagnostic test is now available to diagnose herpes simplex virus encephalitis in patients of all ages and how reliable is it?**

HSV polymerase chain reaction (PCR) on cerebrospinal fluid is considered to be highly sensitive and specific in the diagnosis of HSV encephalitis.

❑❑ **What are the most common organisms found in human bite wounds?**

Staphylococcus aureus, streptococcus and *Eikenella corrodens*. Anaerobes are also commonly seen.

❑❑ Pasteurella multocida **infection from an animal bite is best treated with which antibiotic?**

Penicillin.

❑❑ **What is the most common infectious disease complication of both measles and influenza?**

Pneumococcal pneumonia.

❑❑ **What prophylactic intravenous antibiotic should be given systemically to burn victims?**

None. Prophylactic antibiotics are given topically.

❑❑ **On Tuesday you are driving home from work in rural California and pass a dead squirrel. On Wednesday, taking a different route, you pass two more dead squirrels. The following morning you see a twenty-six year-old male with enlarged tender lymphadenitis and a 105° F fever. What illness do you suspect?**

Cases of human plague (Yersinia pestis) are sometimes heralded by a squirrel die-off. A squirrel die-off occurs when the organism is introduced into a highly susceptible mammalian population, causing a high mortality rate among infected animals. This is referred to as epizootic plague.

❑❑ **What is the epidemiology of necrotizing fasciitis?**

Necrotizing fasciitis is a severe infection distinguished by necrosis of the fascia and subcutaneous tissues, resulting in undermining of the skin. Onset is abrupt and is more common in diabetics, alcoholics and IV drug abusers, usually precipitated by a traumatized area of skin.

❑❑ **What are the clinical findings of necrotizing fasciitis?**

Initial physical findings may mimic cellulitis with swollen, very tender, erythematous skin. Unlike cellulitis, the margins are usually not well demarcated and the involved area typically becomes anesthetic due to the destruction of cutaneous nerves by the inflammatory process. Some patients develop subcutaneous gas and grossly necrotic skin or bulla formation. Very high fever and signs of toxicity disproportionate to the physical findings suggest necrotizing fasciitis. The superficial skin findings can be thought of as the tip of the iceberg.

❑❑ **How is necrotizing fasciitis diagnosed?**

Early diagnosis, which can be made by biopsy of subcutaneous tissue, fascia and muscle, may help decrease the mortality rate (from up to 50% in the untreated patient).

❑❑ **What is the treatment for necrotizing fasciitis?**

Organisms seen with Type I necrotizing fasciitis include streptococci, anaerobes and Enterobacteriaceae. These are treated with penicillin/clindamycin/gentamicin. Type II necrotizing fasciitis is caused by invasive group A streptococci, which is popularly referred to as the "flesh-eating bacteria." Penicillin and clindamycin are the agents of choice. Systemic involvement may occur with type II infection, resulting in streptococcal toxic shock syndrome. Assertive surgical debridement is necessary for both types.

❑❑ What are the extracutaneous manifestations of chickenpox in the adult?

Varicella pneumonia occurs in up to 1 out of 400 adult cases of chickenpox. CXR findings include diffuse interstitial or nodular infiltrates. Cough, dyspnea, hemoptysis and respiratory failure may develop. Sputum Tzanck smear may be positive. Encephalitis, myocarditis and hepatitis may also complicate the infection. Treatment is IV acyclovir.

❑❑ How does a subphrenic abscess present?

It follows surgery for a ruptured viscus, cholecystitis or penetrating abdominal wound. Patients may complain of right upper quadrant or shoulder pain in addition to fever and chills. Subphrenic abscesses occur far more commonly on the right. The chest x-ray typically reveals an elevated hemidiaphragm and may show a pleural effusion or an air/fluid level below the diaphragm in more advanced cases. CT is diagnostic.

❑❑ What is the treatment for influenza?

Amantadine or rimantadine should ideally be initiated within 48 to 72 hours from the onset of symptoms. Complicating bacterial pneumonias are common, especially *Streptococcal pneumoniae* and *Staphylococcus aureus* and need to be specifically treated as well.

❑❑ What mechanism is felt to be responsible for the association of aminoglycoside and muscle weakness?

Aminoglycosides can prevent calcium uptake into the presynaptic membrane at the neuromuscular junction, which can inhibit acetylcholine release. They also can blunt the effects of acetylcholine at the postsynaptic membrane.

The likelihood of muscle weakness is increased in patients who have received neuromuscular blockers, in patients who have muscle disorders or are hypocalcemic or hypomagnesemic. Calcium channel blockers may potentiate this effect.

❑❑ What are the characteristics of drug fever?

Patients with a drug related fever often will appear relatively well, despite a high temperature. Usual temperatures are in the range of 102 to 104 degrees Fahrenheit, though low grade and extreme elevations may also be seen. Sustained fevers and a relative bradycardia are typical. Besides antibiotics, other common causes of drug fever include amphotericin, procainamide, salicylates, barbiturates, phenytoin, quinidine and interferon. Drug fever is not always accompanied by rash.

❑❑ What are the signs and symptoms of diphtheria infection?

Infection is heralded by acute onset of exudative pharyngitis, high fever and malaise. A pseudomembrane may form in the oropharynx with possible respiratory compromise. A circulating exotoxin has direct effects on the heart, kidneys and nervous system. Diphtheria infection may lead to paralysis of the intrinsic and extrinsic eye muscles.

❑❑ What is the most common cause of endocarditis in IV drug abusers?

Staphylococcus aureus, most commonly involving the tricuspid valve.

❒❒ What does the India ink test stain for?

Cryptococcus neoformans.

❒❒ What strain of influenza is more common in adults? In children?

Adults: Influenza A. Children: Influenza B.

❒❒ What strain of influenza is most virulent?

Influenza A.

❒❒ A 34 year-old female presents with a maculopapular rash on her palms and soles. She complains of headaches and general weakness. On examination, you find she has multiple condyloma lata and lymphadenopathy. What is the diagnosis?

Secondary syphilis. This develops 6 to 9 weeks after the syphilitic chancre, which will have resolved by this time. If it goes untreated, tertiary syphilis will develop. This can affect all the tissues in the body, including the CNS and the heart. Treatment is with penicillin.

RHEUM/IMMUNOLOGY PEARLS

"SUCCESS FOUR FLIGHTS THURSDAY MORNING ALL AGAINST TWENTY ONE MILE WIND STARTED FROM LEVEL WITH ENGINE POWER ALONE AVERAGE SPEED THROUGH AIR THIRTY ONE MILES LONGEST 57 SECONDS INFORM PRESS HOME CHRISTMAS."
Telegram from Orville Wright to his father, 12/17/1903

❑❑ **What is the treatment of choice for a patient in anaphylactic shock?**

Epinephrine 0.3-0.5 mg IV of 1:10,000 solution. If no IV access, then inject into the venous plexus at base of the tongue.

❑❑ **What is the most common cause of anaphylactoid reactions?**

Radiographic contrast agents.

❑❑ **For how long should a patient with a generalized anaphylactic reaction be observed?**

24 h. Recurrence and delayed reactions are possible. Patients should be treated with oral antihistamines and corticosteroids for at least 72 h.

❑❑ **What percentage of patients with relapsing polychondritis can be expected to have airway involvement?**

Approximately 50% have airway involvement. They frequently present with acute onset of pain, oropharyngeal tenderness over cartilaginous structures, and hoarseness. Erythema and edema of the nose and oropharynx is also common.

❑❑ **What is the appropriate treatment of a patient presenting with acute onset of relapsing polychondritis with airway involvement?**

Admit for observation and high dose steroids. These patients may develop dyspnea, stridor, or cough. Repeated exacerbations may lead to asphyxiation .

❑❑ **A RA patient presenting with painful speaking or swallowing, hoarseness, or stridor requires what type of diagnostic procedure?**

Urgent laryngoscopy to evaluate involvement of the paired cricoarytenoid joints. These may become fixed in the closed position, resulting in airway compromise.

❑❑ **What percentage of SLE patients will develop signs and symptoms of pleurisy during the course of their disease?**

Approximately half. Pleurisy is also common in RA, but is often asymptomatic. All pulmonary effusions in patients with rheumatic disease require thoracentesis to distinguish from infectious processes.

❑❑ **Myocardial infarction can be related to which two rheumatic diseases?**

Kawasaki disease and polyarteritis nodosa.

❑❑ **What percentage of patients with Kawasaki disease who do not receive proper therapy will develop coronary artery aneurysms?**

20%. 2-3% will go on to die from MI during the resolution phase of the disease.

❑❑ **A patient presents with fever, acute polyarthritis, or migratory arthritis a few weeks after a bout of Streptococcal pharyngitis, they should be evaluated for what disease?**

Rheumatic fever. Approximately 30% will have subcutaneous nodules, erythema marginatum, or chorea.

❑❑ **What is the Rx of choice for the fever and arthritis of rheumatic fever?**

Salicylates and bedrest until signs and symptoms return to normal.

❑❑ **What clinical sign do the following often have in common; rheumatic fever, bacterial endocarditis, Schönlein-Henoch-purpura, prodromal pulmonary** Mycoplasma, **or fungal infections?**

Migratory arthritis.

❑❑ **What pathological process should be considered in a patient treated with steroids, who presents with weakness, depression, fatigue, and postural dizziness?**

Adrenal insufficiency. Treatment consists of stress steroids - dexamethasone is preferred because it does not interfere with testing of adrenal steroids levels.

❑❑ **Name a common complication of SLE, RA, & JRA.**

Pericarditis.

❑❑ **What is the normal atlantodental distance on lateral flexion views of the C-spine?**

3.5 mm in adults.
4 mm in the child under 12 yr.

❑❑ **What might a change in bladder or bowel function, limb paresthesias, or new weakness indicate in a patient with RA or ankylosing spondylosis?**

Destruction of the C-spine ligamentous structures - this can lead to atlantoaxial subluxation.

❑❑ **What is Lhermitte's sign, found in patients with RA or ankylosing spondylosis?**

The sensation of an electric shock radiating down the back with neck flexion. A classic sign of C-spine instability.

❑❑ **What is another name for granulomatous arteritis of the thoracic aorta, and branches? (Hint: usually presents with tender scalp, new headache, fluctuating vision, reduced or lost brachial pulse, and pain in the tongue or jaw while talking or chewing).**

Temporal arteritis.

❑❑ **Polymyalgia rheumatica coexists in 10-30% of patients with which disease affecting the vascular system?**

Temporal arteritis.

❑❑ **What rheumatic syndrome may lead to corneal irritation, ulceration, and infection?**

Sjögren's syndrome.

❒❒ What is the most common pathogen found in osteomyelitis and septic arthritis of the foot?

Pseudomonas.

❒❒ How does the time course of the onset of joint pain help differentiate between gout and pseudogout?

Patients with gout develop joint pain over a few hours, while pseudogout usually evolves over a day.

❒❒ The finding of rhomboid shaped crystals under a polarizing scope in an aspirate of a painful joint indicates what type of synovitis?

Pseudogout (calcium pyrophosphate).
Yellow needle shaped crystals indicate gout (urate).

❒❒ What is the first priority in the workup of a patient suspected of having gout?

Exclusion of septic arthritis.

❒❒ Name a complication of RA that mimics a DVT?

Ruptured Baker's cyst. The ruptured cyst may be differentiated from a DVT by absence of swelling in the foot, and a crescent sign (a purplish discoloration below the malleoli).

❒❒ How may an olecranon bursitis be differentiated from arthritis of the elbow?

Bursitis will not affect pronation or supination.

❒❒ What is the treatment of choice if there is any clinical suspicion of a septic olecranon bursa?

Appropriate antibiotic therapy should be started. Using a large bore needle the bursa should be drained completely.

❒❒ What uncommon musculoskeletal disorder of children must be considered in a child that refuses to sit or walk, and holds themselves rigidly stiff?

Discitis. Any attempts to maneuver the child will elicit guarding, and plain films will often reveal an abnormal lordosis.

❒❒ Toxic synovitis affects what age group of patients?

School age children. Treatment is to rule out sepsis, and relieve synovial pressure through aspiration.

❒❒ What disease entity should be investigated in a child with joint swelling following minor trauma.

JRA. Minor trauma may cause intra-articular bleeding. The joint should not be immobilized.

❒❒ What is the appropriate management for a child with normal x-rays and tenderness over the end of a long bone after trauma.

Immobilization and orthopedic evaluation for Salter-Harris type I fracture. These fractures may be occult.

❒❒ What pathologic process must be considered in a patient with painless progressive weakness in a C-spine distribution?

Cervical ventral root compromise by a degenerative disk. The dorsal and ventral nerve roots remain discrete in the C-spine in over half the population.

❑❑ **Complaints of bilateral upper extremity pain may involve what pathologic process?**

A C6 spinal radiculopathy.

❑❑ **What pathological process is suggested in a patient with a reduction of the radial pulse when the shoulder is passively abducted? Hint - a patient with this syndrome may also have a subclavian bruit.**

Thoracic outlet syndrome.

❑❑ **Tenderness over the ulnar nerve at the elbow may indicate a cervical radiculopathy at what level?**

C8 - T1.

❑❑ **Numbness or tingling in the long finger may be the only presenting symptom of a radiculopathy at what level?**

C7.

❑❑ **Hyperreflexia and a Hoffmann's sign in the upper extremities with neck pain indicate a lesion where?**

Above C5.

❑❑ **Where does cervical disk prolapse most often occur?**

C6-7 (on the left), and C5-6 (on the right). Most often in the fourth decade.

❑❑ **Angina-like chest pain, Horner's syndrome, painless upper extremity weakness, and severe radicular symptoms without neck pain may all be caused by what pathologic cervical process?**

Spurious cervical osteophytes.

❑❑ **What pathology should be presumed when there is a sudden loss of bladder control, onset of lumbosacral pain, and associated bilateral leg pain?**

Midline herniation of a thoraco-lumbar disk. With these symptoms comes the threat of paraparesis.

❑❑ **What constitutes immediate admission criteria for a patient with acute low back pain?**

Paraparesis, bowel or bladder incontinence, intractable L-S pain and spasticity, inability to sit or stand, upright sleeping position, metastatic cancer, 2nd ED visit, or X-ray film with defects.

❑❑ **An inability to walk on the toes indicates a radiculopathy where?**

S1. An L5 radiculopathy manifests as inability to walk on the heels.

❑❑ **A painful "strum" sign in the presence of a progressive inability to extend the knee on the affected side is pathognomic of what pathology?**

A herniated disk with nerve root impaction.

❑❑ **Compromise of which nerve roots can mimic the muscular calf pain of thrombophlebitis or the anterior tibial compartment pain of "shin splints"?**

L5 and S1 root compromise.

❒❒ What are the two most common causes of fatal anaphylaxis?

#1 = Drug reactions, 95% to penicillin. Parenteral most dangerous. 300 people/y.
#2 = Hymenoptera stings. 100 people/y.

❒❒ Which type of hypersensitivity reaction is responsible for anaphylaxis?

Type I, (IgE mediated).

Hypersensitivity Reaction	Mediator	Example
Type 1 - Immediate	IgE binds allergen, includes mast cells and basophils	Food allergy. Asthma in children.
Type 2 - Cytotoxic	IgG & IgM antibody reactions to antigen on cell surface activates complement and killers	Blood transfusion rxn. ITP, hemolytic anemia, ITP.
Type 3 - Immune complex, Arthus	Complexes activate complement	Tetanus toxoid in sensitized persons. Poststreptococcal glomerulonephritis.
Type 4 - Cell mediated, delayed hypersensitivity	Activated T-lymphocytes	Skin tests

❒❒ Food-mediated hypersensitivity reactions are due to what component of the immune system?

IgE. Dairy products, nuts and eggs are the most common.

❒❒ When do the clinical manifestations of a drug allergy reaction usually become apparent?

The first or second week following administration of the drug.

❒❒ Generalized malaise, fever, arthralgias, and urticaria are common to what type of allergic reaction?

Drug allergy. Allergic reactions to drugs may involve any or all of the four types of hypersensitivity reactions.

❒❒ What drug is the most common pharmaceutical cause of true allergic reactions?

Penicillin

❒❒ How long after exposure to an allergen does anaphylaxis occur?

Seconds to 1 hour.

❒❒ After penicillin, what is the most common cause of anaphylaxis-related deaths?

Insect stings. Approximately 100 deaths occur in the US annually because of anaphylaxis induced by insect stings.

❒❒ A patient on a beta-blocker who develops anaphylactic cardiovascular collapse may not respond to epinephrine or dopamine infusions. What drug can be used in this setting?

Glucagon.

❒❒ Cite an example for each of the four major types of allergic reactions: Type I (immediate hypersensitivity); type II (cytotoxic); type III (Arthus reaction); and type IV (delayed hypersensitivity).

Type I: Asthma, food allergies (IgE).
Type II: Transfusion reaction (IgG and IgM).
Type III: Serum sickness, post streptococcal glomerulonephritis (complex activates complement).
Type IV: Skin testing (activated T-lymphocytes).

❑❑ Which of the four types of allergic reactions can be caused by a drug allergy?

All of them.

❑❑ Myocardial infarction can occur with which two rheumatic diseases?

Kawasaki disease and polyarteritis nodosa (PAN).

❑❑ What diagnostic procedure is indicated for a patient with rheumatoid arthritis who presents with dysphagia, hoarseness and stridor?

Urgent laryngoscopy to assess the paired cricoarytenoid joints. These joints can cause airway compromise if they become fixed in a closed position.

❑❑ What is the treatment of choice for a patient in anaphylactic shock?

Epinephrine intravenously.

❑❑ A patient on chronic steroids presents with weakness, depression, fatigue and postural dizziness. What pathological process should be suspected? What is the treatment?

Adrenal insufficiency. The treatment is to administer large "stress doses" of steroids.

❑❑ What cardiac complication commonly occurs with SLE, juvenile rheumatoid arthritis and rheumatoid arthritis?

Pericarditis.

❑❑ What causes fatality in hereditary angioedema?

Edema of the larynx.

❑❑ What neurologic disorders, if present, serve as diagnostic criteria for SLE?

Seizures and psychosis.

❑❑ What pharmacologic agents are most commonly associated with drug-induced lupus?

Anticonvulsants, hydralazine and isoniazid.

❑❑ An 18 year-old female presents with complains of fever and malaise one week prior to the development of 1 to 3 cm painful, red, ovoid nodules on her shins bilaterally. Bilateral hilar lymphadenopathy is demonstrated on chest x-ray. What is the diagnosis?

Erythema nodosum associated with sarcoidosis.

PSYCHIATRIC PEARLS

"It is difficult to say what is impossible, for the dream of yesterday is the hope of today and the reality of tomorrow."
Robert H. Goddard, at his high school graduation, 1904.

❑❑ **Describe a patient with generalized anxiety disorder.**

Patients appear apprehensive, restless, irritable and easily distracted. Patients may experience muscle tension and fatigue as well as various autonomic symptoms such as palpitations, shortness of breath, chest tightness, nausea or diffuse weakness and numbness.

❑❑ **Name a few substances that may mimic generalized anxiety when ingested.**

Nicotine, caffeine, amphetamines, cocaine, anticholinergics; alcohol and sedative withdrawal.

❑❑ **What is the epidemiologic difference between suicide attempters and suicide completers?**

Suicide completers tend to be older males with medical problems, living alone or with a poor social network.

❑❑ **Name 2 Axis I disorders commonly associated with suicidal ideation.**

Alcohol abuse and affective (mood) disorder.

❑❑ **What happens when one combines EtOH with an anxiolytic (benzodiazepine)?**

Death! (Due to their combined respiratory depressive effects).

❑❑ **Name another contraindication to benzodiazepine use.**

Known hypersensitivity, acute narrow angle glaucoma, pregnancy especially 1st trimester.

❑❑ **Why have mono-amine oxidase (MAO) inhibitors been prescribed less frequently?**

Why don't you try a tyramine-free diet sometime! Mmm Mmm good! Tyramine containing substances can cause hypertensive crisis - such foods include pickled herring, snails, chicken liver, beer, red wine and cheese.

❑❑ **Name some drugs <u>contraindicated</u> for a patient taking MAO inhibitors.**

Toxic reactions that include excitation and hyperpyrexia can occur with meperidine (Demerol) and with dextromethorphan. The effects of indirect acting adrenergic drugs are potentiated, including ephedrine, sympathomimetic amines in cold remedies, amphetamines, cocaine and methylphenidate (Ritalin).

❑❑ **Name the three common MAO inhibitors (chemical and Brand name).**

Phenelzine (Nardil).
Isocarboxazid (Marplan).
Tranylcypromine (Parnate).

❑❑ **How does one treat hypertensive crisis caused by combining MAO inhibitors with a known toxin, cheese pizza?**

An α- and ß-adrenergic antagonist such as labetalol.
Also consider nifedipine or nitroglycerin. If unsuccessful, consider sodium nitroprusside or IV phentolamine.

❑❑ **A 27 year-old male arrives somnolent with vitals of P 130, R 26, BP 170/80 T of 105 °F. You note diffuse muscular rigidity and intermittent focal muscle twitching/jerking lasting 1-2 seconds. As you 'work him up', your faithful nurse returns from the waiting area with news from the family that the patient has had a progressive decline of mental status for 2 d after seeing his psychiatrist. The patient has had a history of 'psychosis' for almost one year. What process should be included in your differential diagnosis at this time?**

Neuroleptic malignant syndrome.

❑❑ **Psychiatrists use a multiaxial diagnostic system to describe a particular patient's medical problem list; discuss.**

Axis I: Symptoms and syndromes comprising a mental disorder, includes substance abuse/addiction.
Axis II: Personality and developmental disorders (underlying the Axis I diagnosis).
Axis III: Physical medical problems/conditions which may or may not contribute to Axis I diagnosis.
Axis IV: Psychosocial factors.
Axis V: Adaptive ability/disability.

❑❑ **What is organic brain syndrome?**

Reversible or nonreversible mental condition thought to be caused by disease process or substance use which interrupts normal anatomical, physiological or biochemical brain functions.

❑❑ **Describe dementia.**

Disturbed cognitive function resulting in impaired memory, personality, judgment and/or language. Insidious onset, but may present as acute worsened mental state while facing other physical or environmental stressors.

❑❑ **Describe delirium.**

"Clouding of consciousness" resulting in disorientation, decreased alertness and impaired cognitive function. Acute onset, visual hallucinosis, fluctuating psychomotor activity; all symptoms variable and may change over hours.

❑❑ **Neuroleptic medications come in three flavors: low, medium and high potency. Can you name some of these meds and their category?**

Low potency: Chlorpromazine (Thorazine).
Medium potency: Perphenazine (Trilafon).
High potency: Haloperidol, droperidol (Inapsine), thiothixene (Navane), fluphenazine (Prolixin), trifluoperazine (Stelazine).

❑❑ **So, what's the big deal?**

Neuroleptics act to block dopamine receptors. Receptor blockade within the mesolimbic area of the brain provides their antipsychotic effect. Dopaminergic receptor blockade throughout the CNS and anticholinergic effect produce many side effects observed in the ED.

❑❑ **Which neuroleptics produce which side effects?**

Low potency: Sedative, orthostatic hypotension, anticholinergic effects.

High potency: Less sedating, profound extrapyramidal reactions.

❒❒ **What are extrapyramidal reactions?**

Dopamine receptor blockade within the nigrostriatal system results in involuntary and spontaneous motor responses including: dystonia, akathisia and Parkinson's-like syndrome.

❒❒ **What is a dystonic reaction?**

Very common side effect of neuroleptics seen in the ED. Muscle spasm of tongue, face, neck and back are seen. Severe laryngospasm and extraocular muscle spasm may occur also. Patients may bite the tongue leading to potential airway compromise either by inability to open the mouth or by tongue edema or hemorrhage.

❒❒ **How do you treat a dystonic reaction?**

Diphenhydramine (Benadryl), 25-50 mg IM or IV or benztropine (Cogentin), 1-2 mg IV or PO. Remember that dystonias can recur acutely. The patient is generally sent home with oral benztropine for a few days to avoid this problem.

❒❒ **Describe symptoms of alcohol withdrawal.**

Autonomic hyperactivity: tachycardia, hypertension, tremors, anxiety, agitation; 6-8 h after drinking.

Hallucinations: auditory, visual, tactile; 24 h after drinking.

Global confusion: 1-3 d after drinking.

❒❒ **List some life-threatening causes of acute psychosis.**

WHHHIMP: Wernicke's Encephalopathy, Hypoxia, Hypoglycemia, Hypertensive encephalopathy, Intracerebral hemorrhage, Meningitis/Encephalitis, and Poisoning.

❒❒ **Characteristics of schizophrenia?**

Delusional disorder, hallucinations, (usually auditory), disorganized thinking, loosening of associations, disheveled appearance, lack of insight in realizing thoughts and behavior are abnormal, onset age usually less than 40, and duration of symptoms longer than 6 mo.

❒❒ **What is the difference between schizophrenia and schizophreniform disorder?**

Very little. In schizophreniform disorder, schizophrenic symptoms have lasted less than 6 mo.

❒❒ **What is a brief reactive psychosis?**

Acute psychotic break, usually after an emotional or traumatic event. Short duration, usually less than 2 weeks.

❒❒ **Signs and symptoms suggestive of organic source of psychosis.**

Acute onset, disorientation, visual or tactile hallucinations, evidence suggesting overdose or acute ingestion, such as abnormal vital signs, pupil size and reactivity, nystagmus, and age less than 10 or older than 60.

❒❒ **Name some symptoms of major depression.**

IN SAD CAGES: Interest, sleep, appetite, depressed mood, concentration, activity, guilt, energy, suicide.

❒❒ Name some vegetative symptoms.

Loss of appetite, lack of concentration, chronic fatigue, agitation, restlessness, inability to sleep, weight loss.

❒❒ What are common neuroleptic-induced side effects?

Oculogyric crisis, akathisia, tardive dyskinesia and dystonia.

❒❒ Describe risk factors for tardive dyskinesia.

Tardive dyskinesia occurs in about 20% of patients receiving traditional antipsychotics for long periods of time and in up to 50% of high risk patients such as the elderly. Other risk factors include total duration of exposure to antipsychotics, female sex, history of extrapyramidal side effects and a mood disorder diagnosis. Spontaneous dyskinesias are seen in 1-2% of antipsychotic naive patients.

❒❒ Describe factors associated with suicide in schizophrenia.

Ten percent of patients with schizophrenia commit suicide, primarily in the first ten years of the illness. Risk factors include male gender, age under 30 years, college education, paranoid subtype, comorbid substance use, depressive symptoms, unemployment, frequent exacerbations of the disease, prior suicide attempts, living alone, and recent hospital discharge.

❒❒ Describe the onset of schizophrenia.

Schizophrenia typically becomes manifest in adolescence or early adulthood and has a rather heterogeneous natural history. About half of cases present with the insidious onset of subtle progressive impairment of function in personal, social, school or work areas lasting weeks to years, prior to the onset of psychosis. However, a rapid onset of psychosis may also be seen in persons with no prior disturbance of personal or social functioning.

❒❒ Discuss the management of acute dystonic reactions.

Parenteral administration of anticholinergic medications or benzodiazepines produce dramatic responses. Maintaining or assuring the patient's airway is imperative, and reassurance and support is essential. Oral anticholinergic maintenance is often necessary.

❒❒ When monitoring blood counts during treatment with clozapine, when should clozapine be discontinued?

As agranulocytosis is a serious side effect of clozapine, daily monitoring should occur when the white blood cell count (WBC) drops to < 5,000 and the absolute neutrophil count (ANC) should be closely followed. When the WBC is < 3,500 or the ANC is <1500, clozapine should be discontinued immediately.

❒❒ What is neuroleptic malignant syndrome (NMS)?

The syndrome consists of the development of severe muscle rigidity and elevated temperature with exposure to neuroleptic medications at any time during the course of treatment. Autonomic and metabolic instability can lead to tachycardia, hypertension, hypotension, leucocytosis, and elevated creatine phosphokinase associated with muscle break down. Other symptoms of this potentially lethal condition include diaphoresis, dysphagia, tremor, incontinence, delirium, mutism, and coma.

❒❒ Neuroleptic malignant syndrome occurs how frequently?

0.5% - 1% of patients taking neuroleptics develop NMS.

❑❑ Describe the treatment of NMS.

Antipsychotic medications should be withdrawn immediately. Supportive and symptomatic treatment consists of correcting fluid and electrolyte imbalances, treating fevers, and managing blood pressure instability. Studies have indicated that the treatment with dantrolene, bromocriptine, or amantadine may be helpful. In a number of cases, ECT has been shown to effectively treat NMS.

❑❑ How do you differentiate delusional disorder from schizophrenia?

In contrast to schizophrenia, the delusions of delusional disorder are non-bizarre in that they involve situations that could occur in real life. Also, there is not the deterioration in functioning that usually occurs in schizophrenia. Patients with delusional disorder do not have negative symptoms or loose associations, but olfactory and tactile hallucinations may occur in delusional disorder in the context of the delusion.

❑❑ What are the most common side effects of tricyclic antidepressants? Sedation, weight gain, anticholinergic effects (dry mouth, constipation, urinary retention, confusion), tremor, orthostatic hypotension, excessive sweating, and impotence. Generally these side effects are dose related. Additionally, tricyclics have the tendency to slow intracardiac conduction by quinidine-like effects, and may be associated with decreased heart rate variability. A screening ECG is warranted on patients with suspected cardiac disease and all patients above the age of 40 before initiating treatment with tricyclics. Bifascicular block, left bundle branch block, and a prolonged QT interval are considered as strong relative contraindications to tricyclic use. Sexual dysfunction can also be seen with tricyclic use.

❑❑ What are the symptoms of serious tricyclic toxicity?

Antimuscarinic symptoms (dry mucous membranes, decreased bowel motility, mydriasis, blurry vision, urinary retention, confusion), CNS depression from drowsiness to coma, cardiac arrhythmias and conduction block, hypotension, and seizures. Death often occurs from arrhythmia, hypotension, or seizures. The minimum fatal dose of tricyclics is considered to be between 1-2 grams. Thus, it is not advisable to prescribe more than one week supply of TCA to a depressed patient at risk for suicide.

❑❑ What is the treatment of a significant tricyclic overdose?

Intubate and administer gastric lavage if the patient is stuporous or comatose. To block absorption of tricyclic, activated charcoal (30 mg) is given as well. Intravenous sodium bicarbonate is the main stay of therapy for most of the toxicity seen with tricyclic overdose. Ventilatory support and vasopressors may be required. Arrhythmias may require emergent treatment, and continuous telemetry is indicated for patients who experience arrhythmias. QRS duration above 0.1 second is an indication for immediate alkalinization. Seizures may require intravenous anticonvulsants.

❑❑ What is the potentially fatal consequence of combining MAOI's with SSRI's, tryptophan, venlafaxine, meperidine and certain other serotonin agonists?

Serotonin syndrome, which ranges from mild tremor, hypertension, tachycardia, and fever to a dangerous cluster of severe hyperthermia, seizures, coma, and even death. Because of this risk, SSRI's should not be used concomitantly with MAOI's. In fact, fluoxetine should be "washed out" for five weeks prior to initiating treatment with an MAOI, and shorter-acting SSRI's and venlafaxine should be "washed out" for the equivalent of about four to five half-lives (or two weeks) to play it safe. When switching from an MAOI to an SSRI, the MAOI should be "washed out" for two weeks prior to initiating SSRI treatment. Because the tricyclic, clomipramine, is predominantly serotonergic, similar restrictions apply with this medication as with the shorter acting SSRI's. Other tricyclics can be used with caution with MAOI's if indicated.

❑❑ What other medications should be rigorously avoided in patients being treated with MAOI's?

Hyperadrenergic crisis can occur when MAOI's are co-administered with sympathomimetics including amphetamines, methylphenidate, pseudoephedrine, phenylpropanolamine, levodopa, and others. Opiates must be used with caution; meperidine and dextromethorphan should be avoided due to reports of delirium, autonomic instability, and death associated with the use of these agents with MAOI's.

❐❐ **What is a panic attack? How long does it last?**

Panic attacks are episodes of sudden, intense periods of anxiety. The severity of symptoms leads to the fear of having a heart attack, fainting, "going crazy", or dying. These episodes usually abate within 10 minutes and rarely last more than an hour, but for the person experiencing the attack, it may seem like a very long time.

❐❐ **What foods, drugs, and maneuvers can precipitate panic attacks?**

Caffeine, alcohol, marijuana, thyroid supplements, sympathomimetics, stimulants, and Yohimbine can precipitate panic attacks. Sodium lactate infusion provokes panic attacks in approximately 70% of patients with panic disorders. Exercise, carbon-dioxide inhalation, and cholecystokinin administration can also precipitate panic attacks.

❐❐ **What cardiac disorders are associated with panic disorder?**

Mitral valve prolapse is seen in approximately 50% of patients with panic disorder. There is also a high association between cardiac arrhythmia, hypertension, and panic disorder.

❐❐ **Which endocrine disorders may be associated with panic attacks?**

Diabetes, hypothyroidism, hyperthyroidism, parathyroid disease, Cushing's disease, and pheochromocytoma.

❐❐ **Can buspirone be used in the treatment of alcohol or benzodiazepine withdrawal?**

No. Buspirone is ineffective in the treatment of alcohol or benzodiazepine withdrawal.

❐❐ **What are the side effects of propranolol?**

Bronchospasm, worsening of congestive heart failure, hypotension, peripheral vasospasm, depression, confusion, and hallucinations.

❐❐ **What are the indications for using benzodiazepines?**

Generalized anxiety disorder, insomnia, panic disorder, agitation, akathisia, and alcohol withdrawal.

❐❐ **Which antihistamine is sometimes used as an anxiolytic?**

Hydroxyzine (Vistaril)

❐❐ **Are there any sex differences in prevalence of factitious disorders?**

Yes. Contrary to popular belief that the factitious disorders are more common in males (probably because of the well known example of Munchausen's syndrome), a number of old and new reviews of literature including a ten year retrospective study of patients, revealed that factitious disorders are more common in females.

❐❐ **What are the characteristics of factitious disorder with predominantly psychological symptoms?**

These highly suggestible patients commonly present symptoms according to their own concept of mental illness. They may endorse symptoms mentioned in a review of systems, and their symptoms appear to worsen when under perceived observation. They may present with symptoms of bereavement, dissociation, or psychosis.

Finally, these individuals may be pleasant and overly cooperative or they may be extremely uncooperative and negativistic.

❒❒ **What are the characteristics of factitious disorder with predominantly physical symptoms?**

As the name implies, physical symptoms dominate the clinical picture suggesting the presence of a general medical condition(s). Patients may seem to spare no effort at attempts to secure admission or stay in hospital. They may present with a multitude of physical symptoms limited only by the patient's sophistication and imagination. They may show multiple scars and commonly present with acute abdominal pain, hematuria, fever, seizures, rashes, abscesses and any other combination of symptoms.

❒❒ **How are factitious disorders differentiated from acts of malingering?**

The underlying motives for patient behavior distinguish these disorders from each other. However, the symptoms are intentionally produced in both cases. In factitious disorders, it is the psychological need for assumption of the sick role, while in malingering there is usually an obvious external incentive, e.g., avoidance of conscription, or a prisoner feigning illness to avoid physical labor. Factitious disorders are always considered to be psychopathological in nature, while malingering may be an adaptive response in certain circumstances, e.g., a person held hostage simulates illness to avoid physical labor

❒❒ **What features characterize Munchausen by proxy?**

In this disorder, a care provider intentionally feigns or produces signs and symptoms of an illness in the person under her or his care. Typically, a parent (usually mother) causes illness in her child to indirectly assume the sick role.

❒❒ **In Munchausen by proxy, who is most frequently the perpetrator?**

The mother is reported to be the perpetrator in 95% of the cases, and in the remaining 5% of the cases, it may be the father or baby sitter.

❒❒ **What is the usual profile of a parent perpetrator in Munchausen by proxy?**

The usual profile of a parent perpetrator is that of an apparently very caring, overly concerned, articulate and intelligent person (usually mother) with knowledge and sophistication commensurate with that person's experience in health and childcare fields.

❒❒ **What psychiatric disorders are often seen in perpetrators of Munchausen by proxy?**

Depression, personality disorders and factitious disorders are commonly found in perpetrators of Munchausen by proxy.

❒❒ **How high is the mortality rate in child victims of Munchausen by proxy?**

Mortality rates as high as 9% have been reported in these cases.

❒❒ **Is Munchausen by proxy is considered a form of child abuse?**

Yes. And it is reportable within the limits of state and local laws. A treating physician who fails to report a child victim of this disorder is liable for medical malpractice.

❒❒ **What is the key factor in diagnosing Munchausen by proxy in children?**

If the symptoms disappear promptly once the child victim is removed from the custody of a suspected perpetrator, this should prompt any physician to consider the diagnosis of Munchausen by proxy.

❐❐ In order of frequency, what are the most common presenting symptoms in cases of Munchausen by proxy?

According to the literature review by D. A. Rosenberg, the most common presenting symptoms are bleeding (44%), seizures (42%), CNS depression (19%), apnea (15%), diarrhea (11%), vomiting (10%), fever (10%), and rash (9%).

❐❐ What special challenges are encountered in the treatment of patients with Munchausen by proxy?

Once the diagnosis is suspected, treatment will be similar to any other child abuse case. Treatment priorities include prevention of further abuse, treatment of the victim, and counseling of the perpetrator, usually the mother. Parents must be informed, and the case must be reported to authorities. As the perpetrator usually becomes depressed, and even suicidal after acknowledging child abuse, particular care should be taken in providing proper counseling and follow up. Treatment of the victim will depend upon the type and severity of symptoms. Hospitalization for an intensive work up is usually indicated, while the placement issues are carefully considered. The child is usually removed from the family. Long-term follow up studies of these cases indicate a poor prognosis, and many children reportedly themselves develop factitious disorders in adult life.

❐❐ What are the essential criteria for a diagnosis of anorexia nervosa?

Weight less than 85% of expected; intense fear of fat; disturbance in body image; and amenorrhea for at least 3 cycles.

❐❐ What are the two subtypes of anorexia nervosa?

Restricting type and binge eating/purging type.

❐❐ What are the essential criteria for a diagnosis of bulimia nervosa?

Recurrent episodes of binge eating, recurrent inappropriate compensatory behavior, self-evaluation unduly influenced by body shape & weight, and frequency of binge/purge episodes of at least twice a week for three months.

❐❐ What is the mortality rate for anorexia nervosa?

10-20% over 10-30 years.

❐❐ What are the most common causes of death secondary to anorexia nervosa?

Severe and chronic starvation, sudden death due to cardiac failure, and suicide.

❐❐ What psychiatric disorders have a high rate of comorbidity with bulimia nervosa?

Major depression, substance abuse, and anxiety disorders.

❐❐ What are the criteria for hospitalization in a patient with an eating disorder?

Substantial weight loss (>30%), inability to gain weight during outpatient treatment, metabolic crises, and suicidal crises.

❐❐ What cardiac changes occur with anorexia nervosa?

Cardiac changes include loss of cardiac muscle, and cardiac arrhythmias, including atrial and ventricular premature contractions, prolonged His bundle transmission (prolonged QT interval), and ventricular tachycardia.

❒❒ **What is "Russell's sign"?**

Russell's sign is the presence of calluses on the knuckles secondary to repeated, self-induction of emesis.

❒❒ **What changes occur in the teeth with bulimia nervosa?**

Dental erosion, especially of the front teeth, with corresponding decay (perimolysis).

❒❒ **What changes occur in amylase levels with bulimia nervosa?**

Mild elevation in salivary subtype of amylase.

❒❒ **What are the most common electrolyte disturbances with bulimia nervosa?**

Hypokalemia, hyponatremia, and hypochloremic alkalosis occur in bulimia nervosa secondary to excessive emesis and consequent loss of hydrogen and chloride ions.

❒❒ **What is the most common skin change that is associated with anorexia nervosa?**

Presence of lanugo hair.

❒❒ **What changes in the gastrointestinal system are seen in anorexia nervosa?**

Diminished motility, delayed gastric emptying, bloating, constipation, acute gastric dilation or gastric rupture, and abdominal pain.

❒❒ **What role may fluoxetine play in the treatment of anorexia nervosa?**

Fluoxetine may reduce the risk of relapse among patients with anorexia nervosa who have gained weight. It may also be used to treat comorbid depression.

❒❒ **What event usually precedes the onset of both anorexia nervosa and bulimia nervosa?**

Both illnesses typically follow a period of dieting.

❒❒ **What medical complications may develop if ipecac is ingested?**

Cardiomyopathy and toxic myopathy. Cardiac failure caused by cardiomyopathy from ipecac intoxication may occur and usually results in death.

❒❒ **What are the signs and symptoms of ipecac intoxication?**

Symptoms of precordial pain, dyspnea, generalized muscle weakness associated with hypotension, tachycardia, abnormalities in the electrocardiogram, elevated liver enzymes and elevated erythrocyte sedimentation rate.

❒❒ **If an alcoholic patient comes into the ER, which should you give first, thiamine or glucose?**

It doesn't matter even if thiamine is administered first, it takes longer for it to enter cells. The immediate order of these two AMS antidotes is not a clinically issue.

❒❒ **If a patient has a blood alcohol level of 200mg% how long would it take to reach zero?**

The answer is 14.3 hours. Alcohol will decrease approximately 15 mg% per hour. As a rule of thumb, avoid treating alcohol withdrawal at a blood alcohol level greater than 150 mg%.

❒❒ **What is delirium tremens?**

Delirium tremens is an acute, reversible organic psychosis beginning approximately 72 hours after the last drink. It is associated with hallucinations, disorientation and seizures, and may last 2-6 days.

❒❒ **Name the most common causes of death related to cocaine.**

The most common causes of cocaine–related deaths include sudden death by myocardial infarction, cerebral vascular accident, and sequelae of the Muelleris maneuver (pneumothorax caused by exhaling against a closed glottis).

❒❒ **If a patient describes flashbacks, what is the most likely drug used?**

PCP. In the DSM IV, the term for flashbacks is hallucinogen persistent perceptual disorder.

❒❒ **Describe the treatment of common medical problems associated with PCP.**

For tachycardia and hypertension associated with PCP, administer a beta-blocker. Lorazepam is useful for agitation, while haloperidol can be used to treat psychotic symptoms. For intoxication, use ammonia chloride to acidify the urine, and to increase the excretion of PCP. Lasix can be added to cause diuresis.

❒❒ **Name substances in which acidification and alkalization of the urine is used to increase elimination from the body.**

Acidification is never recommended!
Use alkalinization: phenobarbital and salicylates.

❒❒ **A teenager is brought to the emergency room by his/her parents, and during the exam you discover a strange odor on his/her breath. What do you make of it?**

You need to consider inhalant abuse, i.e., huffing. Also look for a rash near the nose and mouth.

❒❒ **A patient is noted to have conjunctival injection. What drug of abuse should you suspect?**

Marijuana.

❒❒ **What is tachyphylaxis?**

Tachyphylaxis is the development of tolerance after a single dose (or repeated doses) of a substance. It particularly pertains to nicotine.

❒❒ **What is the most addicting substance of abuse?**

Nicotine.

❒❒ **Discuss the relationship of age to suicide risk.**

Suicide rates increase steadily with age, with the highest rates among older white males. In the U.S. , the suicide rate for individuals over the age of 65 is 50% higher than that of the general population. While the highest rates occur among older people, it is important to note that suicide rates have been increasing among adolescents and young adults (15-24 years). Higher rates among the elderly may be associated with increased medical problems and the emotional losses common in these later years of life.

❒❒ **Discuss the incidence of suicide among adolescents.**

Suicide is the third leading cause of death among adolescents 15-19 years old (gunshot wounds and motor vehicle accidents being the first and second leading cause of death). The rate of suicide among this age group has tripled in last three decades, and is attributed to an increase in alcohol abuse and greater availability of firearms.

❏❏ List important risk factors for suicide.

A useful mnemonic for suicide risk factors is the phrase SAD PERSONS.

S= Sex: Men are three times as likely as women to complete suicide, however women are four times more likely than men to attempt.
A= Age: Suicide rates are higher among older persons.
D= Depression: 10-15% of persons with a major affective disorder commit suicide.

P= Previous Attempts: Persons with previous suicide attempts are more likely to complete suicide.
E= Ethanol/Drug Abuse: Alcohol and drug use are associated with 50% of all suicides.
R= Rational Thinking Loss: The risk of suicide increases with the presence of psychosis or confusion.
S= Social Supports: Lacking or inadequate.
O= Organized Plan: Individuals with an organized plan are more likely to complete suicide.
N= No Spouse: Suicide rates are higher among those who are divorced, widowed, or never married.
S= Sickness: The presence of a chronic medical condition, particularly when there is significant loss of function or decrease in quality of life increases the risk of suicide.

❏❏ What is the most consistent predictor of suicidal behavior?

A previous suicide attempt.

❏❏ What is confidentiality?

Confidentiality is the long standing, ethical/moral principle that the patient has the right to expect that information provided to a physician will be kept secret and not shared with others.

❏❏ To whom does the duty of confidentiality extend?

The duty of confidentiality extends to the patient. If a physician shares this information they may be liable for breach of that duty and may be sued by the patient. The expectation of confidentiality does not extend to other caregivers and consultants as they require information to treat the patient. The supervision of physicians in training, especially psychiatrists, presents an interesting issue about the extent of the duty.

❏❏ When, if ever, may you breach confidentiality?

Confidentiality may be breached when a patient tells a physician about plans to murder or harm a specific person (doesn't apply to past crimes); when there is a life-threatening emergency, at which time information necessary to maintain the patient's life may be provided to another provider; when subpoenaed by a court of law to provide testimony; when given permission, preferably in writing, by the patient; and when child abuse is suspected.

❏❏ If you receive a call from a hospital about a patient you are treating, can you acknowledge that they are your patient and provide information about their diagnosis, medication and treatment?

Usually you can not disclose or even acknowledge that you are treating a patient for a mental disease or defect without the prior consent of the patient. Most courts will carve out an exception for the provision of emergency information to treat a patient in an emergency situation (e.g., types and dosages of a patient that is unable to provide the information or may be having a drug reaction). It good practice to obtain the patient's consent to such disclosure as soon as possible afterwards.

❏❏ May you disclose the diagnosis and medications of a patient who is covered by an insurance company, so that you can be reimbursed for your services already rendered to the patient?

You can not disclose such information to a third party such as an insurance company or employer, even if it means you will not be paid for your services, unless you have a prior written consent from your patient for the disclosure of such information to that particular party.

❑❑ What are the diagnostic criteria for neuroleptic malignant syndrome (NMS)?

The diagnostic criteria for NMS include treatment with a neuroleptic medication within the last seven days (or 2-4 weeks for depot neuroleptics), hyperthermia ($\geq 38^\circ$ C), muscle rigidity, and three of the following seven sets of symptoms: mental status changes, tachycardia, hypertension or hypotension, tachypnea or hypoxia, elevation of CPK or myoglobinuria, leukocytosis, and metabolic acidosis. Finally the presence of a drug-induced, systemic or neuropsychiatric illness should be excluded.

❑❑ What other agents can cause a syndrome similar to NMS?

Lithium (especially in combination with neuroleptics), tricyclic antidepressants, monoamine oxidase inhibitors, sympathomimetics (amphetamines, cocaine, and fenfluramine), psychedelics (PCP, LSD), anticholinergics, dopamine depleting agents (such as tetrabenazine and reserpine) and dopamine antagonists (such as metoclopramide) can cause NMS-like syndromes. In addition, patients with Parkinson's disease and other basal ganglia disorders can exhibit an NMS-like syndrome when abruptly withdrawn from dopamine agonists like levodopa.

❑❑ Fatal hyperthermia is associated with what medication group?

Fatal hyperthermia is associated with neuroleptics, especially those with high anticholinergic side effects. Hot weather, alcohol ingestion, and CNS disorders are also risk factors for this condition.

❑❑ What neuroleptics lower the seizure threshold?

Chlorpromazine and clozapine significantly reduce the seizure threshold.

❑❑ Which antidepressants have a relatively higher incidence of seizures associated with them?

Bupropion, clomipramine, and maprotiline.

❑❑ How should neuroleptic-induced acute akathisia be treated?

Akathisia can be treated by reducing the antipsychotic dosage, or by addition of propranolol, benzodiazepines, or clonidine. Anticholinergics, amantadine, or clonidine can also be tried.

❑❑ How should neuroleptic-induced tardive dyskinesia be treated?

Reduce or stop the antipsychotic if possible. Switching to clozapine may be indicated. One could also try vitamin E, or high dose buspirone. For treatment of both the psychosis and tardive dyskinesia, use of lithium, carbamazepine, or benzodiazepines is possible.

❑❑ What are the risk factors for neuroleptic malignant syndrome?

Young males; use of high potency, conventional antipsychotics; use of high doses of antipsychotics; and rapid increases in the dose.

❑❑ What is the mortality rate with neuroleptic malignant syndrome?

15 to 30%.

❑❑ How should neuroleptic malignant syndrome be treated?

Discontinue the antipsychotic, cool the patient, provide supportive therapy, and monitor carefully (including vitals, urine output). Use of bromocriptine (dopamine receptor agonist) and dantrolene (direct acting skeletal muscle relaxant) to reduce muscle spasms may be indicated.

GU PEARLS

Trust only movement. Life happens at the level of events not of words. Trust movement.
Alfred Adler

❑❑ **Describe acute glomerulonephritis (GN).**

Hematuria.
Proteinuria.
Oliguria or Anuria.
Edema.
Hypertension.

❑❑ **Let us mention some diseases that cause glomerular dysfunction (skip this one if you are in a hurry!) -**

Goodpasture's syndrome - pulmonary hemorrhage with hemoptysis followed by anti-glomerular basement membrane antibody induced glomerulonephritis.

Post-infectious GN - most commonly post-streptococcal (group A, ß- hemolytic) but may follow other infections with GN secondary to immune complex deposits in glomeruli.

Polyarteritis Nodosa (PAN)- A systemic necrotizing vasculitis affecting primarily medium and small caliber arteries particularly at bifurcations and branchings. PAN occurs from infancy to old age with a peak incidence near age 60. 90% of patients with PAN develop renal involvement.

Systemic Lupus Erythematosus - Autoimmune disorder resulting, in part, in necrotizing vasculitis of primarily small vessels complicated by direct immunoglobulin deposits in glomeruli; mortality range 18-58% depending on histologic type.

Henoch-Schönlein Purpura (HSP) - another systemic necrotizing vasculitis of small vessels with typical renal presentation of nephrotic syndrome without edema or hypertension, or with hematuria.

Hemolytic Uremic Syndrome (HUS) - microangiopathic hemolytic anemia, thrombocytopenia and renal dysfunction with rapid onset in children about 1 wk after gastroenteritis or URI. May occur in adults, most commonly complicating pregnancy or postpartum period. Acute renal failure develops in ~ 60% of children with HUS, most of which resolve in weeks with only supportive therapy.

Thrombotic Thrombocytopenic Purpura (TTP) - closely related to HUS with higher occurrence in young adults and association with fevers, more neurologic problems and less renal involvement, usually with hematuria and proteinuria. TTP prognosis is much worse than HUS with 75% 3-mo mortality.

❑❑ **What is the mortality for patients with acute renal failure?**

About 65%.

❑❑ **ATN resulting from 2 different mechanisms is the <u>most common</u> cause of intrinsic renal failure. Name the 2 mechanisms.**

Ischemic injury and nephrotoxic agents.

❑❑ **Name some common drugs/substances that can contribute to renal failure.**

Aminoglycosides, NSAIDs, contrast agents, myoglobin.

❑❑ Can a selected group of women with a UTI probably be treated safely with single dose or short-course (3 d) antibiotic therapy with TMP/SMX?

Yes; those with few "priors", short period of UTI symptoms and no risk factors for subclinical pyelonephritis.

❑❑ What are the risk factors for subclinical pyelonephritis?

Those are the things that make someone more likely to have it. They include multiple prior UTIs, longer duration of sx, recent pyelonephritis, diabetes, anatomic abnormalities, immunocompromised patients and in those who are indigent.

❑❑ The "rule of twos" is a wonderful pearl described by Dr. David S. Howes of the University of Illinois which explains outpatient management for appropriate women who present at that institution with uncomplicated pyelonephritis. Outline the "rule of twos."

Give 2 L of IV fluid.
Give 2 Tylenol #3.
Give 2 g ceftriaxone.
If patient can tolerate 2 glasses of water and fever decreases by 2 degrees:
Give TMP/SMX Double strength bid for 2 weeks, plan f/u in 2 d for progress check.

Ed. note: Not exactly my practice, but a great rule! JNA

❑❑ About what percentage of patients with epididymitis will have pyuria?

24%.

❑❑ Contrast the pain associated with epididymitis to that of prostatitis.

Epididymitis -pain begins in scrotum or groin radiates along spermatic cord, often intensifies quickly after onset, may be associated with dysuria and may be relieved by scrotal elevation.
Prostatitis -acute prostatitis is associated with more frequency, dysuria and urgency, bladder outlet obstruction and retention, low back and perineal area pain associated with fever and chills, and with arthralgias and myalgias.

Patients with either of these disorders may become toxic and require admission.

❑❑ T/F: Incidence of testicular torsion is bimodal with peak occurrence rates in the first year of life and again near puberty.

True.

❑❑ T/F: Testicular torsion often occurs after exertion or during sleep.

True.

❑❑ T/F: About 40% of patients with testicular torsion have a history of a similar pain that resolved spontaneously.

True.

❑❑ With what condition is the "blue dot" sign associated?

Torsion of the testicular appendage, also of the epididymis.

❑❑ What is the eponym for idiopathic scrotal gangrene?

Fournier's gangrene.

❑❑ A penile fracture is actually a rent of the tunica albuginea and requires surgery to appose the ends of the tunica and to evacuate the hematoma. Is a retrograde urethrogram necessary in the evaluation of a patient with this injury?

Yes, though uncommon, the urethra can be disrupted.

❑❑ What is the initial treatment for priapism?

Terbutaline 0.25-0.5 mg SQ q 4 - 6 h.

❑❑ What are most renal calculi made out of?

70% of renal calculi are composed of calcium oxalate.

❑❑ About what percentage of renal stones are radiopaque?

90%.

❑❑ About what percentage of renal calculi will pass spontaneously?

90%.

❑❑ What is the most common infectious cause of the hemolytic uremic syndrome?

E. coli (O157:H7).

❑❑ What is the diagnostic triad for HUS?

Microangiopathic anemia, acute renal failure and thrombocytopenia.

❑❑ What is the prognosis for patients with acute renal failure secondary to HUS?

Over 90% survival with many patients eventually recovering normal renal function.

❑❑ What is the role of corticosteroids in the treatment of HUS?

None.

❑❑ What are the indications for emergency hemodialysis?

Elevated potassium with ECG changes, decreased pH, pericarditis, mental status changes and severe volume overload.

❑❑ What are the most common etiologies of chronic renal failure leading to dialysis in the U.S.?

Hypertensive and diabetic renal disease.

❑❑ What is the most common cause of acute renal failure?

Acute tubular necrosis. This occurs after toxic or ischemic renal injuries.

❑❑ What is Fournier's gangrene?

Fournier's gangrene is a polymicrobial infection of the subcutaneous tissue of the perineum characterized by widespread tissue necrosis. Treatment consists of broad-spectrum parenteral antibiotics and immediate surgical debridement.

❒❒ **What clinical findings are seen with acute glomerulonephritis (GN)?**

1) Oliguria
2) Hypertension
3) Urine sediment containing RBCs, WBCs, protein and RBC casts
4) Edema

❒❒ **What is the most common cause of post-infectious GN?**

Post streptococcal Group A beta-hemolytic glomerulonephritis. The GN is caused by immune complex deposition in glomeruli. Most patients completely recover normal renal function, spontaneously, within a few weeks.

❒❒ **What syndrome is characterized by an anti-glomerular basement membrane antibody induced GN that is preceded by pulmonary hemorrhage and hemoptysis?**

Goodpasture's syndrome.

❒❒ **What are some causes of false positive hematuria?**

Food coloring, beets, paprika, rifampin, phenothiazine, phenytoin, myoglobin or menstruation.

❒❒ **A urinalysis reveals RBC casts and dysmorphic RBCs. What is the probable origin of hematuria?**

Glomerulus.

❒❒ **What are the admission criteria for patients with renal calculi?**

Infection with concurrent obstruction, a solitary kidney and complete obstruction, renal insufficiency, uncontrolled pain, intractable emesis or large stones. Only 10% of stones > 6 mm pass spontaneously.

❒❒ **What is the most common cause of nephrotic syndrome in children? In adults?**

Children: Minimal change disease. Adults: Idiopathic glomerulonephritis.

❒❒ **What are some common nephrotoxic agents?**

Aminoglycoside, NSAIDs, contrast dye and myoglobin.

❒❒ **When is a retrograde urethrogram necessary to evaluate a patient with a penile fracture?**

Patients with hematuria, blood at the urethral meatus or the inability to void should undergo this procedure to rule out a urethral injury. A penile fracture is rupture of the corpus cavernosum with tearing of the tunica albuginea. It occurs as a result of a blunt trauma to the erect penis. Urethral injury occurs in approximately 10% of patients with a penile fracture.

❒❒ **What are the causative organisms of prostatitis?**

E. coli (80%), *Klebsiella, Enterobacter, Proteus* and *Pseudomonas.*

❒❒ **What is the anatomical approach to ARF?**

Ask whether the site is pre-, intra-, or post-renal. Pre-renal is due to hypovolemia, intra-renal is mostly due to ATN or toxins and post-renal is due to obstruction.

❒❒ **What is the most common cause of intrinsic (intra-) renal failure?**

Acute tubular necrosis (80 to 90%), resulting from an ischemic injury (the most common cause of ATN) or from a nephrotoxic agent. Less frequent causes of intrinsic renal failure (10 to 20%) include vasculitis, malignant hypertension, acute GN or allergic interstitial nephritis.

❒❒ If a urine dipstick is positive for blood, but a urine analysis is negative for RBCs, what is the likely explanation?

Rhabdomyolysis. Severe muscle damage results in free myoglobin in the blood. Very high levels lead to acute renal failure when myoglobin is filtered in the kidneys.

❒❒ What is the most common manifestation of Goodpasture's disease?

Hemoptysis. These patients usually develop pulmonary hemorrhage before any signs of renal failure develop.

❒❒ What is the diagnostic triad of the nephrotic syndrome?

Edema, hyperlipidemia and proteinuria with hypoproteinemia.

❒❒ What do patient's with sickle cell trait most commonly present with?

Hematuria and decreased urine concentrating ability. AKA (isosthenuria).

EMS PEARLS

"Houston, Tranquillity Base here. The Eagle has landed."
Neil Armstrong, radio transmission to Mission Control, at the moment of the first manned landing on the moon, 7/20/1969.

❒❒ **About what percentage of normal coronary blood flow is achieved during CPR?**

5%.

❒❒ **About what percentage of normal cardiac output is achieved during CPR?**

20-25%.

❒❒ **What is the currently favored theory explaining how CPR works?**

The thoracic pump theory - that blood flow is induced by a pressure gradient between the intrathoracic and extrathoracic compartments.

❒❒ **About what percentage of patients who undergo cardiac resuscitation attempts recover and are neurologically intact?**

10%.

❒❒ **About what percentage of patients who undergo cardiac resuscitation attempts survive, but are not functionally and neurologically intact?**

25%.

❒❒ **Intracellular accumulation of what electrolyte is currently thought to initiate a cascade of events that lead to cell death?**

Calcium.

❒❒ **EOA is contraindicated in patients less than how old?**

16 years.

❒❒ **Catheter over needle puncture/ventilation, rather than cricothyroidotomy is recommended for patients under how many years of age?**

10 years.

❒❒ **Uncuffed ET tubes should be selected for patients under how old?**

6 years.

❒❒ **What is the most common complication of EOA use?**

Insertion into the trachea (about 10%).

❑❑ **T/F: When a patient arrives in the ED with an EOA the first thing the ED physician should do is remove the EOA and replace it with an endotracheal tube.**

False - an endotracheal tube should be placed with the EOA still in position.

❑❑ **What recent development, in the pre-hospital setting, has been documented to show improvement in cardiac arrest outcome?**

Automatic External Defibrillator.

❑❑ **EMS systems had an emphasis in their development of managing cardiac arrests. What percent of EMS calls are cardiac arrests?**

<5%.

❑❑ **What percent of an EMS system's call are pediatric?**

10%.

❑❑ **What act or law authorized the U.S. Dept. of Transportation to fund ambulance communication & training programs for pre-hospital medical services?**

1966 National Highway Safety Act. In 1973, Public Law 93-154 defined a goal to improve EMS services on a national scale. This law identified 15 elements.

❑❑ **What are the 3 emergency medical technician levels recognized nationally?**

EMT-A (ambulance), EMT-I (intermediate), EMT-P (paramedic).

❑❑ **What are the 3 main duties of EMS off-line medical director?**

Development of protocols, of medical accountability (quality assurance), and of ongoing education.

❑❑ **How does the American College of Emergency Physicians define a medical disaster?**

Destructive effects of natural or man-made forces that overwhelm the ability of a given area or community to meet health care demands.

❑❑ **What are the 3 phases of a disaster response?**

Activation, implementation, recovery.

❑❑ **What are the 4 categories for a typical triage system?**

Severe, Moderate, Minor, Dead or Expectant Death. Remember, triage is a dynamic process that is ongoing; each patient should be reassessed numerous times.

❑❑ **Who is in command of a disaster scene?**

The chief executive officer or commander. The EMS director acts in support, not command, of public safety agencies with overall scene control.

❑❑ **Who requires hospitals to have a disaster plan? How often should it be tested?**

The Joint Commission on Accreditation of Health Organizations (JCAHO). Test it twice per year.

❑❑ **What are the key points when dealing with a disaster?**

Do the most good for the most number of potential survivors. Don't become a victim yourself. Prioritize patient care. Triage is an ongoing process. Make your plan as close to every day operating procedures as possible. EMS is not in overall scene command.

❒❒ What is the EMT-Intermediate's role in regard to transportation of patients?

He must direct and coordinate the transport of the patient by selecting the best available method(s) in conjunction with medical command authority.

❒❒ After the conclusion of patient transport, what additional duties does the EMT-Intermediate have?

Recording in writing or dictation the details related to the patient's emergency care and the incident, and directing the maintenance and preparation of emergency care equipment and supplies.

❒❒ What are the essential items that citizens need to know about their EMS System?

What care is available from EMS; what EMS is; cost of service; accessing services; first aid.

❒❒ What are the essential items that citizens need to know about first aid?

CPR; hemorrhage control; don't move patient.

❒❒ T/F: Prehospital care is an extension of hospital care.

True.

❒❒ Who may provide on-line medical control?

The medical control physician or physician designee.

❒❒ Who is ultimately responsible for run reviews and quality assurance in an ALS service?

The medical control physician.

❒❒ Every ambulance call consists of three main elements. What are they?

Pre-incident planning, immediate field care, incident follow-up.

❒❒ All EMS vehicles must come up to a specific standard. What is this standard known as?

KKK Standards.

❒❒ All ambulances should be equipped with certain equipment. What is this list known as?

The American College of Surgeons Committee on Trauma Essential Equipment List.

❒❒ What types of circumstances require ambulances to carry additional equipment?

Environment, rescues, geography, special services.

❒❒ The National Standard Curriculum for EMT-Ambulance covers ten skills and knowledge areas. What are they?

CPR; airway and ventilation; hemorrhage control; fracture stabilization; emergency childbirth; extrication; special rescue skills; diagnosis and management; PASG; communication.

❑❑ **The National Standard Curriculum for EMT-Intermediate covers seven skills and knowledge areas. What are they?**

All of EMT-A curriculum content; patient assessment and initial management; EOA; endotracheal intubation and defibrillation (optional); recognition and management of shock; ventilation management; intravenous fluid therapy.

❑❑ **The National Standard Curriculum for EMT-Paramedic covers five skills and knowledge areas. What are they?**

All of EMT-A and EMT-I curriculum content; advanced airway management; medical, including cardiac (AHA-ACLS) and other medical emergencies; advanced trauma management as identified by the American College of Surgeons and American Academy of Orthopedic Surgeons; optional skills and therapeutics.

❑❑ **What knowledge should the EMS dispatcher have?**

He should be knowledgeable of EMT-Intermediate skills and telephone first aid until help arrives.

❑❑ **What three elements go into the decision to dispatch a specific unit?**

Distance, time, and appropriate level of care.

❑❑ **What ranges of frequencies are used for EMS dispatch?**

UHF and VHF.

❑❑ **What types of radio systems are used for physician to EMT communication?**

Simplex, Duplex and Multiplex.

❑❑ **In addition to radio, what other devices can physicians and EMT use to communicate?**

Telemetry, telephone.

❑❑ **In what ways can the EMS system and hospital interface?**

Drug and supply exchange; housing for unit; emergency department observation; education.

❑❑ **What are the first three things the EMT must do on arrival at the scene?**

Scene assessment, patient evaluation, management of life threatening conditions.

❑❑ **What information must the EMT and physician exchange on initial contact?**

Description of situation; description of patient; description of care instituted; physician instruction for additional care.

❑❑ **After initial assessment and treatment, what are the next three steps the EMT must complete?**

Completion of physician instructions for patient care; preparation for transportation; transportation (trauma-as soon as possible, medical-usually after initial stabilization).

❑❑ **Under what law does the EMT function?**

Medical Practice Act.

❑❑ Does the EMT function under federal, state or local law?

State and sometimes local.

❑❑ With which particular aspect of the Medical Practice Act should the EMT be particularly familiar?

The delegation of practice.

❑❑ What must the EMT know in relation to the Good Samaritan Act?

How it differs from state to state, its limitations, and the particular state act.

❑❑ What are the four main areas with which state EMS legislation deals?

Scope of practice; licensure, regulations and certification; medical control; protocols and communications.

❑❑ What must the EMT know about motor vehicle laws?

That they vary considerably from state to state. It is mandatory that the EMT-Intermediate is familiar with appropriate state statutes regarding operation of emergency vehicles.

❑❑ What are the six steps in the progression of a typical EMS event?

Occurrence, detection, notification and response, treatment and preparation for transport, transport and delivery, preparation for next event.

❑❑ What are the four communications links in the EMS chain?

Party requesting help and dispatcher; dispatcher and EMT-Intermediate team; dispatcher and public safety units, local hospitals, and other community agencies; EMT-Intermediate in the field and receiving hospital and/or medical control physician.

❑❑ What are two ways in which a party requesting help can communicate with a dispatcher?

Via the public telephone system—preferably 911 or some other widely publicized emergency number, or via non-public telephone or radio from another emergency agency, such as police or fire.

❑❑ In what ways can the dispatcher communicate with the EMT team?

Telephone notification, voice radio communication, or radio paging.

❑❑ What kinds of communication should take place between the EMT team and the receiving hospital and/or medical control physician?

Early alert of hospital to incoming patients; receiving advice regarding transport and orders for medical treatment; telemetry transmissions.

❑❑ Name some of the components of complex radio communications systems.

Remote consoles, high power transmitters; repeaters, satellite receivers; tower mounted antennas; high power, multi-frequency vehicle radios; mobile transmitter steering; vehicular repeaters; mobile encode-decode capabilities; mobile digital terminals; microwave.

❑❑ What is the power output range of the typical base station transmitter?

45 to 275 watts.

❑❑ **Where can you find the maximum allowable base station power rating?**

It is printed on the Federal Communications Commission radio station license.

❑❑ **What is the typical power output range of a mobile transmitter?**

20-50 watts.

❑❑ **What is the typical transmission range for a mobile transmitter over average terrain?**

15-20 miles.

❑❑ **What terrain features increase radio range?**

Flat land or transmissions over water.

❑❑ **What terrain features decrease radio range?**

Mountains, dense foliage, urban areas with tall buildings.

❑❑ **T/F: The term "mobile two-way radio" implies a hand-held device.**

False. Mobile radios are vehicle mounted.

❑❑ **T/F: Radio equipment used for EMS communications typically employs frequency modulation (FM).**

True. FM is less susceptible to interference than AM (amplitude modulation).

❑❑ **What factors can cause interference in the biotelemetry of ECGs?**

Loose ECG electrodes, muscle tremor, 60-cycle hum, and fluctuations in transmitter power.

❑❑ **What is the "echo" procedure in radio communications?**

The "echo procedure" involves the repetition of important information to ensure it has been understood, and should be used when receiving directions from the dispatcher or physician orders. Another term for this is "mirroring."

❑❑ **How can you be sure a radio message was received?**

When completing a transmission, obtain confirmation that your message was received.

❑❑ **Who should develop written protocols?**

The medical group responsible for medical control.

❑❑ **T/F: Written protocols vary greatly from system to system.**

True.

❑❑ **There are twelve sequential items to be covered in the radio report to the receiving physician. What are they?**

Unit call name and number or name of the EMT
Description of scene
Patient's age, sex and approximate weight (if pertinent for drug orders)
Patient's chief complaint and associated symptoms

Brief, pertinent history of the present illness
Pertinent past medical history
Medications and allergies
Physical exam findings
Treatment given so far
Estimated time of arrival at hospital
Name of private medical physician
Await further questions and orders from base physician.

❒❒ **What seven areas should the radio report on the physical exam cover?**

Level of consciousness; vital signs; neuro exam; general appearance and degree of distress; ECG (if applicable); trauma index or Glasgow Coma Scale (if applicable); other pertinent observations, significant positive and negative findings.

ENVIRONMENTAL PEARLS

"He who possesses virtue in abundance may be compared to an infant.
Poisonous insects will not sting him. Fierce beasts will not seize him.
Birds of prey will not strike him....
He may cry all day without becoming hoarse,
This means that his natural harmony is perfect."
Tao-te Ching, 55; Lao Tzu

❒❒ **Above what altitude does acute mountain sickness typically develop?**

8,000 feet.

❒❒ **What organ is most commonly affected in a radiation accident?**

The skin. Burns may take up to two weeks to become clinically apparent.

❒❒ **What is the LD_{50} for a radiation victim?**

The dose causing death in 50% of patients at 60 days is 450 rads; the LD_{90} is 700 rads.

❒❒ **What is the clinical significance of fixed and dilated pupils in a drowning victim?**

Don't give up the ship! 10% to 20% of patients presenting in coma with fixed and dilated pupils recover completely. Asymptomatic patients should be observed for a minimum of 4 to 6 hours.

❒❒ **What blood gas findings are expected in a drowning victim?**

Poor perfusion and hypoxia result in metabolic acidosis.

❒❒ **Are abdominal thrusts (Heimlich maneuver) indicated in a drowning victim?**

No. Drowning victims usually aspirate small quantities of water and no drainage procedure has been found helpful.

❒❒ **What percentage of dog and cat bites become infected?**

About 10% of dog and 50% of cat bites become infected. *Pasteurella multocida* infects 30% of dog and 50% of cat bites.

❒❒ **A six year-old child presents with headache, fever, malaise, and tender regional lymphadenopathy about a week after a cat bite. A tender papule develops at the site. Diagnosis?**

Cat-scratch disease. Usually develops 3 days to 6 weeks following a cat bite or scratch. The papule typically blisters and heals with eschar formation or a transient macular or vesicular rash may develop.

❒❒ **What is the most likely cause of an infection from an animal bite that develops in less than 24 hours? More than 48 hours?**

Less than 24 hours is typically *P. multocida* or *streptococci*. More than 48 hours is usually *S. aureus.*

❒❒ A patient presents with two minute puncture wounds, a halo lesion is present with a circular area of pallor surrounded by a ring of erythema. Diagnosis?

Black widow spider envenomation.

❒❒ Describe the presentation of a black widow spider versus a scorpion envenomation?

Black widow victims typically stay in one position for a few seconds to minutes before moving, they also have a halo lesion. Scorpion victims present with a constant writhing and abnormal eye movements.

❒❒ What are the indications for giving antivenin in a black widow spider envenomation?

Severe pain, dangerous hypertension, pregnant women with moderate to severe envenomations, and pregnant women threatening abortion who are mildly symptomatic after an envenomation. Antivenin should be avoided in patients taking beta-adrenergic blocking agents as if anaphylaxis occurs, it will be difficult to treat.

❒❒ When is calcium used in the treatment of black widow envenomations?

Recent literature suggests that calcium provides little if any benefit.

❒❒ Can a scratch from a rattlesnake result in a serious envenomation?

A single puncture wound or scratch has resulted in serious envenomation. Up to 25% of bites do not result in envenomation.

❒❒ At what point should fasciotomy be considered in a rattlesnake bite victim?

Only after documented increased compartment pressure unresponsive to limb elevation, antivenin (5-10 vials), and mannitol (1-2 g/kg IV).

❒❒ Which rattlesnake patients will develop serum sickness following antivenin administration?

Most patients who receive more than five vials will develop serum sickness. Symptoms may range from a mild viral-like to severe urticarial rash and arthralgias. Treatment includes antihistamines, corticosteroids, and analgesics.

❒❒ Is horse serum allergy an absolute contraindication to antivenin administration in a rattlesnake victim?

No. When necessary, antivenin is administered along with intravenous antihistamines and corticosteroids in serious envenomizations)despite horse serum allergy).

❒❒ A patient is brought to the ED with a history of a bite wound inflicted at a mental ward. What bacterium is likely?

Eikenella corrodens is more common in hospitalized and institutionalized patients. Most human bite infections are due *to Staphylococcus aureus* or *Streptococcus.*

❒❒ What is the frequency of eye injuries in lightning strike victims?

Half develop structural eye lesions. Cataracts are the most common and develop within days to years. Unreactive dilated pupils may not signify death as transient autonomic instability may occur.

❒❒ What is the most common otologic injury in a lightning strike victim?

50% have tympanic membrane rupture. Hemotympanum, basilar skull fracture, and acoustic and vestibular deficits may also occur.

❑❑ What is the most common arrhythmia found in a patient with hypothermia?

Atrial fibrillation. Other ECG findings include PAT, prolongation of the P-R, QRS, or Q-T, decreased P-wave amplitude, T-wave changes, PVCs, or humped ST segment adjacent to the QRS complex (Osborne wave).

❑❑ What is the first-line treatment of ventricular fibrillation in a hypothermic patient?

Bretylium NOT lidocaine.

❑❑ A near-drowning victim presents to the ED. What electrolyte abnormalities are expected?

Electrolyte abnormalities are usually not significant.

❑❑ What antibiotics and what steroid dose are indicated in the ED for a near-drowning victim?

Trick question. Prophylactic antibiotics and steroids are not useful for preventing aspiration pneumonia or pulmonary edema. Steroids may be used for increased ICP.

❑❑ A 14 year-old football player presents to the ED with a history of light-headedness, headache, nausea, and vomiting. On exam, the patient has a HR of 110, RR 22, BP of 90/60, and is afebrile. Profuse sweating is noted. Diagnosis?

Heat exhaustion. Treat with 0.9% NS IV fluid.

❑❑ A 23 year-old marathon runner presents confused and combative. Temperature is 105° C. Why must renal function be monitored?

This patient has heatstroke. Rhabdomyolysis may occur 2-3 d post-injury. Recall that in heatstroke volume depletion and dehydration may not always occur.

❑❑ Treatment of heatstroke?

Cool sponging, ice packs to groin and axilla, fanning, and iced gastric lavage. Antipyretics are not useful.

❑❑ A 12 year-old male presents with complaints of fatigue, fever, headache, itching rash, and joint aches. Exam reveals multiple sites of lymphadenopathy. The patient cannot recall any past medical problems. Just as you are about to leave the room, scratching your head, mom says "Oh doctor, he was stung by a bee 2 wk ago. Is that important?" Diagnosis?

Serum-sickness-like delayed reaction.

❑❑ How should a honeybee's stinger be removed?

Scrape it out. Squeezing with a tweezers or finger may increase envenomation.

❑❑ A 4 year-old presents with an itching lesion on the legs and waist. On exam, you find hemorrhagic puncta surrounded by urticarial and erythematous patches following a zigzag pattern. Treatment?

Starch baths at bedtime are used to treat pruritus of flea bites.

❑❑ A 16 year-old presents with intense itching of the penis and the web spaces of his hands. Diagnosis?

Scabies frequently attacks the web spaces of the hands and feet. Small vesicles and papules may be present. Scabies does not occur above the neck region in adults (it may in children).

❑❑ **A 6 year-old in Texas presents with a history of being bitten by a caterpillar. The child has tense rhythmic pain. Edema and a red blotchy rash are apparent at the site as well as a white vesicle. Diagnosis and treatment?**

Megalopyge opercularis larva (puss caterpillar) sting. Remove remaining spines with sticky-tape and treat with 10 mL of 10% calcium gluconate IV.

❑❑ **A color blind 36 year-old Texan presents with a history of snake bite. He says the snake was as big as a telephone pole, had fangs like a lion, and was striped like a zebra. On exam, you find ptosis, slurred speech, dysphagia, myalgia, and dilated pupils. What snake bit this man?**

Most likely a coral snake (Micrurus sp.).

❑❑ **Should blisters be débrided for a burn victim?**

YES. They contain vasospastic agents and should be drained.

❑❑ **An Osborne (J) wave seen on ECG is associated with what disorder?**

Hypothermia.

❑❑ **Hypothermia is defined as a core temperature below:**

35° C.

❑❑ **Heat loss can occur via radiation, convection, conduction and evaporation. Which of these accounts for the greatest loss?**

Radiation, followed by convection when not perspiring.
If immersed, conduction causes the greatest heat loss.

❑❑ **A 4 year-old bites into an extension cord and receives a burn on the lips. What specific concern do you have?**

Delayed rupture of the labial artery may occur 3-5 d post-injury.

❑❑ **Compare the entrance and exit wounds of AC and DC.**

AC - Entrance and exit wounds same size.
DC - Small entrance and large exit.
NB. - Not all texts agree!

❑❑ **How is a sodium metal wound débrided?**

Cover with mineral oil and excise retained metal fragments. Never rinse with water! Sodium metal will ignite when it comes in contact with water.

❑❑ **Is lightning AC or DC?**

DC. May cause asystole and respiratory arrest.

❑❑ **What type of arrhythmia is expected with AC shock?**

V-fib.

❒❒ **Can lightning strike twice in the same place?**

Yes. Yes.

❒❒ **Why should the ears be examined in a lightning strike victim?**

TM rupture (50%). Associated with basilar skull fracture.

❒❒ **For how long should an asymptomatic lightning strike victim be monitored?**

Several hours as CHF may be delayed. Serial enzymes if EKG changes or chest pain.

❒❒ **What neurologic injury may be expected in a lightning injury?**

Lower and upper extremity paralysis due to vascular spasm.

❒❒ **What lab work-up should be considered in a lightning victim?**

CBC, BUN/Cr, UA (Check myoglobin), CPK -MM & MB, EKG, and CT if change in sensorium.

❒❒ **What eye finding is associated with lightning strike?**

Cataracts.

❒❒ **A patient presents with a history of headache, nausea, vomiting, and weakness. They also feel lightheaded. In addition to gastroenteritis, what other diagnosis should always be considered?**

CO poisoning.

❒❒ **What is the most common cause of death with CO poisoning?**

Cardiac arrhythmias.

❒❒ **How is topical phenol exposure treated?**

Water and olive oil can be useful in the field. Isopropyl alcohol, glycerol, or polyethylene glycol mixture in the ED for carbolic acid exposure.

❒❒ **In what two plant ingestions is ipecac contraindicated?**

Jequirity bean (alkaline) and hemlocks sp. (may induce seizures).

❒❒ **How is frostnip treated?**

Frostnip is the only form of frostbite that can be treated at the scene. It is treated by warming the affected area(s) by hand, by breathing on the skin or by placing the exposed extremities in the armpit. The affected part should not be rubbed because this action does not thaw the tissues completely.

❒❒ **What is appropriate treatment for frostbite?**

The exposed extremity should be rewarmed rapidly by immersing the affected area in 42° C circulating water for 20 minutes or until flushing is observed. Do not use dry heat. Refreezing thawed tissue greatly increases damage. Remember to provide tetanus prophylaxis. Débride white or clear blisters because toxic mediators (prostaglandin and thromboxanes) may be present. However, leave hemorrhagic blisters intact. Topical antibiotics, such as silver sulfadiazine, may be used.

❑❑ **What are some common complications of frostbite?**

Rhabdomyolysis, permanent depigmentation of the extremity, an increased probability of a subsequent injury caused by cold conditions, and cold intolerance.. Extremity frostbite may result in later x-ray findings of irregular, fine, punched-out lytic lesions on the MTP, PIP and DIP joints.

❑❑ **What are the four degrees of frostbite?**

First degree:	Erythema and edema.
Second degree:	Blister formation.
Third degree:	Necrosis.
Fourth degree:	Gangrene.

❑❑ **What complications are associated with hypothermia?**

Coagulopathy, confusion, disorientation, decreased immune response, platelet dysfunction, reduced cardiac function, decreased cardiac output, vasoconstriction and hypotension.

❑❑ **What measures can be instituted to treat hypothermia?**

Increasing the room temperature, using intravenous fluid and blood warmers, heating ventilator gases and using warming blankets.

❑❑ **As the patient re-warms, what problems can arise?**

Development of metabolic acidosis, shivering, hypotension, tachycardia, and DIC.

❑❑ **A patient's temperature is 30° Celsius. During cardiac arrest defibrillation was unsuccessful. What treatment is recommend?**

Active warming should precede further defibrillation attempts and medication administration.

❑❑ **What are the effects of hypothermia on the central nervous system?**

Mild hypothermia (32 to 35° C) will decrease cerebral metabolic rate by 15 to 20%, which combined with general anesthesia will provide some degree of protection against hypoxia and ischemia. The MAC of volatile agents is reduced by approximately 5% for every degree centigrade reduction in body temperature. Hypothermia is associated with delayed emergence from general anesthesia. Body temperatures of less than 30° C can produce narcosis.

❑❑ **What are the cardiovascular side effects of hypothermia?**

When temperature falls below 35° C there is significant vasoconstriction, increasing central blood volume. Further falls in temperature to below 32° C are associated with a decrease in cardiac output and delays in electrical conduction. At temperatures less than 30° C increased ventricular irritability is encountered, with increased danger for ventricular fibrillation. Hypothermia below 28° C is associated with decreased contractility and further reductions to below 20° C results in cardiovascular collapse because of decreased peripheral resistance.

❑❑ **Is respiratory function compromised by hypothermia?**

There are a variety of pulmonary changes associated with hypothermia including a decrease in hypoxic ventilatory drive, attenuation of hypoxic pulmonary vasoconstriction, increased bronchiolar tone and respiratory depression. Hypothermia has been cited as one of the reasons for reintubation in the recovery room following anesthesia.

❑❑ **How does hypothermia affect the metabolism of anesthetic drugs?**

Hypothermia impairs both hepatic and renal functions. Any drug that is dependent on either of these organs for clearance will accumulate. The duration of action of vecuronium and pancuronium are prolonged by hypothermia.

❑❑ **What are the hematologic consequences of hypothermia?**

As body temperature falls, vasomotor tone increases resulting in a increase in plasma volume. This results in a diuresis, the loss of free water resulting in a increase in viscosity. Because of this there tends to be sludging with an increased risk of vascular occlusion. Additionally there is a reversible sequestration of platelets by the reticular endothelial system and decline in platelet function. These two factors together with an inhibition of the coagulation cascade, lead to an increased risk in bleeding.

❑❑ **What are the metabolic consequences of hypothermia?**

There is a temperature dependent decrease in metabolic rate. In addition hypothermia is associated with increased protein catabolism and decreased insulin secretion.

❑❑ **How is renal function affected by hypothermia?**

Renal blood flow is decreased to a greater extent than cardiac output. Initially, there is a cold-induced diuresis because of a decreased secretion of antidiuretic hormone AKA (arginine vasopressin) and an impaired renal reabsorption of sodium. As temperatures fall further, both urine output and renal concentrating ability become impaired.

❑❑ **What are the consequences of shivering?**

Shivering is the rhythmical contraction and relaxation of small muscle groups. It results in a significant increase in oxygen consumption and CO_2 production. If this increase in metabolic activity is not met by increased minute ventilation, respiratory acidosis ensues. If cardiac output is not increased, to meet the increased O_2 demand, then mixed venous oxygen levels will decrease and the patient will possibly develop tissue hypoxia.

❑❑ **Which modalities are available in order to treat shivering?**

The most reliable method to prevent shivering is to prevent intraoperative hypothermia. Conservation of radiant heat loss can prevent shivering. Another method that can be used for skin warming is the forced air exchange blanket. There are pharmacological methods to treat shivering, the most popular being meperidine.

❑❑ **Can warming fluids aid in the prevention of hypothermia?**

Yes. Cold banked blood should always be warmed. Rapid and large volumes of crystalloid or colloid should be warmed. If a massive transfusion is anticipated then a rapid infusion system that can deliver blood at 37°C at rates of 250 to 500 mL/min should be used.

❑❑ **What distinguishes heat stroke from heat exhaustion?**

Heat exhaustion is progressive loss of electrolytes and body fluid depletion. Therapy is rehydration.

Heat stroke occurs when temperatures are above 42° C and enzyme systems cease to function normally. As a result, there is necrosis, denaturing and organ failure. Heat stroke requires much more aggressive treatment than simple fluid rehydration.

Remember - in patients with an altered sensorium and a core temperature above 42° C, always suspect heat stroke. Half of patients will be diaphoretic.

❑❑ **What lab abnormalities may be found with heat stroke?**

Elevations in SGOT, SGPT, LDH, BUN, creatinine, CPK and other indices of rhabdomyolysis. There is almost always some evidence for a bleeding diathesis when the patient truly has heat stroke.

❒❒ **How should a patient with heat stroke be treated?**

1) Cool the patient with cool water and fans.
2) Pack the axillae, neck and groin with ice.
3) Maintain euvolemia.
4) Treat shivering with chlorpromazine (Thorazine) IV.

❒❒ **What complications can result from heat stroke?**

Renal failure, rhabdomyolysis, DIC and seizures. Remember antipyretics will not help.

HEM/ONC PEARLS

"Nature does nothing without a purpose."
Aristotle

❑❑ **Vitamin K dependent factors of the clotting cascade include:**

X, IX, VII and II. REMEMBER 1972.

❑❑ **An adult patient receives a major head injury. He also suffers from classic hemophilia, what treatment should be given?**

Give Factor VIII 50 U/kg.

❑❑ **What is von Willebrand's disease?**

It is an autosomal dominant disorder of platelet function.
It causes bleeding from mucous membranes, menorrhagia and increased bleeding from wounds.
Patients with vW disease have less (or dysfunctional) vW factor.
vW factor is a plasma protein secreted by endothelial cells. vW factor serves two functions - it is required for platelets to adhere to collagen at the site of vascular injury (initial step in forming a hemostatic plug) and it forms complexes in plasma with factor VIII which are required to maintain normal factor VIII levels.

❑❑ **Describe the laboratory features of von Willebrand's disease (PT, PTT, Plt Ct, BT, and Factors).**

PT	- Normal.
PTT	- Prolonged (usually slightly reflecting low factor VIII level).
Plt Ct	- Normal.
BT	- Prolonged.
Factors	- Levels low of VIII-C (coagulation activity), vWF:Ag (immunologic activity) and vWF: activity (platelet aggregation).

❑❑ **What is the treatment for a bleeding patient with von Willebrand's disease (usual type 1 form)?**

Use a vasopressin analog, D-amino-8, D-arginine vasopressin (DDAVP) that stimulates release of vW factor from endothelial stores. This results in increased serum factor VIII levels. (DDAVP is not effective in severe vW disease and is not indicated for the rare type II or type III form, in these cases use cryoprecipitate or Factor VIII).

❑❑ **What lab abnormalities does DIC cause?**

Increased PT, elevated fibrin split products, decreased fibrinogen and thrombocytopenia.

❑❑ **What type of hemophilia results from a deficiency of factor 9, is sex linked and has a positive family history?**

Christmas disease or hemophilia B.

❒❒ **What type of hemophilia has a factor 8 deficiency, is sex linked and may present without a family history?**

Classic hemophilia. Also called hemophilia A, about 1/2 have a family Hx!

❒❒ **What type of hemophilia is autosomal dominant and has a deficiency in factor 8?**

von Willebrand's.

❒❒ **What are the two most common tumors causing ischemic dysfunction of the spinal cord?**

Lymphoma and multiple myeloma.

❒❒ **What is the most effective way to control the bleeding induced by warfarin therapy?**

Fresh frozen plasma provides fast response. Also give vitamin K, intramuscularly. May want to check test dose first.

❒❒ **What laboratory abnormalities would be expected in a patient with platelet dysfunction?**

Abnormal bleeding time with normal PT, normal PTT and normal platelet count. NSAIDs are a common cause of abnormal platelet function.

❒❒ **What are common features of thrombocytopenic purpura?**

Thrombocytopenia, micro-angiopathic hemolytic anemia, fever, renal failure and fluctuating neurologic symptoms. Coagulation studies are typically normal.

❒❒ **What clotting study is typically abnormal with thrombocytopenia?**

Bleeding time.
Usually thrombocytopenia is an acquired disorder secondary to infections, drugs or autoimmune disease. As platelets are not involved in the intrinsic or extrinsic clotting pathways, both PT and PTT remain normal.

❒❒ **Name four conditions that may cause reactive thrombocytosis.**

Iron deficiency, post-splenectomy, malignancy and infection.

❒❒ **Name a special feature of von Willebrand's disease which allows differentiation from classic hemophilia.**

von Willebrand's disease has both a prolonged bleeding time and prolonged PTT, whereas classic hemophilia has only prolonged PTT.

❒❒ **What electrolyte abnormalities are seen in acute tumor lysis syndrome?**

Hyperuricemia secondary to breakdown of nucleic acids.
Hyperkalemia from massive cell lysis.
Hyperphosphatemia because of protein breakdown.
Hypocalcemia secondary to hyperphosphatemia.

❒❒ **What is the treatment for acute tumor lysis syndrome?**

Hydration, alkalinization, allopurinol, and hemodialysis.
The hypocalcemia associated with acute tumor lysis syndrome is secondary to increased phosphate, and should not be treated with calcium. Additional calcium could cause widespread precipitation of calcium phosphate.

❐❐ A patient with lung cancer presents with complaints of nausea, vomiting, weakness, anorexia, and is also experiencing polydipsia and polyuria. What diagnosis is suspected?

Hypercalcemia. The patient has GI, CNS, and renal symptoms which are commonly associated with hypercalcemia in a cancer patient.

❐❐ A cancer patient presents with a history of constipation, decreased mental status, and back pain. What diagnosis is suspected?

Hypercalcemia.

Remember - the signs and symptoms of hypercalcemia include nausea, vomiting, anorexia, constipation, polyuria, hypertension and decreased mentation.

❐❐ What is appropriate treatment for a life threatening level of hypercalcemia of 16 mg per deciliter?

Start giving the patient 0.9 NS at 5 to 10 liters per day. In addition, administer furosemide. A typical dose of Lasix would be 80 mg IV every 1 to 2 h. Watch out for hypokalemia. Consider glucocorticoids if the patient is obtunded or comatose.

The admitting internist may also administer agents to counteract parathyroid hormone which include calcitonin and mithramycin.

❐❐ What factors are deficient in Classic hemophilia, Christmas disease, and von Willebrand's disease, respectively?

Classic hemophilia -	Factor VIII.
Christmas disease -	Factor IX.
Willebrand's disease -	Factor VIIIc + von Willebrand's cofactor.

❐❐ Which pathway involves factors VIII and IX?

Intrinsic pathway.

❐❐ What effect does deficiency of factors VIII and IX have on PT and on PTT?

Deficiency leads to increase in PTT.

❐❐ What pathway does the PT measure and what factor is unique to this pathway?

Extrinsic, factor VII.

❐❐ How may hemophilia A be clinically distinguished from hemophilia B?

Hemophilia A is not clinically distinguishable from Christmas disease (Hemophilia B).

❐❐ Which blood product is given when the coagulation abnormality is unknown?

FFP.

❐❐ What agent can be used for treating mild hemophilia A and von Willebrand's disease type 1?

D-Amino-8, D-arginine vasopressin (DDAVP) induces a rapid rise in factor VIII levels.

❐❐ Major cause of death in hemophiliacs?

Blood component infections (HIV).

❑❑ **What diagnostic tests are available to distinguish SSA from sickle cell trait in the ED?**

None. Sickledex, Sik-L-Stat, SickleScrene, and SCAT are unable to distinguish between trait and disease.

❑❑ **What are the common pathogens causing pneumonia in sickle cell patients?**

S. pneumoniae, *H. influenzae*, alpha-hemolytic streptococcus and salmonella.

❑❑ **What is the most common cause of pneumonia in sickle cell disease?**

Streptococcus pneumoniae.

❑❑ **Below what platelet count is spontaneous hemorrhage likely to occur?**

< 10,000/mm^3.

❑❑ **It is generally agreed that most patients with active bleeding and platelet counts < 50,000/mm^3 should receive platelet transfusion. How much will the platelet count be raised for each unit of platelets infused?**

5,000 to 10,000/mm^3.

❑❑ **How can an overdose of warfarin be treated? What are the advantages and disadvantages of each treatment?**

Fresh frozen plasma (FFP) or vitamin K. If there are no signs of bleeding, temporary discontinuation may be all that is necessary.
FPP advantages: Rapid repletion of coagulation factors and control of hemorrhage.
FPP disadvantages: Volume overload, possible viral transmission.
Vitamin K advantages: Ease of administration.
Vitamin K disadvantages: Possible anaphylaxis when given IV. Delayed onset of 12 to 24 hours. Effects may last up to 2 weeks, making anticoagulation of the patient difficult or impossible.

❑❑ **Which laboratory studies are most helpful in diagnosing DIC?**

1) PT and PTT (prolonged)
2) Platelet count (usually low)
3) Fibrinogen level (low)
4) Presence of D-dimers

❑❑ **What is the most common inherited bleeding disorder?**

Von Willebrand's disease.

❑❑ **Seventy to eighty percent of patients with Von Willebrand's disease have type I. What is the current approved mode of therapy for bleeding in these patients?**

DDAVP.

❑❑ **What is the most common hemoglobin variant?**

Hemoglobin S (valine substituted for glutamic acid in the sixth position on the beta chain).

❑❑ **Which is the most common type of sickle-cell crisis?**

Vaso-occlusive.

❐❐ What percentage of patients with sickle-cell disease have gallstones?

75%.

❐❐ What is the only crystalloid fluid compatible with RBCs?

Normal saline.

❐❐ What condition should be suspected in a patient with multiple myeloma who presents with paraplegia and urinary incontinence?

Acute spinal cord compression. This condition occurs primarily with multiple myeloma and lymphoma and it is also encountered with carcinomas of the lung, breast and prostate.

❐❐ What are the two most common neoplasms that cause pericardial effusion and tamponade?

Carcinoma of the lung and breast.

❐❐ A 48 year-old male smoker presents with a headache, swelling of the face and arms and a feeling of fullness in his face and neck. He is noted to have JVD upon physical examination and papilledema upon funduscopic examination. What is the most likely diagnosis?

Superior vena cava syndrome.

❐❐ What is the most common cause of hyperviscosity syndrome?

Waldenström's macroglobulinemia (IgM myeloma).

❐❐ What should be considered in a patient who presents in a coma and has anemia and Rouleaux formation on the peripheral blood smear?

Hyperviscosity syndrome.

❐❐ What are the major causes of GI bleeding in cancer patients?

Hemorrhagic gastritis and peptic ulcer disease.

❐❐ Pheochromocytomas produce what compounds?

Catecholamines. This group of chemicals result in hypertension, perspiration, palpitations, anxiety and weight loss.

❐❐ If vanillylmandelic acid, normetanephrine and metanephrine are detected in the urine, what is the likely cause?

Pheochromocytoma.

❐❐ What is the rule of "tens" for pheochromocytomas?

10% are malignant, 10% are multiple or bilateral, 10% are extra-adrenal, 10% occur in children, 10% recur after surgical removal and 10% are familial.

❐❐ What are the potential treatment modalities for ITP?

Corticosteroids, gammaglobulin, plasmapheresis and splenectomy.

❐❐ What are the signs and symptoms of splenic sequestration crisis?

Pallor, weakness, lethargy, disorientation, shock, decreased level of consciousness and enlarged spleen.

❑❑ What is the treatment of splenic sequestration crisis?

Rapid infusion of saline and transfusion of red cells.

❑❑ What is the predominant symptom in DIC?

Bleeding.

❑❑ What are some common ischemic complications of DIC?

Renal failure, seizures, coma, pulmonary infarction and hemorrhagic necrosis of the skin.

❑❑ What are the common lab findings in DIC?

Decreased platelets, increased PT and PTT, decreased fibrinogen, increased FDP and D-dimers.

❑❑ G-6-PD deficiency is prevalent in what ethnic groups?

Greeks, southern Italians, Sephardic Jews, Filipinos, southern Chinese, African-Americans and Thailanders.

❑❑ What does Prothrombin Time (PT) measure? How is it performed?

PT measures the extrinsic and common pathways of the coagulation system. The time to clot formation is measured after the addition of thromboplastin. If the concentration of factors II, V, VII, and X are significantly lower than usual, the PT will be prolonged.

❑❑ What does Activated Partial Thromboplastin Time (aPTT) measure? How is it performed?

PTT measures the intrinsic and common pathways of the coagulation cascade. After the blood sample is exposed to celite for activation and a reagent is added, the clot formation is measured. When factors II, V, VIII, IX, X, XI, XII or fibrinogen are deficient, the PTT will be prolonged.

❑❑ What are the indications for the administration of FFP?

1- Replacement of isolated factor deficiencies.
2- Reversal of coumadin effect.
3- Treatment of pathological hemorrhage in patients who have received massive transfusion.
4- Use in antithrombin III deficiency.
5- Treatment of immunodeficiencies.

❑❑ What are the indications for cryoprecipitate administration?

For the treatment of congenital or acquired fibrinogen and factor VIII deficiencies. Cryoprecipitate can also be administered prophylactically for nonbleeding perioperative or peripartum patients with congenital fibrinogen deficiencies or for Von Willebrand's disease that is unresponsive to desmopressin (DDAVP).

❑❑ A patient on chemotherapy for his Burkitt's lymphoma is found to be hyperkalemic, hypocalcemic, hyperphosphatemic and hyperuricemic. What is the presumptive diagnosis?

Tumor lysis syndrome.

❑❑ What are the three phases of type and crossmatch of blood?

The first phase combines recipient serum and donor cells to test ABO group compatibility at room temperature. It identifies M, N, P and Lewis incompatibilities. This phase takes approximately 5 minutes. The second phase incubates the products from the first phase in albumin at 37°C, enhancing incomplete antibodies. The last phase is the antiglobulin test. Antiglobulin serum is added to the previous incubated test tubes. This phase aids in the detection of incomplete antibodies in Rh, Kell, Duffy and Kidd systems.

❏❏ **Which solutions are considered incompatible with PRBC?**

Calcium containing solutions should not be added to blood, particularly at slow infusion rates, because small clots may form due to the presence of calcium in excess of the chelating ability of the citrate anticoagulant.

❏❏ **What are the problems associated with citrate in a massive transfusion?**

Massive transfusions increase citrate levels and decrease ionized calcium levels.

❏❏ **How does renal papillary necrosis that is secondary to sickle cell vaso-occlusion commonly present?**

Painless hematuria.

OB/GYN PEARLS

"A great part, I believe, of the Art is to be able to observe."
Hippocrates (460 - 370 B.C.)

❒❒ **How much blood does a standard size pad absorb?**

20 - 30 mL blood.

❒❒ **How soon after implantation can ß-HCG be detected?**

2-3 days.

❒❒ **What percentage of pregnancies are ectopic?**

1.5%. Ectopic pregnancies are the leading cause of death in the first trimester.

❒❒ **What is the most common presentation of ectopic pregnancy?**

Amenorrhea followed by pain.

❒❒ **How does a spontaneous abortion most commonly present?**

Pain followed by bleeding.

❒❒ **What is the most common finding on pelvic exam in a patient with an ectopic pregnancy?**

Unilateral adnexal tenderness.

❒❒ **Does a negative culdocentesis rule out an ectopic pregnancy?**

No. It only rules out hemoperitoneum.

❒❒ **When can abdominal ultrasound find an intrauterine gestational sac?**

5th week. Fetal pole, 6th week. Embryonic mass with cardiac motion, 7th week.

❒❒ **A 3 mo pregnant patient presents with pelvic pain. On exam, a retroverted and retroflexed uterus is found. What diagnosis should come to mind?**

Incarceration of the uterus. Patients typically complain of rectal and pelvic pressure . Urinary retention may also be found. The knee-chest position or rectal pressure may correct the problem.

❒❒ **What patients with PID should be admitted?**

Pregnant; temperature > 38° C (100.4° F); nausea and vomiting which prohibits po antibiotics; pyosalpinx or tubo-ovarian abscess; peritoneal signs; IUCD present; no response to oral antibiotics; and uncertain diagnosis.

❒❒ **What criteria are necessary for the diagnosis of PID?**

All three of the following: adnexal tenderness, cervical and uterine tenderness, and abdominal tenderness. Also one of the following: T >38° C, endocervix gram stain positive for gram negative intracellular diplococci, leukocytosis greater than 10,000/mm^3, inflammatory mass on US or pelvic, and WBC and bacteria in the peritoneal fluid.

❑❑ **What is the most common cause of toxic shock syndrome?**

The most common cause is *S. aureus*. Other causes which are clinically similar include group A *Streptococci*, *Pseudomonas aeruginosa,* and *Streptococcus pneumoniae.*

❑❑ **What criteria are necessary for the diagnosis of toxic shock syndrome?**

All of the following must be present: T > 38.9° C (102° F), rash, systolic BP < 90 and orthostasis, involvement of three organ systems (GI, renal, musculoskeletal, mucosal, hepatic, hematologic, or CNS), and negative serologic tests for such diseases as RMSF, hepatitis B, measles, leptospirosis, VDRL, etc.

❑❑ **What type of rash is seen with TSS?**

Blanching erythroderma which resolves in 3 d and is followed by a desquamation (full thickness). This typically occurs between the 6th and 14th d with peeling prominent on the hands and feet.

❑❑ **How should a patient with toxic shock syndrome be treated?**

FLUIDS, pressure support, FFP or transfusions, vaginal irrigation with iodine or saline, and antistaphylococcal penicillin or cephalosporin with anti-**ß**-lactamase activity (nafcillin or oxacillin). Rifampin should be considered to eliminate the carrier state.

❑❑ **What anticoagulant should be used in pregnant patients?**

Heparin because it does not cross the placenta.

❑❑ **What antiemetic can be used in pregnant patients?**

Prochlorperazine (Compazine) or trimethobenzamide (Tigan).

❑❑ **What dose of radiation to a fetus increases the risk of inhibiting fetal growth?**

10 rad. A typical abdominal or pelvic film delivers 100 to 350 mrad. A shielded chest x-ray should deliver < 10 mrad to the fetus. Necessary x-rays should not be withheld.

❑❑ **Define preeclampsia.**

HTN after 20 wk EGA with generalized edema or proteinuria.

❑❑ **Define eclampsia.**

Preeclampsia plus grand mal seizures or coma.

❑❑ **Should BP be lowered acutely in a preeclampsia patient?**

Dangerous HTN (>170/110) should be gradually lowered with hydralazine 10 mg IV followed by a drip. Definitive treatment for preeclampsia and eclampsia is delivery.

❑❑ **What level of serum glucose warrants admission in a patient with gestational diabetes?**

Hyperglycemia (>200 mg %) which is persistent requires admission.

❑❑ **Can iodinated radiodiagnostic agents be used in a pregnant patient?**

They should be avoided as concentration in the fetal thyroid can cause permanent loss of thyroid function. Nuclear medicine scans, pulmonary angiography with pelvic shielding, and impedance plethysmography are preferred.

❑❑ What viral or protozoal infections require extensive work-up during pregnancy?

Herpes genitalis, rubella, cytomegalovirus, and Toxoplasma gondii. These patients require full work-ups and referral for genetic counseling.

❑❑ What is the most common cause of vaginitis?

Candida albicans.

❑❑ A 26 year-old female complains of dysuria and mild lower abdominal pain. On pelvic exam, punctate hemorrhages are noted on the cervix. Diagnosis?

Trichomonas vaginitis. The cervix is called "strawberry cervix." The diagnosis can be confirmed by obtaining <u>vaginal vault secretions</u> using the "hanging drip" slide test. The sexual partner must be treated.

❑❑ A wet prep of vaginal secretions reveals clue cells. Diagnosis?

Gardnerella vaginitis. Male partners should be treated.
Sherlock Holmes looks for "clues" in the "Garden."

❑❑ A pregnant patient presents in a coma. The husband indicates the patient has had been itching for a few days, seemed slightly yellow, and earlier in the day her daughter said "Mom was confused". Diagnosis?

Acute fatty liver of pregnancy. Conjugated bilirubin and transaminase levels will be increased.

❑❑ Is appendicitis more common during pregnancy?

No (1/850). Outcome is worse. As pregnancy progresses, the appendix moves, at term it is near the right subcostal margin. The distal end is pointed toward the diaphragm. The WBC count usually does not increase beyond the normal value of 12-15,000. In a pregnant patient, pyuria with no bacteria suggest appendicitis. Pregnant patients may lack GI distress, fever may be absent or low grade.

❑❑ 3 d post-partum a patient presents with fever. On exam, a foul lochia and tender boggy uterus is present. Diagnosis?

Endometritis typically occurs 1-3 d post-partum.

❑❑ Why is Rh status important in a pregnant patient?

Rh negative with Rh positive fetus can result in fetal anemia, hydrops, and fetal loss. Rh immunoglobulin should be given to all Rh negative patients. The usual amount of RhoGAM may be inadequate in the setting of trauma; a Kleihauer-Betke assay can quantitate fetomaternal hemorrhage.

❑❑ What is the expected finding on culdocentesis in a patient with ectopic pregnancy?

Non-clotting blood.

❑❑ When can transvaginal and abdominal ultrasound identify an intrauterine sac?

Transvaginal, 31-32 days. Abdominal, 5 wk.

❐❐ A 24 year-old, 10 w pregnant patient presents with bleeding per vagina. She also complains of nausea, vomiting, and abdominal pain. Physical findings reveal a blood pressure of 150/100 and a uterus which is larger than dates. Lab studies reveal proteinuria. Diagnosis?

Molar pregnancy. Uterus may be larger or smaller than expected dates.

❐❐ An 8 mo pregnant patient presents to the ED with profuse bleeding. What must be ruled out with ultrasound before a pelvic exam is performed?

Placenta previa.

❐❐ Risk factors for placenta previa?

Previous cesarean section, previous placenta previa, multiparity, multiple induced abortions, and multiple gestations.

❐❐ Risk factors for abruptio placenta?

Smoking, hypertension, multiparity, trauma, and previous abruptio placenta.

❐❐ What effect does pregnancy have on: Cardiac output, BP, HR, coagulation, sed rate, leukocytes, blood volume, arterial blood gases, tidal volume, bladder, BUN/CR, and GI.

Cardiac Output	Increases. Moving the uterus off the IVC increases CO 25%.
BP	Falls in second trimester. Returns to normal state in third trimester.
Heart Rate	Increases.
Coagulation	Factors 7, 8, 9, 10, and fibrinogen increase, the others remain unchanged.
Sed Rate	Elevated.
Leukocytes	Increase to as much as 18,000.
Blood volume	Increases, RBC unchanged, dilutional "anemia" is physiologic.
Tidal volume	Increases 40%.
Bladder	Displaced superiorly and anteriorly.
BUN/Cr	Decrease because of increased GFR and renal blood flow.
GI	Gastric emptying and GI motility decrease. Peritoneal signs such as rigidity and rebound are diminished or absent. Alkaline phosphatase is increased.

❐❐ What are the presenting signs and symptoms of abruptio placentae?

Placental separation before delivery is associated with vaginal bleeding (78%), abdominal pain (66%), as well as tetanic uterine contractions, uterine irritability, and fetal death.

❐❐ What dose of oxytocin (Pitocin) should be administered following a postpartum hemorrhage?

20 to 40 units of oxytocin added to 1000 mL normal saline or Ringer's lactate infused at 200 - 500 mL/h.

❐❐ How can ruptured membranes be diagnosed?

Nitrazine paper turns blue and a "ferning" pattern is seen under a microscope in the presence of amniotic fluid.

❐❐ What are the indications for cardiotocography in a trauma patient?

All women past 20 w gestation with indirect or direct abdominal trauma require 4 h of monitoring. Loss of beat-to-beat variability, uterine contractions, or fetal brady- or tachycardia demands immediate obstetrical consultation.

❒❒ Is life threatening hemorrhage due to trauma during pregnancy most often intra- or retroperitoneal?

Retroperitoneal.

❒❒ What type of incision should be used in a post-mortem cesarean section?

Vertical (Classical) incision.

❒❒ What is the normal fetal heart rate?

120 to 160 beats per minute. If bradycardia is detected, position the mother on her left side, give oxygen and an IV fluid bolus.

❒❒ A pregnant patient presents with fetal bradycardia and tetanic contractions. Delivery is not imminent. Treatment?

Tocolytic agents to relax the uterus: magnesium sulfate 4 to 6 g IV over 20 min or terbutaline 0.25 mg subcutaneously.

❒❒ What technique can be used to identify intravaginal semen?

Semen will fluoresce with a Wood's Lamp.

❒❒ How long after intercourse can acid phosphatase be detected?

2-9 hours.

❒❒ How quickly must a patient be treated to provide pregnancy prevention after being raped?

72 hours. Treatment is Ovral, 2 tablets po and 2 tablets 12 hours later.

DERM PEARLS

He: "You have beautiful skin!"
She: "Yes and it covers my whole body."
Woody Allen

❑❑ What type of reaction is erythema multiforme?

Hypersensitivity. Bullae are subepidermal, the dermis is edematous, and a lymphatic infiltrate may be present around the capillaries and venules. In children, infections are the most important cause and in adults, drugs and malignancies. EM is often seen during epidemics of adenovirus, atypical pneumonia, and histoplasmosis.

❑❑ A patient presents with fever, myalgias, malaise, and arthralgias. On exam, findings include bullous lesions of the lips, eyes, and nose. The patient indicates eating is very painful. What should the family be told about the patient's prognosis?

Stevens-Johnson syndrome has a mortality of 5 - 10% and may have significant complications including corneal ulceration, panophthalmitis, corneal opacities, anterior uveitis, blindness, hematuria, renal tubular necrosis, and progressive renal failure. Scarring of the foreskin and stenosis of the vagina can occur. Treatment in a burn unit is supportive; steroids may provide symptomatic relief but are not of proven value, and may be contraindicated.

❑❑ What are the two distinct causes of toxic epidermal necrolysis (scalded skin syndrome)?

Staphylococcal and drugs or chemicals. Both begin with appearance of patches of tender erythema followed by loosening of the skin and denuding to glistening bases. Staphylococcal scalded skin syndrome is commonly found in children less than 5y and is due to toxin that cleaves <u>within the epidermis</u> under the stratum granulosum.

❑❑ What area does Staphylococcal scalded skin syndrome usually affect?

The face around nose and mouth, neck, axillae, and groin. Disease commonly occurs after upper respiratory tract infections or purulent conjunctivitis. Nikolsky's sign is present when lateral pressure on the skin results in epidermal separation from the dermis.

❑❑ How can SSSS be distinguished from scalded skin syndrome caused by drugs or chemicals?

Pull out your microscopes and call in the pathologists trivia fans, in drug or chemical etiologies the skin separates at the dermoepidermal junction. This drug induced TEN carries up to 50% mortality as a result of fluid loss and secondary infection. On microscopic exam of SSSS intraepidermal cleavage occurs with a few acantholytic keratinocytes will be seen. In non-staphylococcal type, cellular debris, inflammatory cells, and basal cell keratinocytes are present.

❑❑ Treatment of SSSS?

Oral or IV penicillinase-resistant penicillin, baths of potassium permanganate or dressings soaked in 0.5% silver nitrate, and fluids. Corticosteroids and silver sulfadine are contraindicated.

❑❑ **What is the most common gram-negative anaerobe found in human feces?**

Bacteroides fragilis. It is also the most common organism found in abscesses involving the perineal region. Its other claim to fame is being the only anaerobe resistant to penicillin.

❑❑ **Where are cutaneous abscesses caused by** *Escherichia coli* **and** *Neisseria gonorrhoeae* **commonly found?**

"Sorry about that chief," but they are not typically seen in cutaneous abscesses.

Staphylococcus aureus is the most common aerobe in cutaneous abscesses, two-thirds are found in the upper torso, 97% are resistant to penicillin G. It is most commonly isolated in axilla abscesses.

❑❑ **What is the most common gram-negative aerobe found in the upper torso?**

Proteus mirabilis, most commonly isolated in the axilla.

❑❑ **What is the most common aerobe seen in stool and intra-abdominal abscesses?**

Escherichia coli. The pus of *E. coli* is odorless. The "sweat succulent" smell of abscesses in the perirectal area is due to anaerobic bacteria.

❑❑ **How may the Toxicodendron species be recognized?**

Poison oak and ivy have leaves with 3 leaflets per leaf. They also have U- or V-shaped leaf scars. The milky sap becomes black when exposed to air.

❑❑ **How quickly will people react to the Toxicodendron antigen?**

Contact dermatitis typically develops within 2 d of exposure; cases have been reported in as quickly as 8 h to as long as 10d. Lesions appear in a linear arrangement of papulovesicles or erythema. Fluid from vesicles does not contain antigen and does not transmit the dermatitis.

❑❑ **How should steroids be prescribed in a patient with poison ivy?**

Prednisone 40 - 60 mg q d tapered over 2 to 3 wk. Short courses may result in rebound.

❑❑ **What are the causes of exfoliative dermatitis?**

Chemicals, drugs, and cutaneous or systemic diseases. Usually scaly erythematous dermatitis involves most or all of the surface skin. It can be recognized by erythroderma with epidermal flaking or scaling. Acute signs and symptoms may include low-grade fever, pruritus, chills, and skin tightness. The chronic condition may produce dystrophic nails, thinning of body hair, and patchy hyperpigmentation or hypopigmentation. Cutaneous vasodilation may result in increased cardiac output and high-output cardiac failure. Splenomegaly suggests leukemia or lymphoma.

❑❑ **What is a furuncle?**

Deeeeep-inflammatory nodule which grew out of superficial folliculitis.

❑❑ **What is a carbuncle?**

Deep abscess that interconnects and extends into the subcutaneous tissue. Commonly seen in patients with diabetes, folliculitis, steroid use, obesity, heavy perspiration, and areas of friction.

❑❑ What is a Bartholin's cyst?

Obstructed Bartholin's duct resulting in an abscess.

❑❑ What is a pilonidal abscess?

Abscess which occurs in the gluteal fold as a result of disruption of the epithelial surface. They do not originate from rectal crypts and bacteria are from the cutaneous surface.

❑❑ Where does a perirectal abscess originate?

Anal crypts and burrows through the ischiorectal space. They may be perianal, perirectal, supralevator, or ischiorectal. Perianal abscesses which involve the supralevator muscle, ischiorectal space, or rectum require operative drainage.

❑❑ What is hidradenitis suppurativa?

Chronic suppurative abscesses found in the apocrine sweat glands of the groin and/or axilla. Proteus mirabilis overgrowth is common.

❑❑ What is the cause of tetanus?

Tetanospasmin, which is an exotoxin produced by a gram-positive anaerobic rod, Clostridium tetani.

❑❑ What is the mechanism of action of tetanospasmin?

Enters peripheral nerve endings and ascends the axons to reach the brain and spinal cord. At this point it binds four areas of the nervous system:

1. Anterior horn cells of the spinal cord - impairs inhibitory interneurons resulting in neuromuscular irritability and generalized spasms.
2. Sympathetic nervous system - resulting in sweating, labile blood pressure, tachycardia, and peripheral vasoconstriction.
3. Myoneural junction - inhibits release of acetylcholine.
4. Binds to cerebral gangliosides - thought to cause seizures.

❑❑ What is the treatment of a tetanus prone wound?

Surgical debridement, 500 units of human tetanus immune globulin [TIG (h), (Hyper-Tet)] IM (Do Not Inject Into Wound), penicillin G or metronidazole.

❑❑ What is the danger of giving tetanus toxoid boosters in a pleonastic fashion (e.g., with only a 9 mo interval)?

Arthus-type hypersensitivity reaction, with onset about 4 - 6 h after injection. History of a severe hypersensitivity reaction or of a severe neurologic reaction are the only contraindications to tetanus toxoid.

❑❑ What is the most common cause of gas gangrene?

C. perfringens. The first symptom is a sensation of weight or heaviness in the muscle followed by severe pain. The DOC is penicillin G, an alternative is chloramphenicol.

❑❑ A patient presents with a raised, red, small, and painful plaque on the face. On exam, a distinct, sharp advancing edge is noted. What is the cause?

Erysipelas is caused by group A streptococci. When the face is involved, the patient should be admitted.

❒❒ Rank these skin conditions in order of decreasing risk for mortality: erythema multiforme minor, toxic epidermal necrolysis and erythema multiforme major (Stevens-Johnson Syndrome).

Toxic epidermal necrolysis > erythema multiforme major (Stevens-Johnson syndrome) > erythema multiforme minor.

❒❒ What is the mortality in erythema multiforme minor?

0 %.

❒❒ T/F: Oral lesions are very common in erythema multiforme minor.

False.

❒❒ T/F: Oral lesions are very common in erythema multiforme major.

True.

❒❒ What disease produces erythematous plaques with dusky centers and red borders resembling bull's eye targets?

Erythema multiforme. This disease can also produce non-pruritic urticarial lesions, petechiae, vesicles and bullae.

❒❒ A mother brings her 17 year-old boy to you a week after you prescribed ampicillin for his pharyngitis. Mom says he developed a rash over his torso, arms, legs and even the palms of his hands. Upon examination, the patient has an erythematous, maculopapular rash. What might the child have other than pharyngitis?

Infectious mononucleosis. In almost 95% of patients with Epstein-Barr viruses that are treated with ampicillin, a rash will develop. The rash and subsequent desquamation will last about a week.

❒❒ Ecthyma most commonly presents on what body parts?

The lower legs. Ecthyma is similar to impetigo but can also be associated with a fever and lymphadenopathy. The most common infecting agent is *Staphylococcus aureus*. This infection is most prevalent in moist, warm climates.

❒❒ What is the most common bullous disease?

Erythema multiforme. The typical erythema multiforme lesion is the iris lesion (a gray center with a red rim). These lesions are symmetrical and most frequently found on the distal extremities spreading proximally. Patients may also have plaques, papules and bullous lesions. The disease most commonly occurs in children and young adults.

PSYCHOSOCIAL PEARLS

Little minds are interested in the extraordinary,
great minds in the commonplace.
Elbert Hubbard

❏❏ Name some over-the-counter and street medications that may produce delirium or acute psychosis.

Salicylates, antihistamines, anticholinergics, alcohols, phencyclidine, LSD, mescaline, cocaine and amphetamines.

❏❏ You are considering chemical restraint. List your options.

Benzodiazepines: lorazepam, (Ativan), 1-2 mg IV, 2-6 mg orally every 30 min.
midazolam, (Versed), 2-4 mg IV every 30 min.
diazepam, (Valium), 5 mg IV or orally every 30 min.

Sedative hypnotics: haloperidol, (Haldol), 1-5 mg IM/IV, titrate to clinical response
droperidol, (Inapsine), 1-2 mg IV every 30 min.

Benzodiazepines may be given in combination with sedative hypnotics above to both hasten and potentiate their effect. Titrate to effect and monitor appropriately, of course.

❏❏ A patient has ingested a phenothiazine and arrives hypotensive. What intervention(s) may be considered?

IV crystalloid boluses usually suffice. Severe cases are best managed with norepinephrine, (Levophed), or metaraminol, (Aramine). These pressors stimulate alpha adrenergic receptors preferentially. Beta agonists such as isoproterenol, (Isuprel), are contraindicated due to the risks of beta receptor stimulated vasodilation.

❏❏ List some potential complications of clozapine therapy.

Clozapine appears to stimulate limbic rather than striated dopaminergic receptors preferentially, reducing the incidence of extrapyramidal symptoms. Well documented complications include oversedation, hypotension, anticholinergic symptoms, EKG changes and agranulocytosis.

❏❏ Why are Type 1A antiarrhythmics best avoided in clozapine or risperidone ingestion?

These medications prolong the QT interval as well as widen the QRS complex. Agents such as procainamide, quinidine and disopyramide can further prolong the QT interval, raising the risk of refractory SVT, VT and cardiovascular collapse.

❏❏ What is Wellbutrin?

Bupropion, (Wellbutrin), is an aminoketone, a different chemical structure than other antidepressants. Mechanism of action remains unknown. Its effect on serotonin and norepinephrine reuptake is minimal as are its anticholinergic effects. It is best avoided in patients with seizure disorder or taking medications known to lower seizure threshold. Use with MAO inhibitors is contraindicated.

❒❒ List some common pathophysiology associated with eating disorders?

Hyponatremia, hypokalemia, hypocalcemia, hypophosphatemia, anemia, hypoglycemia, starvation ketoacidosis, abnormal glucose tolerance, hypothyroidism due to low T3 levels, persistently elevated cortisol due to starvation, low FSH, LH and estrogens, and elevated growth hormone.

❒❒ What are characteristics of failure to thrive syndrome in infants?

Body mass index (BMI) < 5%, irritable, hard to console behavior, increased muscle tone in the lower extremities or hypotonia, and subsequent weight gain in the hospital.

❒❒ When considering failure to thrive syndrome which historical features are important to assess?

History of prematurity, birth weight, maternal use of cigarettes, alcohol, and or drugs during the pregnancy, previous hospitalizations, and parental stature.

❒❒ In what percentage of cases of child sexual abuse is the abuser known by the child?

90%.

❒❒ In what percentage of cases of child abuse is the mother also abused?

50%.

❒❒ What is involved in the genital examination with a history of child sexual abuse?

Unless there is a suspicion of perforating vaginal trauma, genital examination should be confined to an examination of the external genitalia and perianal area. There is no need for a speculum exam unless the victim is an older adolescent.

❒❒ In the case of child sexual assault, what laboratory tests should be done?

As indicated, oral, rectal, vaginal or urethral swabs for GC and Chlamydia. Serological tests for syphilis or HIV testing should be done if there is a history of, or clinical evidence of infection in the assailant or the victim. Urine or plasma ß-HCG should be checked in girls beyond age of menarche.

❒❒ What is considered physical evidence of acute ano-genital trauma in the genital exam of a child?

With acute sexual abuse you may see fissures, abrasions, hematomas, changes in tone (either dilation or spasm), or discharges (semen fluoresces with a woods light, or examine under microscope). Erythema is a sign of inflammation, irritation or manipulation and is not specific for abuse.

❒❒ What is considered physical evidence of chronic ano-genital trauma in the genital exam of a child?

With chronic sexual abuse signs of an STD such as vaginal or anal discharge, venereal warts or vesicles may be observed. Injuries can heal without residual scarring and a lack of physical changes in no way rules out child sexual abuse.

❒❒ In addition to the history, physical, laboratory tests and collection of physical evidence, what else needs to done in the case of child sexual abuse?

File a report with child protective services and law enforcement agencies. Provide emotional support to the child and family. Give a return appointment for follow-up of STD cultures and testing for pregnancy, HIV, Syphilis as indicated. Assure follow up for psychological counseling by connecting the family/child to the appropriate services in your area.

❒❒ What are the most common ages for child physical abuse?

Two thirds of physically abused children are under the age of three and one third are under the age of 6 months.

❒❒ In cases where the mother is abused how often are the children also abused?

Approximately 40% of cases.

❒❒ In addition to an evaluation for child abuse, what laboratory studies should be done in the child with multiple bruises?

CBC with differential, platelet count, PT, and UA.

❒❒ An infant with mental status changes and retinal hemorrhages and/or subdural hematomas who has no evidence of external head injury may be a victim of what type of child abuse?

"Shaken baby syndrome."

❒❒ What is our best knowledge about the frequency of rape?

According to the 1987 Uniform Crimes Report at least one in eight women have been raped and it is estimated that only 25% of all rapes are reported.

❒❒ What is the definition of domestic abuse?

A pattern of assaultive and coercive behaviors including physical, sexual, and psychological abuse designed to gain power and control over an intimate partner.

❒❒ What is the epidemiology of domestic violence?

95% of the victims are women. An estimated 4 million women are battered each year. The life time prevalence of abuse for adult women is about 10%. Domestic abuse is the number one cause of injuries to women. More than half of all women murdered in the U.S. are killed by a current or intimate partner.

❒❒ What are the rates of domestic abuse in the acute care setting?

In an ED, trauma or acute psychiatric setting, prevalence rates of domestic abuse have been reported to range from 15 to 25% with appropriate screening protocols. In the absence of screening protocols, physicians identify less than 5% of cases of domestic abuse.

❒❒ What are characteristics of an abusive relationship?

The abusive relationship evolves over time usually escalating from jealousy and a desire to control a partner's behavior into humiliation, degradation, and use of the fear of physical violence. He may or may not have to actually hit her if she knows that he is capable of hurting her or her children. The end result is low self-esteem, control, isolation and entrapment.

❒❒ What are the socio-economics of domestic abuse?

Anyone can be involved in an abusive relationship, including men and women in same-sex relationships. Domestic abuse crosses all socio-economic, religious, and racial lines.

❒❒ What historical factors have been reported to be associated with a history of domestic abuse?

Young, pregnant, unmarried or separated women appear to be at greater risk. There has also been high prevalence reported in women with HIV, anxiety disorders, substance abuse, chronic pain syndromes (headaches, functional GI complaints, pelvic pain) and mental illness.

❏❏ **In what percentage of domestic abuse are the children also abused?**

In 33 - 50% of the families in which the mother is battered, the partner also abuses the children. An abused mother is also 7 times more likely to abuse her children.

❏❏ **What are clinical clues of domestic violence?**

Any evidence of injury during pregnancy or late entry into prenatal care. Injuries presenting after significant delay or in various stages of healing especially to the head, neck, breasts, and abdomen or those suggesting a defensive posture such as forearm bruises. Vague complaints or unusual injuries such as bites, scratches, burns, and rope marks. Suicide attempts and rapes.

❏❏ **What is the standard of care for victims of domestic violence currently recommended by JCAHO, the AMA, and the CDC?**

Establish an effective confidential system of identification of DV victims. Documentation of the abuse. Collection of physical evidence. Evaluation of the safety issues, potential for lethality, or suicide. Formulation of a safety plan with the victim. Advising the victim of all her options and resources. Referrals for counseling and other services including legal assistance. Coordination with law enforcement. Transportation to a shelter if desired or needed. Appropriate follow-up by a domestic violence advocate.

❏❏ **What are reasons some women stay with abusers?**

Real fear of escalation of the violence. Economics/lack of resources. Low self-esteem. Feelings of isolation. Love for the abuser. Belief that the violence is her fault. Hope that he'll change. Psychological immobilization, depression, substance abuse. Concern about being able to provide for the children. Cultural or religious beliefs in the maintenance of the family at all costs.

❏❏ **What helps an abused woman leave an abusive relationship?**

Leaving is a process. Extrication from an abusive intimate relationship usually takes place over a period of time as the woman ideally builds a network of support, accesses needed resources, and regains confidence in her own strengths. Women leave when they know they have adequate resources. Most women test out those resources several times first before leaving for good.

❏❏ **What is the problem with the medical model in dealing with victims of domestic abuse?**

The medical model of diagnosing, prescribing, treating symptoms has traditionally been paternalistic and controlling. Patients who do tell physicians about abuse have described experiences with physicians who ignore or minimize their feelings, "prescribe" leaving, are judgmental and abandon her if she is not ready. This desire to control her behavior, mirrors her experience with the abuser. A more therapeutic response would include validating her experience, expressing concern for her safety and that of her children and empowering her by providing access to the resources she needs to escape an unhealthy situation when it is safe for her to do so.

❏❏ **What factors contribute to violence in the ED work setting?**

High patient volumes, long waiting times, substance abuse, and lack of adequate security.

❏❏ **What are predictors of a potentially violent patient?**

Male gender, a history of being violent, and a history of substance abuse are the only reliable predictors. Cultural, educational, economic, and language barriers to effective patient/staff communication as well as trivializing a patient or family member's concerns can increase frustrations and lower the threshold for violent episodes.

❏❏ **What are important clinical considerations in handling an intoxicated violent, psychotic, or threatening patient?**

These patients require a careful history and physical with attention to the mental status exam, looking for evidence of trauma, toxic ingestion, or metabolic derangement. Historical sources such as family, paramedics, mental health workers, police, or medical records may need to be accessed. The patient may need to be physically and at times chemically restrained to obtain an adequate examination and for the safety of the patient and ED staff.

❑❑ **What organic problems are associated with violence?**

Organic problems associated with violent behavior include but are not limited to: delirium, dementia, head trauma, CNS infection, seizures, neoplasm, CVA, hypoglycemia, hypoxia, hyperthermia, anemia, AIDS psychosis, electrolyte abnormalities, vitamin deficiencies, endocrinopathies, toxic ingestion of aromatic hydrocarbons, drug reactions, steroids, alcohol and sedative/hypnotic intoxication and withdrawal, anticholinergics, PCP, cocaine, LSD, and amphetamines.

❑❑ **What psychiatric problems are associated with violence?**

Acute schizophrenia, paranoid ideation, catatonic excitation, mania, borderline and antisocial personality disorders, delusional depression, post-traumatic stress disorder, and decompensating obsessive/compulsive disorder.

❑❑ **What are the prodromes of violent behavior?**

Anxiety, defensiveness and volatility, and physical aggression.

❑❑ **What are the best strategies for prevention of violence in the emergency department setting?**

The physical plan in the ED should be one of controlled access with a reasonable but enforced visitation policy. Isolation rooms should be quite and calm settings, safe for both the patient and the staff, with accessible panic buttons and large enough for a team of security guards, should a "show of force" or use of force be necessary. The training of all ED personnel to recognize and defuse potentially violent situations with cooperation and fast response times from security is critical to staff and patient safety.

❑❑ **What is the number one cause of death for African-American males between the ages of 10 and 24 y?**

Firearm injury. The overall homicide rate for young men in the US is over 7 times that of the next developed country. For Hispanic males this rate is 10 times more and for African American males the rates are over 30 times higher than comparable countries.

❑❑ **Which accounts for more firearm related deaths, intentional or unintentional causes?**

Intentional causes account for 94% of firearm deaths - suicide 48% ad homicide 46%. Unintentional firearm injuries account for about 4%. Only 1% of firearm deaths occur as a result of legal intervention. The number of firearm related fatalities has more than doubled over the last 30 years.

❑❑ **What are risk factors for homicide?**

Most homicide victims are killed by someone they know, someone of the same race, and usually during an argument or fight. Drugs and alcohol are important co-factors as is the presence of a handgun.

❑❑ **What are the relative risks for suicide and homicide if a gun is kept in the home?**

If there is a gun in the home, a suicide is 5 times more likely to occur (9 times more likely if a loaded handgun is available). A homicide is 3 times more likely to occur and the victim is 43% more likely to be a member of the family than an intruder. In the case of domestic violence, a gun at home increases the risk of homicide 20 fold.

❒❒ **What is the clinical significance of the increased availability of semi-automatic weapons?**

Between 1982 and 1992 the percentage of gunshot victims with multiple gunshot wounds increased from 5% to 20%. The rate of spinal cord injuries from GSW quadrupled. This trend has resulted in an increased numbers of major organ injuries, complications, surgeries, severity of injury and probability of death.

❒❒ **Describe a patient with generalized anxiety disorder.**

Patients appear apprehensive, restless, irritable and easily distracted. Patients may experience muscle tension and fatigue as well as various autonomic symptoms such as palpitations, shortness of breath, chest tightness, nausea or diffuse weakness and numbness.

❒❒ **Name a few substances that may mimic generalized anxiety when ingested.**

Nicotine, caffeine, amphetamines, cocaine, anticholinergics; alcohol and sedative withdrawal.

❒❒ **What is the epidemiologic difference between those who attempt and those who complete suicide?**

Suicide completers tend to be older males with medical problems, living alone or with a poor social network.

❒❒ **Name 2 Axis I disorders commonly associated with suicidal ideation.**

Alcohol abuse and affective (mood) disorder.

❒❒ **What happens when one combines EtOH with an anxiolytic (benzodiazepine)?**

Death! (Due to their combined respiratory depressive effects).

❒❒ **Name another contraindication to benzodiazepine use.**

Known hypersensitivity, acute narrow angle glaucoma, pregnancy especially 1st trimester.

❒❒ **Name some drugs <u>contraindicated</u> for a patient taking MAO inhibitors.**

Toxic reactions that include excitation and hyperpyrexia can occur with meperidine (Demerol) and with dextromethorphan. The effects of indirect acting adrenergic drugs are potentiated, including ephedrine, sympathomimetic amines in cold remedies, amphetamines, cocaine and methylphenidate (Ritalin).

❒❒ **Name the three common MAO inhibitors (chemical and Brand name).**

Phenelzine (Nardil).
Isocarboxazid (Marplan).
Tranylcypromine (Parnate).

❒❒ **How does one treat hypertensive crisis caused by combining MAO inhibitors with a known toxin, cheese pizza?**

An α- and ß-adrenergic antagonist such as labetalol. Also consider nifedipine or nitroglycerin. If unsuccessful, consider IV phentolamine or sodium nitroprusside.

❒❒ **Psychiatrists use a multiaxial diagnostic system to describe a particular patient's medical problem list; discuss.**

Axis I: Symptoms and syndromes comprising a mental disorder, includes substance abuse/addiction.
Axis II: Personality and developmental disorders (underlying the Axis I diagnosis).
Axis III: Physical medical problems/conditions which may or may not contribute to Axis I diagnosis.

Axis IV: Psychosocial factors.
Axis V: Adaptive ability/disability.

❒❒ What is organic brain syndrome?

Reversible or non-reversible mental condition thought to be caused by disease process or substance use which interrupts normal anatomical, physiological or biochemical brain functions.

❒❒ Describe dementia.

Disturbed cognitive function resulting in impaired memory, personality, judgment and/or language. Insidious onset, but may present as acute worsened mental state while facing other physical or environmental stressors.

❒❒ Describe delirium.

"Clouding of consciousness" resulting in disorientation, decreased alertness and impaired cognitive function. Acute onset, visual hallucinosis, fluctuating psychomotor activity; all symptoms variable and may change over hours.

❒❒ Neuroleptic medications come in three flavors: low, medium and high potency. Can you name some of these meds and their category?

Low potency: Chlorpromazine (Thorazine).
Medium potency: Perphenazine (Trilafon).
High potency: Haloperidol, droperidol (Inapsine), thiothixene (Navane), fluphenazine (Prolixin), trifluoperazine (Stelazine).

❒❒ So, what's the big deal?

Neuroleptics act to block dopamine receptors. Receptor blockade within the mesolimbic area of the brain provides their antipsychotic effect. Dopaminergic receptor blockade throughout the CNS and anticholinergic effect produce many side effects observed in the ED.

❒❒ Which neuroleptics produce which side effects?

Low potency: Sedative, orthostatic hypotension, anticholinergic effects.

High potency: Less sedating, profound extrapyramidal reactions.

❒❒ What are extrapyramidal reactions?

Dopamine receptor blockade within the nigrostriatal system results in involuntary and spontaneous motor responses including: dystonia, akathisia and Parkinson's-like syndrome.

❒❒ Describe symptoms of alcohol withdrawal.

Autonomic hyperactivity: tachycardia, hypertension, tremors, anxiety, agitation; 6-8 h after drinking.

Hallucinations: auditory, visual, tactile; 24 h after drinking.

Global confusion: 1-3 d after drinking.

❒❒ List some life-threatening causes of acute psychosis.

WHHHIMP: Wernicke's Encephalopathy, Hypoxia, Hypoglycemia, Hypertensive encephalopathy, Intracerebral hemorrhage, Meningitis/Encephalitis, and Poisoning.

❒❒ Characteristics of schizophrenia?

Delusional disorder, hallucinations, (usually auditory), disorganized thinking, loosening of associations, disheveled appearance, lack of insight in realizing thoughts and behavior are abnormal, onset age usually less than 40, and duration of symptoms longer than 6 mo.

❒❒ What is the difference between schizophrenia and schizophreniform disorder?

Very little. In schizophreniform disorder, schizophrenic symptoms have lasted less than 6 mo.

❒❒ What is a brief reactive psychosis?

Acute psychotic break, usually after an emotional or traumatic event. Short duration, usually less than 2 wk.

❒❒ Signs and symptoms suggestive of organic source of psychosis.

Acute onset, disorientation, visual or tactile hallucinations, evidence suggesting overdose or acute ingestion, such as abnormal vital signs, pupil size and reactivity, nystagmus, and age less than 10 or older than 60.

❒❒ Name some symptoms of major depression.

In sad cages: Interest, sleep, appetite, depressed mood, concentration, activity, guilt, energy, suicide.

❒❒ Name some vegetative symptoms.

Loss of appetite, lack of concentration, chronic fatigue, agitation, restlessness, inability to sleep, weight loss.

❒❒ What is informed consent?

When the patient knows what will happen and agrees.

❒❒ What is expressed consent?

When the patient gives written or verbal consent.

❒❒ What is implied consent?

When the patient's condition or status leads one to believe the patient would have given consent if able.

❒❒ When a patient refuses consent or treatment, what must you do to protect yourself against future liability?

Document refusal of consent or treatment.

❒❒ Who can give consent for a minor?

A parent or legal guardian. The state may give consent for wards of the state.

❒❒ What is abandonment?

The termination of the provider/patient relationship without making certain that equal services are available.

❒❒ When may you release care of a patient to a lesser level provider?

When the patient's condition does not warrant the higher level.

❒❒ **Define "assault".**

Creating apprehension of immediate bodily harm without consent.

❒❒ **Is assault a criminal or a civil crime?**

It may be criminal or tort.

❒❒ **How can you avoid being accused of assault?**

Inform the patient of your intentions and obtain consent.

❒❒ **Define "battery."**

Touching the patient without consent.

❒❒ **Is battery a criminal or a civil crime?**

It may be either criminal or tort.

❒❒ **How can you avoid being accused of battery?**

Obtain consent to touch a patient.

❒❒ **Define "false imprisonment."**

Intentional and unjustifiable detention.

❒❒ **In conjunction with what types of cases are charges of false imprisonment most frequently raised?**

Psychiatric cases.

❒❒ **What circumstance may justify detention?**

Evidence of medical necessity.

❒❒ **How may you protect yourself against charges of false imprisonment?**

Obtain consent; act in accordance with protocol.

❒❒ **Define "libel."**

Injuring a person's character, name or reputation by false and malicious writings.

❒❒ **How can you protect yourself against being accused of libel?**

Avoid colloquial terms; describe behavior and avoid labels.

❒❒ **Define "slander."**

Injuring a person's character, name or reputation by false and malicious spoken words.

❒❒ **How can you protect yourself against being accused of slander?**

Limit oral reporting to appropriate personnel; avoid colloquialisms and labels.

❒❒ **Does municipal service or institutional immunity protect you?**

Such immunities may not cover individuals on duty, and are usually very limited.

❒❒ **Why is it a good idea to have individual medical liability insurance?**

The policy is written for specific needs and advocates for the policyholder.

IMAGING PEARLS

"Decide promptly, but never give your reasons. Your decision may be right, but your reasons are sure to be wrong."
Lord Mansfield

❑❑ What is the purpose of ultrasound gel?

It serves to displace air and provide a medium for coupling the probe to the skin surface without impedance mismatching.

❑❑ "Duplex" combines what two features?

A high-resolution image and doppler capability.

❑❑ What audible characteristics differentiate arterial from venous flow when using doppler?

Arterial flow is characterized by sharp, brisk changes in pitch throughout the cardiac cycle (higher pitched during peak systole and lower pitched during diastole; also termed multiphasic) whereas venous signals are lower pitched and more consistent throughout the cardiac cycle (monophasic). Venous flow also varies with the respiratory cycle.

❑❑ What is an ABI and what is its significance?

ABI = ankle/brachial index. The ankle systolic pressure (numerator) is compared to the higher of the two brachial arterial pressures (denominator). It is used to determine if arterial obstruction is present.
Normal ABI = greater than or equal to 1
ABI 0.5-0.9 = obstructive disease of a single peripheral arterial segment e.g. claudication
ABI < 0.5 indicates multiple arterial segments are obstructed

❑❑ What technical factors can effect the accuracy of the ABI?

Probe pressure, probe placement (should be longitudinal to the vessel and 30-60 degree angle to the skin surface), the rapid deflation of the BP cuff, and arterial wall calcifications

❑❑ What is the diagnostic test of choice for documenting DVT?

Duplex ultrasound. Although it is highly operator dependent and not utilized in all centers, its sensitivity and specificity are virtually identical to venography. In addition, its benefits include being noninvasive and not utilizing contrast dye. The accuracy of physical examination for DVT is generally quoted to be approximately 50%.

❑❑ List some of the advantages/disadvantages of CT, ultrasound and DPL for assessing trauma patients?

	Advantages	*Disadvantages:*
DPL	low complication rate done at bedside	invasive, time consuming, can't ID retroperitoneal injury, significant false positive rate
CT	IDs location/extent injury including the retroperitoneum	cost, time consuming, interpretation expertise, patient monitoring not optimal, requires moving the patient out of the ED
US	cheap, noninvasive, done at bedside, good for hemoperitoneum, fast	operator dependent, not good for ID'ing specific organ injury

❒❒ **Surgical repair of abdominal aortic aneurysms is generally indicated for those measuring > _______.**

5 cm. Ultrasound is extremely sensitive for detecting AAA but is not sensitive for the detection of ruptured AAA.

❒❒ **Name some ultrasonographic abnormalities seen in patients with acute cholecystitis.**

Wall thickening, gallstones, surrounding fluid, US Murphy's sign, air in the biliary tree.

❒❒ **An intrauterine gestational sac without a fetal pole, yolk sac or cardiac activity can be confused with what structure?**

The pseudosac of ectopic pregnancy (seen with 10-20% ectopics).

❒❒ **What is the most common site for ectopic implantation?**

The ampullae of the fallopian tube.

❒❒ **Name 6 risk factors for ectopic pregnancy.**

Advanced maternal age, PID, prior ectopic, history of pelvic surgery or tubal ligation, IUDs, in vitro fertilization.

❒❒ **What is the primary use of ultrasonography in females with a positive hCG who present with abdominal pain and/or vaginal bleeding?**

To verify the presence of an intrauterine pregnancy. The incidence of simultaneous intrauterine and extrauterine pregnancies is approx. 1 in 30,000. Ultrasound may not be able to definitively verify that an ectopic pregnancy exists.

❒❒ **What is the only true diagnostic sign of en ectopic pregnancy with ultrasound?**

A fetus with cardiac activity outside the uterus. Complex masses and fluid in the cul-de-sac can be seen in other conditions e.g. pelvic abscess, ruptured ovarian cyst.

❒❒ **In early pregnancy, what is the average doubling time of serum hCG?**

1.5-2 d.

❒❒ **What is the role of ultrasound in detecting placenta previa and abruption?**

Ultrasound is not sensitive for detecting placental abruption. However, in the patient with third trimester vaginal bleeding, ultrasound is used primarily to rule out placenta previa. An experienced ultrasonographer can detect a placenta previa. Uterine contraction, incorrect scanning techniques and an overfilled bladder can result in false positives.

❒❒ **What is the incidence of allergic reaction to IV contrast materials?**

Severe allergic reactions occur in approximately 1 in 14,000 patients, whereas fatal reactions occur about 1 in 40,000 cases.

❒❒ **What is the prevalence of adverse reactions to ionic and nonionic contrast materials?**

12.7% with ionic and 3.1% with nonionic.
Nonionic contrast causes hypotension, bronchospasm, arrhythmia and angioneurotic edema, urticaria, flushing, nausea, vomiting, etc. less often than ionic contrast materials. Whether or not nonionic materials are less nephrotoxic is still controversial.

❒❒ T/F: Oral contrast should be avoided in patients with marginal renal function.

False. Little nephrotoxic iodine is absorbed with oral contrast administration. When barium is used, it is inert and not absorbed.

❒❒ What are the contraindications to administration of oral iodine or barium contrast?

Barium cannot be given when complete colon obstruction exists or intestinal perforation is suspected. Severe allergy to iodine is the only contraindication to the oral iodine-containing preparations.

❒❒ T/F: IV contrast material is contraindicated in chronic renal failure.

False. The contrast material can be dialyzed and the kidney is already maximally impaired.

❒❒ Describe the typical shape and vessel origin of subdural hematomas (SDH) and epidural hematomas (EDH)?

SDH are typically crescent-shaped and are most often caused by the tearing of bridging veins. Acute SDH are hyperdense relative to the brain and become isodense to the brain (1-3 weeks). EDH are biconvex (lenticular) is shape and are usually arterial in origin (although they can be related to bleeding from a dural venous sinus). An EDH does not cross intact skull sutures but can cross the tentorium and the midline.

❒❒ What percentage of SDH are bilateral?

About 25%

❒❒ Why does the performance of a DPL make the evaluation of a subsequent CT more difficult?

Air and fluid are introduced during the DPL.

❒❒ What is the test of choice for evaluating and staging renal trauma?

IV contrast-enhanced CT has replaced IVP for this purpose. CT is more accurate as IVP is not sensitive for renal injuries.

❒❒ The magnetic fields of an MRI can be detrimental to patients with______.

Ferrous metal in their body or electrical equipment whose function can be disrupted by strong magnetic fields. Examples include pacemakers, metal foreign bodies in the eye (welders, sheet metal workers, artists who work with metal, etc), ferromagnetic cerebral aneurysm clips (nonmagnetic steel clips are not dangerous), and cochlear implants. Relative contraindications for the MRI include: certain prosthetic heart valves, implantable defibrillators, bone growth and neurostimulators. One might also include patients who are claustrophobic.

❒❒ Technetium 99m-labeled studies of the gallbladder are viewed every 10 minutes for 1 hour. If the gallbladder is not visualized at 1 hour, what does this signify?

Either complete obstruction of the cystic duct due to inflammation and stones (acute cholecystitis) or partial obstruction with a slow filling rate (due to scarring). Delayed images up to 4 hours are obtained to rule out the latter possibility (chronic cholecystitis).

❒❒ Although bone scans are useful for detecting subtle fractures missed on x-ray, why is it not always useful in the emergent setting for recent fractures?

Skeletal uptake is dependent on blood flow and osteoblastic activity, thus a bone scan may not pick up the increased bone turnover until h or d after trauma. A positive scan demonstrates asymmetric skeletal uptake.

❑❑ **Radionuclide studies are most helpful in determining the bleeding site in upper or lower GI bleeds?**

Lower.

❑❑ **What 2 studies can detect testicular torsion and differentiate it from epididymitis, orchitis or torsion of the appendix testis?**

Technetium 99m nuclear studies and (in some centers) duplex ultrasound. However, if the clinical diagnosis is highly suspected, the patient should be taken to the OR for immediate repair to improve the chance for salvage of the testicle. Times delays for diagnostic testing in this circumstance represent an unacceptable risk.

RANDOM PEARLS

Errors, like straws, upon the surface flow;
He who would search for pearls must dive below.
John Dryden 1631-1700, Prologues and Epilogues: Prologue, All for Love.

❒❒ **Cricothyroidotomy is not recommended in children of less than what age?**

10 years.

❒❒ **Name, in order, the 5 Kübler-Ross stages.**

1) Denial.
2) Anger.
3) Bargaining.
4) Depression.
5) Acceptance.

❒❒ **Use of an EOA is contraindicated in patients of less than _____ years of age.**

16.

❒❒ **Is succinylcholine a depolarizing or a non-depolarizing neuromuscular blocking agent?**

It is the only commonly used depolarizing agent.
It binds to post-synaptic acetylcholine receptors causing depolarization.
It is enzymatically degraded by pseudocholinesterase.
Onset within 1 minute with duration of paralysis of 7-10 min.

❒❒ **What is the rationale for pre-treating a patient with a subpolarizing ("defasciculating") dose of a non-depolarizing agent prior to administration of succinylcholine?**

It attenuates fasciculations from succinylcholine induced depolarization - this may decrease subsequent muscle pain. Blunts increased intragastric and intraocular pressure associated with succinylcholine.

❒❒ **What is the appropriate dose of midazolam (Versed) to cause amnesia during a rapid sequence induction?**

0.1 mg/kg.
5 mg seems to work for most people.

❒❒ **What is the appropriate dose of thiopental to induce anesthesia during a rapid sequence induction?**

4 mg/kg.

❒❒ **Onset of loss of consciousness with thiopental usually occurs within 15 s. What is the usual duration of action?**

2-30 min, depending on source.

❒❒ **What is the appropriate dose of vecuronium for "defasciculating" or "priming" dose?**

0.01 mg/kg.

❑❑ **What is the appropriate dose of vecuronium for paralysis (no "priming")?**

0.20 mg/kg.

❑❑ **What is the appropriate dose of pancuronium (Pavulon) for "defasciculating" or "priming" dose?**

0.015 mg/kg.
≈ 1 mg is a common adult dose.

❑❑ Dermacentor andersoni **(wood tick) is a pesky arthropod associated with four tick-borne illnesses! Name each and its cause.**

Rocky Mtn. Spotted Fever caused by *Rickettsia rickettsii* for which *Dermacentor andersoni* is a vector.
Tick paralysis caused by neurotoxin. Its ascending paralysis with decrease or loss of DTRs can be similar to symptoms of Guillain-Barré syndrome.

Q Fever caused by *Coxiella burnetii*.

Colorado Tick Fever from Orbivirus.

❑❑ **What is the most common opportunistic infection of AIDS?**

PCP. It is the initial opportunistic infection in 60% of AIDS patients and eventually affects 80%.

❑❑ **Describe "AIDS dementia" complex (aka HIV-I encephalopathy).**

A progressive disease caused directly by HIV-I present in 1/3 of AIDS patients characterized by impairment of recent memory, concentration deficit, increasing DTRs, seizures and frontal release signs.

❑❑ **What is the most common cause of** focal **encephalitis in AIDS patients?**

Toxoplasma gondii.

❑❑ **Ethylene glycol is the alcohol that may present with hypocalcemia (1/3 of cases). Where does the calcium go?**

Oxalic acid is one of the metabolites of ethylene glycol.
Calcium precipitates with oxalate and forms calcium oxalate crystals.
The weakly positively birefringent calcium oxalate dihydrate crystals are pathognomonic of this ingestion.

❑❑ **What is the LD_{50} for falling in adults?**

48 feet.

❑❑ **A laryngeal fracture is suggested by finding the hyoid bone elevated above what cervical level on x-ray?**

C3.

❑❑ **Describe the action and side effects of diazoxide.**

Diazoxide is a direct arterial vasodilator. The onset of action is within one to two min and lasts up to 12 h. Side effects may include nausea, vomiting, fluid retention and hyperglycemia. Diazoxide is contraindicated in patients with aortic dissection or angina.

❑❑ **What species of plasmodium may be resistant to chloroquine?**

Falciparum.

❑❑ In children greater than one year of age, where are foreign bodies in the airway usually located?

In the lower airway.

❑❑ In a child with malrotation, what is the most likely age of presentation, what is a common complication, and what signs and symptoms are usually present?

Malrotation usually occurs in children under 12 months of age.
Volvulus is a common complication.
Signs and symptoms usually include vomiting, blood streaked stools, and abdominal pain.

❑❑ Name 2 causes of Toxic Epidermal Necrolysis (aka scalded skin syndrome).

1) Drug or Chemical. Usually in adults. Cleavage at dermo-epidermal junction.

2) Staphylococcal. Usually in children < 5 y. SSSS results in intraepidermal cleavage beneath stratum granulosum.

❑❑ Describe the presentation of SSSS.

Disease begins after URI or purulent conjunctivitis. First lesions are tender, erythematous and scarlatiniform, usually found on face, neck, axillae and groin. Skin peels off in sheets with lateral pressure, i.e., a + Nikolsky's sign.

❑❑ What is appropriate treatment for Toxic Epidermal Necrolysis?

Regardless of cause, treat skin loss similarly to partial thickness burns. Do not use silver sulfadiazine. Adults can sustain large fluid losses. Admit patients with >10% BSA to burn unit. For SSSS treat with IV penicillinase-resistant penicillin.

❑❑ In bullous impetigo, which of the following drugs may not be effective: erythromycin, amoxicillin, cefaclor, or doxycycline?

Amoxicillin.

❑❑ Methanol intoxication causes early death by what cause?

Respiratory arrest. Unknown pathophysiology.

❑❑ Reiter's syndrome diagnostic triad:

Conjunctivitis, polyarthritis, and non-gonococcal urethritis.

❑❑ Nerve most commonly injured in glenohumeral dislocation?

Axillary nerve; numb area over lateral deltoid.

❑❑ Permanent pacemakers have a coding system of 5 letters. The first letter signifies the Chamber Paced. What does the second letter signify?

Chamber Sensed.

❑❑ Describe and contrast regional enteritis and ulcerative colitis.

Category	Regional Enteritis	Ulcerative Colitis
Name	Crohn's disease Regional enteritis Terminal ileitis Granulomatous ileocolitis	Ulcerative colitis
Area	**Stem-to-stern** = social to anti-social (mouth to anus) **Segmental** (skip areas) Most common area is ileum	95% rectosigmoid **Contiguous** (no skip areas)
Demographics	15 - 22 y 55 - 60 y Common in Europeans Jews White > Black 10-15 % have family hx	10 - 20 y 20 - 30 y 15 x greater risk with 1st° relative
Bowel	**ALL LAYERS** Thick Bowel Wall Narrow lumen Creeping fat - mesenteric fat over bowel wall "Cobblestone" mucosal appearance **Fissures** **Fistulas** **Abscesses**	**Mucosa and Submucosa** Mucosal ulceration Epithelial necrosis Mild - Mucosa is fine, granular and friable Severe - Spongy, red, oozing ulcerations **Crypt abscesses** **Toxic Megacolon**

❑❑ Describe the mechanism and cause of a boutonniere deformity.

Boutonniere deformity is secondary to rupture of the extensor apparatus of the PIP joint. The result of the injury is a PIP joint which is flexed and a DIP joint which is hyperextended. It is treated by splinting the PIP joint in full extension.

❑❑ A cyanotic patient has a low oxygen saturation measured on ABG. What flavor of cyanosis does this patient have?

Central.

❑❑ What is a peripheral cyanosis?

ABG reveals an oxygen saturation within normal; shunting or increased O_2 extraction is taking place.

❑❑ Name the two primary causes (groups) of peripheral cyanosis.

Cyanosis with a normal SaO_2 can be due to:
1. Decreased cardiac output.
2. Redistribution - may be 2° to shock, DIC, hypothermia, vascular obstruction.

❑❑ Name the causes of central cyanosis.

The causes of cyanosis with a decreased SaO_2 are:

1. Decreased PaO_2, or decreased O_2 diffusion.
2. Hypoventilation.
3. V-Q mismatch, pulmonary shunting.
4. Dysfunctional hemoglobin (includes sickle cell crisis, drug induced hemoglobinopathies).

NOTE: Hb-CO does not cause cyanosis (though the cherry red appearance of skin and mucous membranes could suggest a cyanosis).

❒❒ A pulmonary embolism causes which 'flavor' of cyanosis?

Central cyanosis, although secondary shock and right-heart failure can lead to peripheral cyanosis.

❒❒ What is a positive Chvostek's sign?

Twitch in the corner of the mouth occurring when the examiner taps over the facial nerve in front of the ear.
It is present in approximately 10 to 30 percent of normal individuals. Eyelid muscle contraction with Chvostek's maneuver is generally considered to be diagnostic of hypocalcemia.

❒❒ What is Trousseau's sign and when is it seen?

Trousseau's sign is a carpal spasm induced when a blood pressure cuff on the upper arm maintains a pressure above systolic for approximately three minutes. Fingers become spastically extended at the interphalangeal joints and flexed at the metacarpophalangeal joints.
Trousseau's sign is generally a more reliable indicator of hypocalcemia than is Chvostek's sign.
Positive Trousseau's sign may also be found in hypomagnesemia, severe alkalosis, and strychnine poisoning.

❒❒ Activated charcoal is <u>not</u> effective treatment for what substances?

Alcohols, ions, hydrocarbons, and acids and bases.

❒❒ Permanent pacemakers have a coding system of 5 letters. In this system the letter A refers to the Atrium and V to the Ventricle. What does the letter D refer to?

D = Double, meaning both Atrium and Ventricle.

❒❒ Describe a patient with Sjögren's syndrome.

Sjögren's syndrome is usually seen in women more than 50 years of age. Symptoms often include diminished lacrimal and salivary gland secretions, salivary gland enlargement and arthritis. Sjögren's syndrome predisposes a patient to corneal irritation, ulceration and superimposed infection. It may complicate many rheumatic diseases or may occur independently. The likely cause of Sjögren's syndrome is lymphatic infiltration of the lacrimal and salivary glands, resulting in dry eyes and dry mouth.

❒❒ Describe the DeBakey classification of regions of aortic dissection.

(I) Ascending and descending aorta.
(II) Ascending aorta.
(III) Descending aorta distal to the left subclavian artery.

❒❒ What is the <u>most</u> <u>common</u> conduction disturbance in acute myocardial infarction?

First degree AV block.

❒❒ What is the <u>most</u> <u>common</u> foot fracture?

Calcaneus (60%). The talus is a distant second most common.

❒❒ Where does the <u>most</u> <u>common</u> metatarsal fracture occur?

At the base of the fifth metatarsal, i.e., a Jones fracture.

❑❑ **Which tendons are involved in de Quervain's tenosynovitis?**

1. The abductor pollicis and the extensor pollicis brevis tendons.
2. Diagnosis is confirmed with positive Finkelstein's test.

❑❑ **Describe Dupuytren's (Guillaume, 1777-1835) contracture.**

Contraction of the longitudinal bands of the palmar aponeurosis.

❑❑ **What is the <u>most common</u> form of anorectal abscess?**

Perianal abscess. Anorectal abscesses are usually mixed infections, both gram negative and anaerobic organisms. Fistula formation is a frequent complication.

❑❑ **What is the <u>most common</u> rhythm disturbance in a pediatric arrest?**

Bradycardia.

❑❑ **How long does it take to prepare type-specific saline cross-matched blood?**

Ten minutes.

❑❑ **Describe the common features of a slipped femoral capital epiphysis.**

Injury usually occurs in adolescence. The rupture typically presents with an insidious development of knee or thigh pain, and a painful limp. Frequently hip motion is limited, particularly that of internal rotation. Evaluation is aided by anteroposterior and frogleg lateral films of both hips.

❑❑ **A core temperature of less than 32° C (90° F) is commonly associated with:**

Poor prognosis, complications including arrhythmias resistant to treatment, and loss of the shivering reflex.

❑❑ **What is the treatment for torsade de pointes?**

Treatment includes techniques to accelerate the heart rate, shortening the duration of ventricular repolarization. This may be accomplished with isoproterenol, temporary pacing, or with magnesium sulfate.

Drugs which increase or prolong repolarization, and therefore exacerbate torsade de pointes, include: Class IA antiarrhythmics (quinidine, procainamide, disopyramide), tricyclic antidepressants and phenothiazines.

❑❑ **Dobutamine in moderate doses causes what cardiovascular effects?**

Decreased peripheral resistance and pulmonary occlusive pressure, and inotropic stimulation of the heart.

❑❑ **Permanent pacemakers have a coding system of 5 letters. The first letter refers to chamber Paced, the second to chamber Sensed. What does the third letter refer to?**

Mode or Response. It comes in several flavors including I = Inhibited, T = Triggered, D = Double, R = Reverse and O = nOne.

❑❑ **What are the common concerns with anterior dislocation of the shoulder?**

Axillary nerve injury, axillary artery injury (elderly patients), compression fracture of the humeral head (Hillsack's deformity), a rotator cuff tear, fractures of the anterior glenoid lip (Bankhart lesion), and fractures of the greater tuberosity.

❐❐ Describe a Monteggia fracture/dislocation.

A fracture of the proximal ulna with dislocation of the radial head. Four variants are described in the orthopedic literature (based on the direction of the radial level dislocation). Anterior dislocation of the radial head is the most common direction. The least common form of Monteggia fracture/dislocation includes a fracture of the proximal radius (in addition of the radial head dislocation).

Treatment usually requires open reduction and internal fixation. When a Monteggia fracture is suspected, x-rays should include the forearm, elbow and wrist.

Michigan University Police Department = MUPD

MUPD = Monteggia, Ulnar fracture, Proximal Dislocation.

❐❐ Describe a Galeazzi's fracture/dislocation.

A radial shaft fracture with dislocation of the distal radioulnar joint.

Great Rays Down Deep! = GRDD

GRDD = Galeazzi, Radius fracture, Distal Dislocation

This is a little-known but true story. Galeazzi's fracture/dislocation is named for the famous orthopod who suffered this injury in a fatal diving accident. Dr. Galeazzi, it seemed, was following a large ray off the coast of Cozumel when he smashed his arm into an unseen coral outcropping. The pain caused him to hyperventilate and head up. His last words as he made the surface (before his dysbaric air embolism) were "Great Rays Down Deep!"

❐❐ Describe the clinical characteristics of carboxyhemoglobin concentrations, specifically for ranges of near 10%, 10 - 20%, near 30%, 40%, 50%, 60% and 70%.

Frontal headache usually becomes evident with COHb levels of 10%.
At 10 to 20% COHb may produce symptoms of headache and dyspnea.
30% causes nausea, dizziness, visual disturbance, fatigue, and impaired judgment.
40% leads to syncope and confusion.
Levels of 50 % may produce coma and seizures.
60% causes respiratory failure and hypotension.
70% level may be lethal.

❐❐ What is the appropriate treatment for cyanide poisoning?

Amyl nitrite, sodium nitrite IV, followed by sodium thiosulfate IV.

❐❐ Organisms which produce focal nervous system pathology via an exotoxin include:

C. diphtheria.
C. botulinum.
C. tetani.
wood and dog tick (Dermacentor A&B).
Staph aureus.

❐❐ Signs and symptoms of diphtheria infection include:

Infection is heralded by acute onset of exudative pharyngitis, high fever and malaise. A pseudomembrane may form in the oropharynx with possible respiratory compromise. Powerful exotoxin has direct effects on the heart, kidneys and nervous system. Diphtheria infection may lead to paralysis of the intrinsic and extrinsic eye muscles. Most likely, you will never see such paralysis in your clinical practice, but you may need to differentiate it from bulbar palsy caused by *C. botulinum* on an exam question. Botulism does not cause fever.

❑❑ **Describe botulism intoxication.**

Botulism exotoxin is elaborated by *C. botulinum*. It affects the myoneural junction and prevents the release of acetylcholine. In the United States, it is caused principally by ingestion of foods that have been inadequately prepared. The most common neurologic complaints are related to the bulbar musculature. Neurologic symptoms usually occur within 24 to 48 hours of ingestion of contaminated foods.
Muscle paralysis and weakness usually spread rapidly to involve all muscles of the trunk and extremities. It is important to distinguish between botulism poisoning and myasthenia gravis. This distinction can be made by using the edrophonium (Tensilon) test, usually performed by a neurologist.

❑❑ **What are some of the key features of Guillain-Barré syndrome?**

Guillain-Barré syndrome is a lower motor neuron disease which commonly affects persons in their 30's and 40's. It presents as an ascending weakness involving the legs more than the arms. A sensory component may be present. Bulbar muscles are usually involved late in the course of the disease. Reflexes are affected early. Paralysis can progress rapidly and recovery is usually slow, but almost always complete.

Lower motor neuron.
Ascending.
Bulbar late.
Reflexes early.

❑❑ **What formula should be used to calculate fluid requirements for resuscitation of a burn victim?**

2-4 mL/kg / %TBSA / day.
One-half of this is given in the first 8 hours.

❑❑ **What percentage of total body surface area is burned in a man with a circumferential burn to both arms, the penis and the anterior chest wall?**

37%.

❑❑ **In a patient who is either less than 10 or greater than 50 years of age, with both deep partial thickness and full thickness burns, what percentage of total body surface area must be burned before referral to the burn center is indicated?**

10%.

❑❑ **In a patient who is <u>between</u> the ages of 10 and 50 years, with both deep partial thickness and full thickness burns, what percentage of total body surface area must be burned before referral to the burn center is indicated?**

20%.

❑❑ **In a patient who has full thickness burns, what percentage of total body surface area must be burned before referral to the burn center is indicated?**

5% -independent of age.
NB. -Above are guidelines from one text, burns to hand, face and perineum require extra caution and burn center referral may be appropriate.

❑❑ **Poor prognostic signs <u>on admission</u> of a patient with pancreatitis include:**

Age over 55 years.
Glucose level greater than 200 mg/dl.
LDH level greater than 700 IU/l.
WBC count greater than 16,000.

SGOT level greater than 250 U/l.
NOTICE - NO AMYLASE INVOLVEMENT!

❏❏ **Poor prognostic signs at 48° after admission of a patient with pancreatitis include:**

Hematocrit fallen more than 10% with a rise in BUN more that 5 mg/dl, declining calcium level to less than 8 mg/dl, PaO_2 less than 60 mmHg, large fluid accumulation and base deficit greater than 4 mEq/L.
NOTICE - NO AMYLASE INVOLVEMENT!

❏❏ **What test is considered to be the gold standard in establishing the diagnosis of acute cholecystitis?**

Radionuclide scan of the biliary tree (HIDA SCAN).

❏❏ **What pain medicine is theoretically contraindicated in the treatment of pain from acute diverticulitis?**

Codeine and morphine are contraindicated, as their use may increase intraluminal colonic pressure. Meperidine (Demerol) is a good substitute as it inhibits segmental contraction of the colon.

❏❏ **What test is best to confirm the diagnosis of Boerhaave's syndrome?**

An esophagram using a water soluble contrast medium should be used in place of barium to confirm the diagnosis.

❏❏ **What pseudonyms are associated with regional enteritis (4)?**

Crohn's disease.
Terminal ileitis.
Regional enteritis.
Granulomatous ileocolitis.

❏❏ **What are the other terms used to refer to ulcerative colitis?**

NONE. If any other pseudonym is used it refers to that other similar disease.

❏❏ **A patient presents with Mallory-Weiss syndrome, and a Sengstaken-Blakemore tube is being considered to control hemorrhage. What problem could a patient have by history that would prevent its use?**

Hiatal hernia, since proper placement of the balloon, as well as proper traction, cannot be applied in such persons.

❏❏ **What are the signs and symptoms of a patient with Boerhaave's syndrome?**

Substernal and left sided chest pain with a history of forceful vomiting leading to spontaneous esophageal rupture.

❏❏ **What is the most common cause of intestinal obstruction?**

Adynamic ileus is the most common cause of intestinal obstruction.

❏❏ **What is the most common cause of small bowel obstruction?**

Adhesions (#1) and hernias are the most common causes of small bowel obstruction.

❒❒ **What is the most common cause of large bowel obstruction?**

Carcinoma (#1), volvulus and sigmoid diverticulitis are the most common causes of large bowel obstruction.

❒❒ **What is the single most common cause of upper GI tract hemorrhage?**

Duodenal ulcers.

❒❒ **Which layers of the bowel wall and mesentery are affected by regional enteritis (Crohn's disease, granulomatous ileocolitis)?**

Inflammatory reaction of regional enteritis involves all layers of the bowel wall.

REGIONAL enteritis involves ALL layers, of course!

❒❒ **What is the most common hernia in women?**

Inguinal hernia, as it is in men.
Though not as common overall, femoral hernias are more common in women than in men.

❒❒ **What are Kanavel's four cardinal signs of infectious digital flexor tenosynovitis?**

Tenderness along the tendon sheath.
Finger held in flexion.
Pain on passive extension of the finger.
Finger swelling.

❒❒ **What symptoms are associated with presentation of regional enteritis (Crohn's disease, granulomatous ileocolitis)?**

Patients with regional enteritis may present with fever, abdominal pain, weight loss and diarrhea. Fistulas, fissures and abscesses may be noted.
Ulcerative colitis, on the other hand, usually presents with bloody diarrhea.

❒❒ **The most common cause of subacute infectious endocarditis is:**

S. viridans.

❒❒ **Subacute bacterial endocarditis most frequently affects which valve?**

SBE usually involves the left side of the heart, specifically the mitral valve.
The aortic valve is the second most commonly involved valve. Rheumatic fever is the most likely cause of valvular damage associated with SBE. Mitral stenosis is a very common predisposing factor in SBE. Drug addicts tend to develop right-sided SBE, usually involving the tricuspid valve.

❒❒ **The most common cause of acute infectious endocarditis is:**

S. aureus.

❒❒ **A good initial antibiotic choice for empiric treatment of acute infectious endocarditis is:**

Gentamicin (1.0 - 1.5 mg/kg q 8° for normal adults) and oxacillin (12 gm/d).

❒❒ **A patient presents to your emergency department after being bitten by a wild raccoon. What treatment would you provide?**

Wound care, tetanus prophylaxis, RIG 20 IU/kg (1/2 at bite site and 1/2 IM), and HDCV 1 cc IM.

❒❒ Describe the skin lesions found in a patient with disseminated gonococcemia.

Umbilicated pustule with a red halo.

❒❒ Describe the skin lesions associated with Pseudomonas aeruginosa **infection.**

Pseudomonas aeruginosa bacteremia typically produces pale, erythematous skin lesions that are approximately 1 cm in size with an ulcerated necrotic center (ecthyma gangrenosum for you Zebe-hunters).

❒❒ Defect of sickle cell disease?

Valine is substituted for glutamic acid in the 6th amino acid of the ß-chain.

❒❒ Describe the intracorporeal travel of the rabies virus.

The virus is spread centripetally up peripheral nerve into the CNS. The incubation period for rabies is usually 30 to 60 d with a range of 10 d up to one yr. Transmission is usually by infected secretions, saliva or infected tissue. Stages include the upper respiratory tract infection symptomatology followed by encephalitis, and the final stage involving the brainstem.

❒❒ What animals are the <u>most</u> <u>common</u> vectors of rabies a.) in the world, b.) in the U.S.?

W<u>o</u>rldwide, the d<u>og</u> is the most common carrier of rabies.
In the <u>U</u>nited States, the sk<u>U</u>nk has become the <u>most</u> <u>common</u> source of disease. Bats, raccoons, cows, dogs, foxes and cats (descending order) are also sources.

Recall, parenthetically, that your rodents (Rocky (the flying squirrel), Dale (the chipmunk), Micky and Ratfink) and your lagomorphs (wild wangy wabbits) , are <u>NOT</u> carriers of rabies.

❒❒ A septic appearing adult has multiple 1 cm diameter skin lesions with a necrotic, ulcerated center and an erythematous surrounding region. What is the likely pathogen?

Pseudomonas aeruginosa.

❒❒ What is the IM treatment for adult streptococcal pharyngitis?

1.2 million units of benzathine penicillin G.
0.6 million units of benzathine penicillin G for kids under 27 kg.

Mercedes "Benz" last a long time.

❒❒ What is the <u>most</u> <u>common</u> initial symptom in botulism poisoning?

Visual disturbance. Visual difficulties have been reported in up to 90 percent of cases. Abducent nerve (CN VI) palsy is common and severe cases may show third cranial nerve involvement with dilated and fixed pupils. Other common initial symptoms include headache, dizziness, weakness, malaise and a dry mouth. Nausea and vomiting is found in about 35% of cases. Symptoms usually appear within the first 24 to 72 hours after exposure.

❒❒ Describe the signs and symptoms of spinal shock.

Spinal shock represents complete loss of spinal cord function below the level of injury. Patients have flaccid paralysis, complete sensory loss, areflexia and loss of autonomic function.
Such patients are usually bradycardic, hypotensive, hypothermic and vasodilated.

❑❑ **Active adduction of the thumb tests which nerve?**

Ulnar nerve.

❑❑ **Positive birefringent crystals in synovial fluid analysis is suggest of:**

Pseudogout. If you are POSITIVE, it must be PSEUDOgout - of course!

❑❑ **In a school aged child, where would a patch of atopic dermatitis typically be found?**

Elbows and knees.

❑❑ **Describe the rash found in exanthem subitum (roseola).**

The rash is usually found on the trunk and neck, and is maculopapular.

❑❑ **What is the most common cause of death among children between 1 and 12 months of age?**

SIDS.

❑❑ **Alkali causes what type of necrosis?**

Liquefactive necrosis.

❑❑ **What is the antibiotic of choice in the treatment of Rocky Mountain spotted fever in a patient allergic to tetracycline?**

Chloramphenicol.

❑❑ **A renal dialysis patient suffers a crush injury. She develops an arrhythmia after intubation using succinylcholine assisted rapid-sequence induction. What is the best treatment?**

Calcium and bicarbonate.

❑❑ **Describe the chest x-ray of Mycoplasma pneumonia.**

Patchy densities involving the entire lobe are most common. Pneumatoceles, cavities, abscesses and pleural effusions can occur, but are uncommon. Erythromycin or a newer macrolide, e.g., azithromycin..

❑❑ **What type of bacterial pneumonia is commonly seen with viral illness?**

Staphylococcal infection.

❑❑ **What two types of pneumonia are often seen in the summer months?**

Staph pneumonia and Legionella.

❑❑ **Describe the chest x-ray findings in Legionella pneumonia.**

Early: fine (interstitial) or patchy infiltrate(s).
Late: dense consolidation and bulging fissures. Expect elevated liver enzymes, hypophosphatemia, hyponatremia.

❑❑ **What are the classic signs and symptoms of TB?**

Night sweats, fever, weight loss, malaise, cough, and a green/yellow sputum most commonly seen in the mornings.

❒❒ What are the chest x-ray findings in tuberculosis?

Right upper lobe cavitation is classic.
Lower lung infiltrates, hilar adenopathy, atelectasis, and pleural effusion are common.

❒❒ Where is the most likely location of a Boerhaave's tear?

Left posterolateral region of the mid-thoracic esophagus.

❒❒ How does a coin appear on AP view of the trachea?

On its side.

❒❒ How does a coin in the esophagus appear on AP?

Like a solid circle.

❒❒ Is GI bleeding common with a perforated ulcer?

No.

❒❒ During which trimester is acute appendicitis most common?

Second.

❒❒ What is the most common cause of paralytic ileus?

Surgery.

❒❒ What is the second most common cause of small bowel obstruction?

Incarcerated hernia. The most common cause is adhesions.

❒❒ An elderly female patient presents with the complaint of pain in the knee and also the medial aspect of the thigh. What GI diagnosis might you entertain?

An obturator hernia may produce pain in the knee and thigh.

❒❒ What is the second most common cause of colonic obstruction?

Diverticulitis. Cancer of the sigmoid is the most common cause. Volvulus is the third most common cause.

❒❒ What is the most common site of volvulus?

Sigmoid colon.

❒❒ Describe the location of an indirect inguinal hernia.

Found lateral to the epigastric vessels, protrudes through the inguinal canal.

❒❒ Describe a femoral hernia.

Through the femoral canal and below the inguinal ligament.

❒❒ Describe the location of a Spigelian hernia.

Located 3-5 cm above the inguinal ligament.

❒❒ **What is a Pantaloon hernia?**

A hernia with both direct and indirect inguinal hernia components.

❒❒ **What is a sliding hernia?**

A hernia in which one wall of the hernia sac includes viscus.

❒❒ **Describe a Richter's hernia.**

An incarceration which contains only one wall of viscus.

❒❒ **What is the single most common hernia in children?**

An indirect hernia. Direct inguinal hernia is more common in the elderly.

❒❒ **When do umbilical hernias typically close?**

Age two.

❒❒ **List three other names for regional ileitis.**

Crohn's disease, terminal ileitis, and granulomatous ileocolitis.

❒❒ **What are other names for ulcerative colitis?**

None.

❒❒ **What is the most common site of Crohn's disease?.**

The ileum. It can actually involve any part of the GI tract from the social end to the antisocial end. It is segmental, often involving granuloma formation along with inflammatory reactions. Crohn's disease has two incidence peaks, one in the 15-22 year-old age group and a second in the 55-60 year-old age group.

❒❒ **How many layers of the bowel does Crohn's disease involve?**

All layers. Associated with *fissures, abscesses and fistulas.*

❒❒ **What are the signs and symptoms of Crohn's disease?**

Fever, diarrhea, right lower quadrant pain with mass possible, *fistulas*, rectal prolapse, perianal *fissures*, and *abscesses*. Associated with arthritis, uveitis, and liver disease.

❒❒ **What is the <u>most</u> <u>common</u> <u>complication</u> of Crohn's disease?**

Perianal abscess.
Also ischiorectal *abscess*, *fissures*, rectovaginal *fistulas*, rectal prolapse, and strictures.

❒❒ **Is toxic megacolon commonly associated with Crohn's disease?**

No. Toxic megacolon <u>is</u> a complication of ulcerative colitis.
Cancer is also an uncommon complication of Crohn's disease.

❒❒ **Systemic diseases associated with Crohn's disease?**

Pyoderma gangrenosum, uveitis, episcleritis, scleritis, arthritis, erythema nodosum, and nephrolithiasis.

❑❑ Patient's with inflammatory bowel disease have ankylosing spondylitis what percentage of the time?

20%.

❑❑ What are the expected contrast x-ray findings with Crohn's disease?

Segmental involvement in the colon with abnormal mucosal pattern and fistulas, often without involvement of the rectum. May see small intestinal narrowing.

❑❑ What is the chief clinical feature of ulcerative colitis?

Bloody diarrhea and involvement of the colon and rectum.
Peak incidence is in 20-30 y olds. The most common site is the rectosigmoid colon. Ulcerative colitis typically involves only the submucosal and mucosal layers. May see crypt abscesses and ulcerations present. Pseudopolyps are associated with ulcerative colitis.

❑❑ What are the principal signs and symptoms of ulcerative colitis?

Fever, weight loss, tachycardia, pancolitis, and six bloody bowel movements per day.

❑❑ Is toxic megacolon more commonly seen in ulcerative colitis or Crohn's disease?

Toxic megacolon is a very common, serious complication of ulcerative colitis.

❑❑ What medications may be used in the treatment of Crohn's disease that are absolutely contraindicated in the treatment of ulcerative colitis?

Antidiarrheal agents may be used in Crohn's disease, they should not be used to treat ulcerative colitis.

❑❑ Is ulcerative colitis or Crohn's more commonly associated with perirectal fistulas and abscesses?

Crohn's.

❑❑ Is cancer more commonly seen in ulcerative colitis or Crohn's disease?

Ulcerative colitis. Remember, with ulcerative colitis, think of toxic megacolon and cancer. Avoid antidiarrheal agents.

❑❑ What are the two most common causes of acute diarrhea?

Rotavirus and Norwalk.

❑❑ What is the most common cause of diarrhea in a child less than one year-old?

Rotavirus.

❑❑ What type of diarrhea is most commonly associated with seizures?

Shigella.

❑❑ What type of diarrhea is associated with rose spots and watery diarrhea, as well as high fever and relative bradycardia?

Salmonella. Particularly common in IV drug abusers with new pet turtles! *Salmonella typhi* may not have much diarrhea.

❑❑ **Treatment for Salmonella?**

Supportive care without antibiotics.
Severe fever may require antibiotic therapy.

❑❑ **What bacteria is associated with mesenteric adenitis and pseudoappendicitis?**

Yersinia.

❑❑ **What is the most common food born pathogen?**

Staphylococcus which presents 6-12 h post ingestion with diarrhea and vomiting. Some patients develop these symptoms within 2 hours.

❑❑ **What gastroenteritis with diarrhea is associated with oysters, clams, crabs, and seafood?**

Vibrio parahaemolyticus. Symptomatic treatment is most common.

❑❑ **What type of diarrhea is associated with profuse, bloody diarrhea and no vomiting?**

Entamoeba histolytica. Diarrhea that is not necessarily bloody and that is associated with contaminated meat could be due to *Clostridium perfringens*.

❑❑ **What is the most common parasite in the United States?**

Giardia. Presents with foul smelling floating stools, abdominal pain, and profuse diarrhea. It may be diagnosed with a positive string test, or duodenal aspiration for trophozoites.

❑❑ **What type of diarrhea is commonly seen in AIDS patients?**

Cryptosporidiosis. Diagnosed with a positive acid fast stain. Presents with profuse, watery diarrhea, no blood.

❑❑ **What is the incubation period for Hepatitis A?**

30 days. It is caused by an RNA virus.

❑❑ **How is hepatitis A transmitted?**

Oral fecal route. No carrier state exists.

❑❑ **What does an elevated IgM anti-HBc mean?**

Exposure to hepatitis B with antibody to the core antigen. High titers associated with contagious disease, low titers with chronic hepatitis B. M = might have the disease.

❑❑ **What does elevated IgG anti-HAV mean?**

It confers immunity. G = gone.

In hepatitis B, IgG anti-HBc means gone only along with anti-HBs. IgG anti-HBc along with HBsAg (surface antigen) implies chronic hepatitis B.

❑❑ **What type of hepatitis is caused by a DNA virus?**

Hepatitis B. Incubation period is 90 days.

❑❑ **What does anti-HBs mean?**

Suggests prior infection and immunity. Pt. has antibodies to the surface antigen just waiting for a chance...S = stopped.

❏❏ What type of defects cause left to right shunt murmurs?

ASD, VSD, and PDA.

❏❏ What type of abnormality produces diminished pulses in the lower extremities of a pediatric patient?

Coarctation of the aorta.

❏❏ What are two fairly common conditions in pediatrics which produce cardiac syncope?

Aortic stenosis, which is not cyanotic and tetralogy of Fallot, which is usually cyanotic during a "tet" spell.

❏❏ What are two unique clinical findings of tetralogy of Fallot?

A boot shaped heart on x-ray and exercise intolerance which is relieved by squatting. TOF is treated by placing the patient in the knee chest position and giving morphine.

❏❏ What would be the signs and symptoms of aortic stenosis in a child?

Exercise intolerance, chest pain, and a systolic ejection click with a crescendo, decrescendo murmur, radiating to the neck with a suprasternal thrill. No cyanosis!

❏❏ What are the signs of left sided heart failure in an infant?

Increased respiratory rate, shortness of breath, and sweating during feeding.

❏❏ What is the single most common cause of CHF in the second week of life?

Coarctation of the aorta.

❏❏ What is the most common cause of otitis media?

Strep pneumoniae.

❏❏ What is the most common cause of impetigo?

Group A ß-hemolytic streptococcus.

❏❏ What is the most common cause of bullous impetigo?

Staph aureus.

❏❏ What is the <u>most common</u> cause of sinusitis?

Streptococcus pneumoniae.

❏❏ What is the <u>most common</u> cause of orbital infections?

Staph aureus. Periorbital infections are most commonly caused by *H flu*.

❏❏ What is the <u>most common</u> cause of pediatric bacteremia?

Strep pneumoniae.

❑❑ What are the most common causes of an abscess or pneumatocele in a pediatric patient?

Staphylococcal pneumonia or anaerobic pneumonia.

❑❑ A patient presents with a staccato cough and a history of conjunctivitis in the first few weeks after birth, what type of pneumonia does this patient have?

Chlamydia.

❑❑ Most common cause of viral pneumonia in the pediatric patient?

RSV.

❑❑ What is the most common type of asthma in children?

Extrinsic asthma which is a type I, immediate hypersensitivity reaction mediated by IgE. Common causes are molds and pet dander.

❑❑ How do steroids function in the treatment of asthma?

They increase cAMP, decrease inflammation, and help restore the function of ß-adrenergic responsiveness to adrenergic drugs.

❑❑ What two viral illnesses are prodromes for Reye's syndrome?

Varicella (chicken pox) and influenzae B.

❑❑ Signs and symptoms of Reye's syndrome:

Irritable, combative, and lethargic, right upper quadrant tenderness, history of influenzae B or recent chicken pox, papilledema, hypoglycemia, and seizures.
Lab findings would include hypoglycemia, and an elevated ammonia level greater than 20 times normal. Bilirubin level is NORMAL.

❑❑ Describe stage I and stage II of Reye's syndrome.

Stage I - vomiting, lethargy and liver dysfunction.
Stage II - disorientation, combativeness, delirium, hyperventilation, increased deep tendon reflexes, liver dysfunction, hyperexcitable, tachypnea, fever, tachycardia, sweating and pupillary dilatation.

❑❑ Describe Stages III, IV, and V of Reye's syndrome.

Stage III - coma, decorticate rigidity, increased respiratory rate, mortality rate of 50%.
Stage IV - coma, decerebrate posturing, no ocular reflexes, loss of corneal reflexes, and liver damage.
Stage V - loss of deep tendon reflexes, seizures, flaccid, respiratory arrest, 95% mortality.

❑❑ What are the first, second, and third drugs of choice for treatment of seizures in children?

The first is phenobarbital, second is phenytoin, and third is carbamazepine.

❑❑ What is the drug of choice for absence (petit mal) seizures in a child?

Ethosuximide, valproate, and acetazolamide. An EEG is usually obtained prior to initiating therapy.

❑❑ What is the drug of choice to treat a febrile seizure?

Phenobarbital.

❒❒ **Use of diazepam (Valium) is avoided in neonatal seizures. Is part of the reason for this because it may cause hyperbilirubinemia by uncoupling the bilirubin-albumin complex?**

Yes.

❒❒ **Serious complication of valproic acid?**

Hepatic failure.

❒❒ **Complications of phenytoin use?**

Folate deficiency, osteomalacia, neutropenia, neuropathies, lupus and myasthenia.

❒❒ **What is the most common viral gastroenteritis in children?**

Rotavirus.

❒❒ **What is the most common cause of bacterial gastroenteritis in the world?**

E. coli.

❒❒ **What is the most common cause of diarrhea in infants and young children in day care centers?**

Giardia.

❒❒ **What bacterium is associated with mesenteric adenitis or appendicitis?**

Yersinia.

❒❒ **What enteritis causing bacterium produces watery diarrhea, encephalopathies, and convulsions.**

Shigella = seizures.

❒❒ **A child presents with vomiting and a moderate amount of blood in the stool. What is the diagnosis?**

Malrotation of the mid-gut.

❒❒ **What is the most common cause of painless lower GI bleeding in an infant or child?**

Meckel's diverticulum.

❒❒ **A 16 mo old presents with bilious vomiting, a distended abdomen, and blood in the stool. Diagnosis?**

Malrotation of the mid-gut.

❒❒ **A child presents with abdominal cramps which come and go, current jelly stools, and a sausage like tumor mass in the right lower quadrant. Contrast x-ray shows a coil spring sign. Diagnosis?**

Intussusception.

❒❒ **A child presents with a history of drug ingestion; she now has convulsions, coma, and cardiac collapse. What drug might have caused this?**

Salicylate with secondary hypoglycemia.

❒❒ **What side effect of propranolol may be concerning for a diabetic patient?**

Hypoglycemia.

❒❒ **What are some possible complications of sodium bicarbonate therapy?**

Hypokalemia, paradoxical CSF acidosis, impaired O_2 dissociation, and sodium overload.

❒❒ **What type of lactic acidosis is associated with hypoxia and shock?**

Type A.

❒❒ **Differentiate between non-ketotic hyperosmolar coma and DKA.**

In non-ketotic hyperosmolar coma, glucose is very high, often > 800. The serum osmolality is also very high, with average about 380. Nitroprusside test is negative. In DKA, glucose is more often in the range of 600, the serum osmolality is approximately 350, nitroprusside test is positive.

❒❒ **What focal signs may be present in a patient with non-ketotic hyperosmolar coma?**

These patients may have hemisensory deficits or perhaps hemiparesis. 10-15% of these patients have a seizure.

❒❒ **What is the most common cause of hyperthyroidism?**

Grave's disease (toxic diffuse goiter).

❒❒ **What is the most common precipitating cause of thyroid storm?**

Pulmonary infection.

❒❒ **What is another name for life threatening hypothyroidism?**

Myxedema coma. Commonly seen in elderly women in the winter months and is stimulated by infection and stress.

❒❒ **What is the most common cause of hypothyroidism?**

Over treatment of Grave's disease with iodine or subtotal thyroidectomy.

❒❒ **What is the second most common cause of hypothyroidism?**

Autoimmune Hashimoto's thyroiditis.

❒❒ **How may primary hypothyroidism be distinguished from secondary?**

In primary hypothyroidism the TSH levels are high, patients often have a history of thyroid surgery and may have a goiter; in secondary the TSH levels are low or normal, no hx of surgery and no goiter.

❒❒ **What drugs may make myxedema worse?**

Propranolol and phenothiazines.

❒❒ **What ECG finding would you expect in myxedema coma?**

Bradycardia.

❏❏ What is a common "surgical problem" in myxedema that should be treated conservatively?

Acquired megacolon.

❏❏ What is primary adrenal insufficiency?

Addison's disease, that is, failure of the adrenal cortex.

❏❏ What hormones are produced by the adrenal cortex?

Mineralocorticoids, glucocorticoids and androgenic steroids.
Salt, sugar, sex.

❏❏ What is the major mineralocorticoid?

Aldosterone. Aldosterone is regulated by the renin angiotensin system. Aldosterone increases sodium reabsorption and increased K^+ excretion.

❏❏ What is the major glucocorticoid?

Cortisol.

❏❏ What does the medulla of the adrenal gland produce?

Epinephrine and norepinephrine.

❏❏ A patient presents two weeks after suffering a myocardial infarction. The patient takes warfarin and has sudden onset of hypotension, right flank pain, right CVA pain, epigastric pain, fever, nausea, and vomiting. Diagnosis?

Bilateral adrenal gland hemorrhage - adrenal apoplexy.

❏❏ What is Waterhouse-Fredrickson syndrome?

Septicemia secondary to meningococcemia with associated bilateral adrenal gland hemorrhage. The patient will have a petechial rash, purpura, shaking chills, and severe headache.

❏❏ What effect does Addison's disease have on cortisol and aldosterone levels?

Cortisol and aldosterone levels are low.
Low cortisol levels mean nausea, vomiting, anorexia, lethargy, hypoglycemia, water intoxication, and inability to withstand even minor stress without shock.
Low aldosterone levels means sodium depletion, dehydration, hypotension, and syncope.

❏❏ What are the signs and symptoms of Addison's disease?

Hyperpigmentation, hyperkalemia, alopecia, and ascending paralysis secondary to hyperkalemia.
Lab findings in Addison's disease include hypoglycemia, hyponatremia, hyperkalemia, and azotemia.

❏❏ What ECG findings are expected in Addison's disease?

Because of the hyperkalemia, expect peaked T-waves.

❏❏ What are the principal signs and symptoms in adrenal crisis?

Abdominal pain, hypotension and shock. The common cause is withdrawal of steroids. Treatment of adrenal crisis is hydrocortisone (Solu-Cortef), 100 mg IV bolus and 100 mg added to a the first liter of D_5 0.9 NS.

❒❒ **Does cyanide cause cyanosis?**

No, except secondarily when bradycardia and apnea precede asystolic arrest.
Consider cyanide in an acidotic comatose patient without cyanosis and no hypoxia on ABG.

❒❒ **What key lab findings are expected in SIADH?**

Serum sodium would be low and urine sodium would be high, greater than 30.

❒❒ **What is the most common cause of a cerebral infarct?**

Atherosclerosis, and the most common site is in the internal carotids.

❒❒ **What is the typical anatomic source of an epidural hematoma?**

The middle meningeal artery.

❒❒ **What is the most common anatomic source of a subdural hematoma?**

Bridging veins.

❒❒ **What is the most common source of a subarachnoid bleed?**

A saccular aneurysm.

❒❒ **If the lesion is in the right hemisphere, which way will the eyes deviate?**

Eyes will deviate toward the lesion.

❒❒ **If there is a lesion in the brain stem, which way will the eyes deviate?**

They will deviate away from the lesion in the brain stem.

❒❒ **What is the single most common intraparenchymal site of intracranial bleeding?**

The putamen.

❒❒ **In the pediatric esophagus, what is the most common site of a foreign body?**

Cricopharyngeal narrowing.

❒❒ **Most common hernia in population?**

Inguinal.

❒❒ **Do household pets transmit** Yersinia**?**

Yes.

❒❒ **What is the most common cause of conjunctivitis in the newborn?**

Chlamydia.

❒❒ **Most common cause of meningitis after the first month of life?**

H. influenzae.

❑❑ **Most common cause of urinary tract infection in a female child?**

E. coli.

❑❑ **First line of treatment of a seizure in a five year-old?**

Phenobarbital.

❑❑ **What is the most common cause of intrinsic renal failure?**

Acute tubular necrosis.

❑❑ **What is the most common cause of cardiac arrest in an uremic patient?**

Hyperkalemia.

❑❑ **A "blue dot" sign suggests:**

Torsion of the epididymis or appendix testis.

❑❑ **What is the first cardiac finding in cyclic antidepressant overdose?**

Sinus tachycardia.

❑❑ **What is the most common cause of right sided endocarditis in IV drug addicts?**

Staph aureus.

❑❑ **Which is the most common valve affected in IV drug addicts?**

Tricuspid.

❑❑ **What is the most common cause of osteomyelitis or septic arthritis in an IV drug addict?**

Serratia marcescens.

❑❑ **What is the most common cause of chronic heavy metal poisoning?**

Lead. Arsenic is most common acute.

❑❑ **What is the most commonly injured area of the mandible?**

Angle.

❑❑ **What is the most commonly fractured area of the maxilla or mandible?**

Alveolar process.

❑❑ **Most common cause of Erysipelas:**

Group A streptococci.

❑❑ **Are steroids effective in treatment of toxic epidermal necrolysis?**

No.

❐❐ **Erythema nodosa is associated with which type of gastroenteritis?**

Yersinia. I've a particular YEN for this answer!!

❐❐ **Thyrotoxicosis may be treated with:**

Support and hydration, IV propylthiouracil 1 gram, sodium iodine IV 1 g q 12 h or IV propranolol 1 mg/min up to 10 mg.

❐❐ **What is the most reliable method of diagnosing a posterior shoulder dislocation?**

Physical exam. Order a "Y-view" x-ray - it may be helpful.

❐❐ **The mortise view of the ankle is important in the diagnosis of:**

Medial (deltoid) ligament disruption of the ankle.

❐❐ **A fracture of the proximal fibular shaft is commonly associated with:**

Medial ankle fracture or sprain. This is a Maisonneuve fx; it may be present with a widened mortise and no fx seen in the ankle.

❐❐ **What is the best x-ray view for diagnosing lunate and perilunate dislocations?**

Lateral x-ray views of the wrist.

❐❐ **What is the formula for calculating the serum osmolarity?**

$$CalculatedOsmol(mOsm/l) = 2(Na) + \frac{\text{glucose}}{18} + \frac{BUN}{2.8}$$

❐❐ **What is a good way to remember the signs and symptoms of anticholinergic toxicity?**

Think of atropine, as most of the signs and symptoms of atropine use are similar.
Tachycardia, hyperthermia, mydriasis, Ø sweat, dry mucosa, blurred vision for near objects (poor accommodation), decreased GI activity, urinary retention, aberration of mentation including delirium, lethargy and hallucinations, seizure and coma.

Dry as a bone,
Red as a beet,
Mad as a hatter,
Hot as a stone,
Blind as a bat.

❐❐ **What are common anticholinergic compounds?**

Atropine, tricyclic antidepressants, antihistamines, phenothiazines, antiparkinsonian drugs, belladonna alkaloids, and some Solanaceae plants (eg. deadly nightshade , jimson weed).

❐❐ **For how long should a patient with TCA overdose demonstrating tachycardia and conduction disturbances be monitored?**

24 hours.

❐❐ **For how long will naloxone typically reverse opioid toxicity?**

$T_{1/2}$ is 1 h with a duration of action of 2-3 h per Tintinalli.

$T_{1/2}$ is 12-20 min with little effect after 45 min per Rosen.

❒❒ A baby is brought to the emergency department with persistent crying for two hours and vomiting. On exam, a testicle is tender and enlarged. What is the most common cause?

Testicular torsion.

❒❒ A child is seen with bluish discoloration of the gingiva. What diagnosis do you suspect?

Chronic lead poisoning. You would also expect erythrocyte protoporphyrin level to be elevated in chronic Pb poisoning.

❒❒ What is the most common cause of periorbital cellulitis in a two year-old child?

The most common cause is *H. influenzae*. The second most common cause is *S. aureus*.

❒❒ What is the most appropriate drug for a patient with low cardiac output and pulmonary congestion?

Dobutamine.

❒❒ What is the anatomical weakness of the esophagus?

Lack of a serosa.

❒❒ In a humeral shaft fracture, what nerve is most commonly injured?

Radial nerve.

❒❒ What is the most common hip dislocation?

Posterior.

❒❒ What disorder is most likely to be confused with erythema nodosum?

Cellulitis.

❒❒ What is erythema nodosum?

An inflammatory disease of skin and subcutaneous tissue characterized by tender red nodules. Nodules are most commonly found in the pretibial area.
Most commonly affects young adults.
Most common cause in children - UTI, especially with streptococci.
Most common cause in adults - Streptococcal infections and sarcoidosis.
Other causes - leprosy, TB, psittacosis, ulcerative colitis, drug reaction.

❒❒ Galeazzi's fracture implies:

Fracture of the shaft of the radius with dislocation of the distal radioulnar joint.
"GREAT RAYS DOWN DEEP!"

❒❒ What is the most common dysrhythmia in a child?

Paroxysmal atrial tachycardia.

❒❒ On an upright chest x-ray, what is the earliest radiographic sign of left ventricular failure?

Apical redistribution of the pulmonary vasculature.

❑❑ What is the most common cause of hyponatremia?

Dilution.

❑❑ Of the following, which is not a common cause of large bowel obstruction: diverticulitis, adhesions, sigmoid volvulus or neoplasms?

Adhesions.

❑❑ A fracture of the acetabulum may be associated with damage to what nerve?

The sciatic nerve.

❑❑ What are some common causes of increased anion gap?

Aspirin, methanol, uremia, diabetes, idiopathic (lactic), ethylene glycol and alcohol are reasonably common.

Numerous etiologies may produce the entity above listed demurely as "lactic." Lactic acidosis may be the result of shock, seizures, acute hypoxemia, INH, cyanide, ritodrine, inhaled acetylene, carbon monoxide and ethanol. Sodium nitroprusside, povidone-iodine ointment, sorbitol and xylitol can cause an anion gap acidosis.

Other causes of anion gap acidosis include toluene intoxication, iron intoxication, sulfuric acidosis, short bowel syndrome (D-lactic acidosis), formaldehyde, nalidixic acid, methenamine and rhubarb (oxalic acid). Inborn errors of metabolism such as methylmalonic acidemia and isovaleric acidemia may also cause a gap acidosis.

Recall some pearls for sorting out the differential diagnosis:

Methanol-	visual disturbances and headache common. Can produce quite wide gaps as each 2.6 mg/dL of methanol contributes 1 mOsm/L to gap. Compare this with alcohol, each 4.3 mg/dL adds 1 mOsm/L to gap.
Uremia-	is quite advanced before it causes an anion gap.
Diabetic Ketoacidosis-	usually has both hyperglycemia and glucosuria; alcoholic ketoacidosis (AKA) often has a lower blood sugar and mild or absent glucosuria.
Salicylates-	high levels contribute to gap.
Lactic Acidosis-	can check serum level. Itself has broad differential as above.
Ethylene glycol-	causes calcium oxalate or hippurate crystals in urine. Each 5.0 mg/dl contributes 1 mOsm/L to gap.

A reasonably comprehensive mnemonic device for recalling causes of anion gap acidosis is A MUDPILE CAT.

A = alcohol,	M = methanol,	C = carbon monoxide,
	U = uremia,	A = ASA (aspirin),
	D = DKA,	T = toluene.
	P = paraldehyde,	
	I = iron and isoniazid,	
	L = lactic acidosis,	
	E = ethylene glycol,	

❑❑ What are the causes of normal anion gap metabolic acidosis?

Causes include diarrhea, ammonium chloride, renal tubular acidosis, renal interstitial disease, hypoadrenalism, ureterosigmoidostomy, and acetazolamide.

❑❑ What are some common causes of respiratory alkalosis?

Respiratory alkalosis is defined as a pH above 7.45 and a pCO_2 less than 35. Common causes of respiratory alkalosis include any process that may cause hyperventilation including shock, sepsis, trauma, asthma, PE, anemia, hepatic failure, heat stroke and exhaustion, emotion, salicylate poisoning, hypoxemia, pregnancy and inappropriate mechanical ventilation. Alkalosis shifts the O_2 disassociation curve to the left. It also causes cerebrovascular constriction. Kidneys compensate for respiratory alkalosis by excreting HCO_3^-.

❑❑ Causes of right shift of O_2 disassociation curve:

"CADET! Right face!!"

Right = Release to tissues.

Hyper	Carbia,
	Acidemia,
2,3	DPG,
	Exercise,
and increased	Temperature.

❑❑ How should a patient with hypertrophic cardiomyopathy be treated who presents with chest pain and normal vital signs except for a heart rate of 140?

ß-antagonists are the primary treatment for hypertrophic cardiomyopathy. ß-antagonists are first-line treatment for any symptomatic patient even without tachycardia present. Calcium channel blocking drugs are second-line therapeutics.

❑❑ What is the adult dose of epinephrine in acute anaphylactic shock?

0.3 - 0.5 mg of 1:10,000 IV.

❑❑ How should neurogenic shock be best managed?

Neurogenic shock is treated with replacement of volume deficit followed by vasopressors.

❑❑ What is the most appropriate medication to treat a hypertensive patient with an acute aortic dissection?

Trimethaphan. Trimethaphan reduces hydraulic stress on the aortic wall and as a consequence, minimizes further dissection. The mechanism of action is via decreasing myocardial contractility. Trimethaphan also functions as a vasodilator and therefore reduces intra-aortic pressure and concomitant total peripheral resistance. Esmolol, a new titratable short acting ß-blocker, may also be a valuable alternative.

❑❑ An elderly male presents to your emergency department with ataxia, confusion, amnesia and ocular paralysis. The patient is apathetic to his situation and has an otherwise normal neurologic exam. What is the likely cause of the patient's problem?

Vitamin B deficiency associated with Wernicke-Korsakoff's syndrome.

❑❑ How is SVR calculated?

$$\frac{(MAP - CVP) \times 80}{CO} \qquad Nl = 800 - 1400\ dyn \cdot s^{-1} \cdot cm^{-5}$$

❒❒ **What is the most common dysrhythmia associated with excess digitalis?**

PVCs.

❒❒ **What is the order of appearance of CHF on chest x-ray?**

Initially cephalization and redistribution of blood flow is seen, followed by interstitial edema with evident Kerley B lines, as well as a perihilar haze. This is followed by alveolar infiltrates in the typical butterfly appearance. Finally, flagrant pulmonary edema and effusions are present.

❒❒ **The most common cause of sporadic encephalitis?**

Herpes simplex virus.

❒❒ **What are the classic EKG findings of a patient with a posterior MI.**

A large R-wave and ST depression in V1 and V2.

❒❒ **What are the classic EKG findings in Wolff-Parkinson-White syndrome?**

A change in the upstroke of QRS, the delta wave, plus a short PR interval.

❒❒ **The most common cause of endemic encephalitis?**

Arbovirus.

❒❒ **What is the best treatment for an unstable patient with Wolff-Parkinson-White syndrome presenting with rapid atrial fibrillation?**

Synchronized cardioversion.

❒❒ **What is the most common dysrhythmia seen with digitalis?**

PVCs are the most common.
AV block and PSVT with block are second most common.
V-tach and junctional tachycardia are the least common arrhythmias associated with digitalis.

❒❒ **What is the best treatment for a verapamil induced bradycardia?**

Calcium chloride 10%, give 10 - 20 mL IV.

(This is about 10 - 20 mg/kg, use 10 - 30 mg/kg in children).

❒❒ **The most common cause of pelvic pain in adolescent females?**

Ovarian cyst.

❒❒ **What is the most common cause of valvular induced syncope in the elderly?**

Aortic stenosis is the most common valvular cause of syncope in the elderly.
Vasovagal mechanisms are the most common mechanism overall.

❒❒ **Describe the signs, symptoms and ECG finding associated with lithium toxicity.**

Tremor, weakness, and flattening of the T-waves.

❒❒ **How many days after a measles vaccine might a fever and a rash be expected to develop?**

Seven to ten days.

❑❑ **The most common complication of acute otitis media?**

Tympanic membrane perforation. Other complications include mastoiditis, cholesteatoma, as well as intracranial infections.

❑❑ **Compare and contrast the rashes and associated symptoms and signs of roseola and rubella.**

With roseola, a child usually develops a fever up to 40° C (104° F) which lasts for three to five days. The child does not look particularly ill during the symptoms, although adenopathy may be noted. As the fever falls, the child may develop a maculopapular rash which usually appears within 48 hours after the fever disappears and may last from a few hours to a few days.

Rubella (measles) usually begins with a prodrome of three to four days of fever, conjunctivitis and upper respiratory tract symptoms. The characteristic rash is also maculopapular, confluent, but distinctively begins on the face and moves down the body. Koplik's spots are diagnostic (pathognomonic).

❑❑ **What is appropriate treatment for a non-immunized individual exposed to hepatitis B?**

Treat with immune globulin, specifically HBIG. Consider vaccination.

❑❑ **What is the most common cause of sigmoid volvulus in the elderly?**

Constipation.

❑❑ **The most common complications of Varicella infections in adults:**

Encephalitis, pneumonia, *Staph* and *Strep* cellulitis.

❑❑ **The anterior drawer test of the ankle is used to test what ligament?**

The anterior talofibular ligament.

❑❑ **A patient presents with a shortened, internally rotated right leg after an accident. What injury is suspected?**

Posterior hip dislocation.

❑❑ **Describe a mallet finger deformity.**

Mallet finger deformity is produced by forced flexion of the DIP joint when the finger is in full extension. The deformity is a result of either rupture of the distal extensor tendon, or an avulsion fraction of the tendon insertion on the distal phalanx with a dorsal plate avulsion.

❑❑ **The most common cause of laryngotracheitis?**

Parainfluenza virus type I. *Staph aureus* is the most common bacterial pathogen.

❑❑ **A patient has a fracture of the proximal 1/3 ulna; what associated injury should be ruled out?**

Dislocation of the radial head. This is also known as a Monteggia fracture. Anterior dislocation is most common.

Michigan University Police Department = MUPD

MUPD = Monteggia, Ulnar fracture, Proximal Dislocation.

Little known fact, this fracture/dislocation is named after the now world-famous quarterback, Joe Monteggia who suffered this injury during a scuffle with the Michigan University PD.

❑❑ A patient has an orbital floor fracture; what symptoms and signs might be seen?

The most common symptom would be diplopia due to entrapment of the inferior rectus and inferior oblique muscles, and resultant paralysis of upward gaze. In addition, one would worry that the inferior orbital nerve could be damaged with paresthesia resulting to the lower lid, infraorbital area and side of the nose.

❑❑ What gynecological infection presents with a malodorous, itchy, white to grayish sometimes frothy vaginal discharge?

Trichomoniasis.

❑❑ What are the signs of an upper motor neuron lesion?

Upper motor neuron lesion involves the corticospinal tract. The lesion usually gives paralysis with:
1. Initial loss of muscle tone and then increased tone, resulting in spasticity.
2. Babinski sign.
3. Loss of superficial reflexes.
4. Increased deep tendon reflexes.

A lower motor neuron lesion is associated with the anterior horn cells' axons. The lesion gives paralysis with decreased muscle tone and prompt atrophy.

❑❑ What condition commonly presents with ocular bulbar deficits?

Botulism poisoning.
Patients with myasthenia gravis may present similarly.
Diphtheria toxin may rarely produce similar deficits.

❑❑ What is the best diagnostic procedure to diagnose ectopic pregnancy?

Laparoscopy.

❑❑ Describe the symptoms and signs of myasthenia gravis.

Weakness and fatigability with ptosis, diplopia and blurred vision are the initial symptoms in 40 to 70 percent of patients. Bulbar muscle weakness is also common with dysarthria and dysphagia.

❑❑ Describe the presenting symptoms of botulism poisoning.

Botulism poisoning often presents with ocular bulbar deficits. Symmetrical descending weakness, usually with no sensory abnormalities, classically develops. Common associated symptoms include dysphagia, dry mouth, diplopia, dysarthria. Deep tendon reflexes may be decreased or absent.

❑❑ Describe the signs and symptoms of Guillain-Barré disease.

Guillain-Barré disease classically presents with symmetric weakness in the leg which ascends to include the arms or trunk. Distal weakness is usually greater than proximal. Onset rarely involves the cranial nerves.

❑❑ Which nerve provides sensation to both dorsum and volar aspects of hand?

Ulnar. Radial is primarily dorsum, and median is primarily volar.

❑❑ Describe the key features of Ménière's disease, also known as endolymphatic hydrops.

Vertigo, hearing loss and tinnitus are the hallmarks of Ménière's disease. Ménière's disease typically presents with rapid onset of vertigo, often with associated nausea and vomiting that lasts for hours to one day. Nystagmus may be spontaneous during the critical stage. Tinnitus may be present and is louder during the attacks. Sensorineural hearing loss may be present. There may also be an aura with a sensation of fullness in the ear during the attack. Symptoms are unilateral in over 90 percent of patients, and recurring attacks are typical.

❏❏ **Describe the key features of benign positional vertigo.**

Violent positional vertigo is usually provoked by certain head positions or movement. Nystagmus is also always positional, of brief duration with fatigability.

❏❏ **What are the key features of viral labyrinthitis or vestibular neuritis?**

Vertigo is severe, usually lasting three to five days, with nausea and vomiting. Symptoms usually regress over three to six weeks. Nystagmus may be spontaneous during the severe stage.

❏❏ **What is a major concern in a patient that presents with unilateral Parkinsonian features?**

Intracranial tumor.

❏❏ **Describe the key features of acoustic neuroma.**

Symptoms and signs may include unilateral high tone sensorineural hearing loss and tinnitus. Other signs and symptoms include decreased corneal sensitivity, diplopia, headache, facial weakness and positive radiographic findings. Vertigo usually appears late, more often presenting as a progressive feeling of imbalance. Vertigo may be provoked by changes in head movement. Nystagmus is frequently present and is usually spontaneous. The CSF may have elevated protein.

❏❏ **Describe the key features of vertebrobasilar insufficiency.**

Vertigo is nearly always positional, provoked by certain head positions. Nystagmus usually accompanies the vertigo. Other signs of arteriosclerosis may be found. Vertebrobasilar insufficiency is usually seen in older persons and may occur with other symptoms of brainstem ischemia, visual symptoms being the most common.

❏❏ **What's that little bone seen behind the tympanic membrane?**

The malleus.

❏❏ **What disease would you expect in a patient with a two week history of lower limb weakness?**

Guillain-Barré is usually an ascending weakness which begins in the lower extremity.
With botulism poisoning, the weakness is descending.
Cranial nerves are typically affected first with myasthenia gravis.

❏❏ **What is the mortality rate of Wernicke's encephalopathy?**

10-20%. Treat with thiamine IV. Symptoms include ocular palsies, nystagmus, confusion, and ataxia.

❏❏ **Deep tendon reflexes are usually maintained in which of the following diseases: Myasthenia gravis, Guillain-Barré or Eaton-Lambert syndrome?**

Myasthenia gravis.
Reflexes are usually depressed in Eaton-Lambert syndrome and absent in Guillain-Barré.

❏❏ **On IVP, what is most indicative of severe urinary tract obstruction?**

A hyperdense nephrogram. Delayed filling may also be an indicator of obstruction.

❑❑ **How might a patient present with a hydatidiform mole?**

Hydatidiform mole presents with a larger than expected uterus and a positive pregnancy test.

❑❑ **Of the major tranquilizers, which one displays the most hypotensive tendency?**

Thorazine.

❑❑ **What is the most common cause for pain of odontogenic origin?**

Dental caries.

❑❑ **What factors and substances are known to decrease theophylline metabolism and increase theophylline levels?**

Age greater than 50, prematurity, liver and renal disease, pulmonary edema, CHF, pneumonia, obesity and viral illness in children. Drugs which increase theophylline levels include cimetidine, erythromycin, allopurinol, troleandomycin, BCP's, and quinolone antibiotics.

In smokers, however, theophylline half-life is decreased, causing decreased levels of serum theophylline. In addition to smoking, phenobarbital, phenytoin, rifampin, carbamazepine, marijuana smoking and exposure to environmental pollutants can decrease serum theophylline levels. Eating charcoal broiled foods may cause lowered theophylline levels.

❑❑ **What narcotic has the shortest half-life?**

Fentanyl has a half-life of about one half hour.

❑❑ **What therapy should be used for a patient with hemophilia A who suffers a head injury?**

Treat this patient with cryoprecipitate or lyophilized factor VIII. Keep total volume as low as possible. Cryoprecipitate has an increased concentration of factor VIII complex and has less volume than fresh frozen plasma.

❑❑ **What is the most serious complication of abscessed anterior maxillary teeth?**

Septic cavernous sinus thrombosis. Results from extension of infection into the canine space and facial venous system.

❑❑ **What is the first therapy to initiate for a bleeding patient on warfarin with a high PT?**

D/C warfarin. Then administer a water soluble form of vitamin K. Give IV slowly, consider test dose. Rapid administration of parenteral vitamin K (>1mg/min) has been associated with hypotension. It may also cause anaphylaxis. Reversal of warfarin's effect with vitamin K requires several hours. If the bleeding is severe, fresh frozen plasma should be given containing active factors X, IX, VII and II (REMEMBER 1972).

❑❑ **What is a common electrolyte abnormality associated with transfusion of packed red blood cells?**

Hypocalcemia secondary to citrate toxicity. Citrate, when rapidly infused, binds ionized calcium and therefore decreases the calcium level. Hyperkalemia may also develop with rapid packed red blood cell transfusion, especially if the patient is in renal failure or if the blood products are old.

❑❑ **What invasive measurement should be performed to evaluate a patient with swelling of the face, neck and arms?**

CVP. Swelling of the face, neck and arms is suggestive of superior vena cava syndrome. To confirm superior vena cava syndrome, increased CVP pressure in the upper body and normal pressure in the lower extremities must be documented. Chest x-ray will detect only about 10 percent of the masses causing superior vena cava syndrome.

❒❒ **Describe Leriche's syndrome.**

Leriche's syndrome is characterized by buttock, calf, and back pain with impotence. It is usually seen with aortoiliac disease.

❒❒ **What diagnosis should be suspected for a patient who has suffered loss of vision and whose fundus is pale?**

Central retinal artery occlusion usually presents with acute, painless loss of vision.

❒❒ **What is the most common cause of otitis media in children?**

Strep pneumoniae and *H. influenza.*

❒❒ **Describe a patient with sigmoid volvulus.**

Patients with sigmoid volvulus are typically either psychiatric patients or elderly who suffer from severe chronic constipation. Symptoms include intermittent cramping, lower abdominal pain and progressive abdominal distention.

❒❒ **Describe a typical patient with intussusception.**

Intussusception typically occurs in children of ages 3 months to 2 years. The majority are in the 5 to 10 mo age group. It is more common in boys. The area of the ileocecal valve is usually the source of the problem.

❒❒ **What are the common symptoms and signs of hyperthyroidism?**

Symptoms include weight loss, palpitations, dyspnea, edema, chest pain, nervousness, weakness, tremor, psychosis, diarrhea, hyperdefecation, abdominal pain, myalgias and disorientation. Signs include fever, tachycardia, wide pulse pressure, CHF, shock, thyromegaly, tremor, weakness, liver tenderness, jaundice, stare, and hyperkinesis. Mental status changes include somnolence, obtundation, coma, or psychosis. Pretibial myxedema may be found (a true misnomer!).

❒❒ **A patient suffers a rotational knee injury and hears a pop. Within 90 minutes hemarthrosis develops. What is the suspected location of the injury?**

The anterior cruciate.

❒❒ **What are radiological and laboratory findings of duodenal injury?**

Retroperitoneal air and increased serum amylase.

❒❒ **A patient has a fracture of the radial shaft. What associated injury should be ruled out?**

Distal radius-ulna joint dislocation, also known as a Galeazzi's fracture/dislocation.
Great Rays Down Deep! = GRDD.

GRDD = Galeazzi, Radius fracture, Distal Dislocation.

❒❒ **G-6-PD is the first enzyme in the hexose monophosphate shunt pathway that generates NADPH. NADPH helps maintain reduced glutathione. In G-6-PD deficiency, which affects 11% of black American males, this enzyme deteriorates with age. So?**

Glutathione serves to protect hemoglobin from injury due to oxidants. If such injury occurs, denatured Hb or hemolysis may follow.

❐❐ What drugs should be avoided in G-6-PD deficiency?

ASA, phenacetin; primaquine, quinine and quinacrine; nitrofurans; sulfamethoxazole and sulfacetamide; and methylene blue are all associated with hemolysis. These are all oxidants.

❐❐ What is the current therapeutic regimen for treatment of meningitis in a neonate?

Initially, ampicillin and aminoglycoside were favored for treating the neonate with meningitis. However, today recommendations include ampicillin and cefotaxime.
A combination used in infants up to 2 months of age will cover coliform, Group *B streptococci*, *Listeria*, and *enterococcus*. Over 2 months of age up to 6 years, cefotaxime alone is indicated.

❐❐ What is the formula for calculating a change in potassium with changes in pH?

For each pH increase of 0.1, expect the potassium to drop by 0.5 mmol/l.

❐❐ A patient has alcoholic ketoacidosis (aka AKA); what is appropriate treatment?

Alcoholic ketoacidosis usually presents with nausea, vomiting and abdominal pain occurring 24 to 72 h after cessation of drinking. No specific physical findings are typically evident, though abdominal pain is a common complaint/finding. Many patients have alcohol-induced gastritis. AKA is thought to be secondary to increased mobilization of free fatty acids with lipolysis to acetoacetate and ß-hydroxybutyrate. A significant component of metabolic alkalosis with hypochloremia and hypokalemia may be present.

Treatment usually includes normal saline and glucose. As acidosis is corrected, K^+ may drop. Sodium bicarbonate should not be given unless pH drops below 7.1.

❐❐ A patient presents to the emergency department and is very sick. Your diagnosis is alcoholic ketoacidosis. Urine dip is trace **positive for ketones. Now what do you think?**

God, I LOVE biochemistry!! I expect urine ketones to be few to none in some patients with AKA, as the nitroprusside test (Acetest®) is the common method used to test for ketones. I recall that this test measures positive for Acetoacetate and is less reactive to Acetone and is not affected by ß-hydroxybutyrate. *I know that ß-hydroxybutyrate is preferentially produced in AKA,* thus it is both possible and likely to obtain a negative or weakly positive test for serum ketones in the presence of clinically significant AKA.

2 Acetyl Co-A

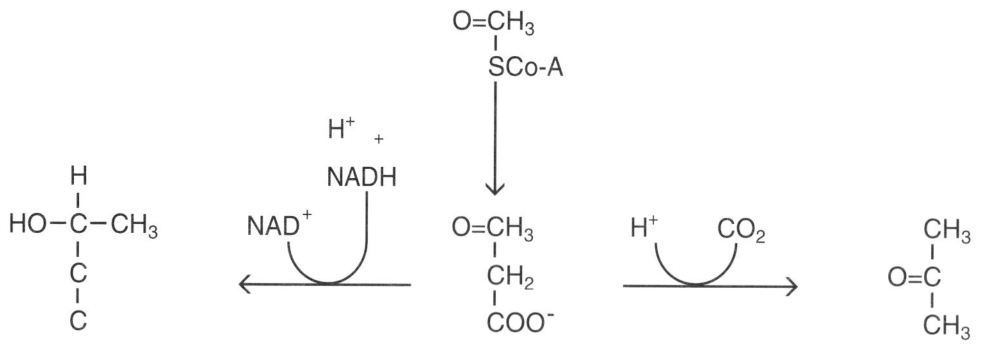

ß-Hydroxybutyrate **Acetoacetate** **Acetone**

❑❑ **Describe the symptoms of optic neuritis.**

The patient suffers a variable loss of central visual acuity with a central scotoma and change in color perception. The patient also has eye pain. The disk margins are blurred from hemorrhage and the blind spot is increased.

❑❑ **Compare and contrast primary and secondary myxedema.**

Primary:	Secondary :
Source: Thyroid	Pituitary
Frequency: Common, 95%	Ø common, 5%
+ Coarse voice	Ø Coarse voice
+ Goiter	Ø Goiter
Heart Big	heart small
+ Pubic hair	Ø Pubic hair
TSH elevated	TSH low
Iodine <2µg/dl	Iodine >2µg/dl

❑❑ **Which renal calculi are radiolucent and which renal calculi are radiopaque?**

Uric acid stones and blood clots are radiolUcent ureteral obstructions. 90% of all stones are radiopaque, composed of calcium oxalate, cysteine, calcium phosphate, or magnesium ammonium phosphate.

❑❑ **Antidote for arsenic?**

British Anti-Lewisite (BAL) 5 mg/kg IM.

❑❑ **Antidote for clonidine?**

Naloxone, tolazoline, and yohimbine may help. Care is primarily supportive.

❑❑ **Cyanide's harmful effects are due to its propensity to bind to metals and to disrupt the function of metal containing enzymes. Which is the most important of these?**

Cytochrome A_3, aka cytochrome oxidase, necessary for aerobic metabolism.

❑❑ **Antidote for cyanide?**

Amyl nitrite followed by sodium nitrite followed by sodium thiosulfate.

❑❑ **Why give nitrites for cyanide?**

Theory says nitrites form methemoglobin and methemoglobin strongly binds cyanide, decreasing binding to cytochrome A_3.

❑❑ **Why give sodium thiosulfate for cyanide?**

Rhodanase, an intrinsic enzyme, transfers cyanide from its attachment to methemoglobin to sulfur, forming thiocyanate. Thiocyanate is excreted. Sodium thiosulfate acts as a sulfur donor for this process.

❑❑ **Antidote for ethylene glycol?**

Ethanol and dialysis.

❑❑ **Antidote for gold?**

BAL.

❑❑ **Antidote for iron?**

Deferoxamine.

❑❑ **Antidote for lead?**

Dimercaptosuccinic acid (DMSA) or calcium EDTA.

❑❑ **Antidote for mercury?**

BAL.

❑❑ **Antidote for methanol?**

Ethanol and dialysis.

❑❑ **Antidote for nitrites?**

Methylene blue 1% 0.2 mL/kg IV over 5 minutes.
Severe methemoglobinemia requires exchange transfusion.

❑❑ **Antidote for organophosphates?**

Atropine with 2-PAM as indicated.

❑❑ **What are the common features of organic brain syndrome?**

Onset may be at any age. Symptoms include visual hallucinations and perception of the unfamiliar as familiar. Signs include mental status changes such as disorientation, clouded sensorium, asterixis or mild clonus and focal neurologic signs. Vital signs are most often within normal limits.

❑❑ **Describe the features of functional syndromes.**

Onset is usually at age less than 40. Symptoms include auditory hallucination and perception of the familiar as unfamiliar. Patients are usually oriented, cognitive function is usually normal and the sensorium is usually clear. Asterixis or myoclonus is not a feature of functional disease. Vital signs are usually normal without focal neurologic deficit.

❑❑ **Is the stomach more commonly injured with penetrating trauma or blunt trauma?**

The stomach is more commonly injured with penetrating trauma.

❑❑ **What is the most common body area affected in trauma that results in death?**

The head.

❑❑ **What is the <u>most</u> <u>common</u> cause of airway obstruction in trauma?**

CNS depression.

❑❑ **What is the <u>most</u> <u>common</u> wound associated with pericardial tamponade?**

Right ventricular injury.

❑❑ **What are the signs and symptoms of acute pericardial tamponade?**

Triad of hypotension, elevated CVP, and tachycardia is usually indicative of either acute pericardial tamponade or a tension pneumothorax in a traumatized patient. Muffled heart tones may be auscultated.

❑❑ Which EKG finding is pathognomonic of pericardial tamponade?

Total electrical alternans. Pulsus paradoxus is nonspecific. Muffled heart tones are subjective findings and are difficult to appreciate.

❑❑ What is the formula for correct infusion of peritoneal lavage fluid in a child?

10 cc/kg of lactated Ringer's solution should be infused to allow accurate interpretation of cell counts.

❑❑ Name 2 retroperitoneal organs which may be injured without producing a positive DPL.

Pancreas and duodenum.

❑❑ Name 2 organs that do not tend to bleed enough to produce a positive DPL when injured.

Bladder and small bowel.

❑❑ What RBC count is considered positive in peritoneal lavage fluid analysis of a patient with blunt abdominal trauma?

RBC counts of more than 100,000 per mm^3 are considered positive for both penetrating and blunt trauma to the abdomen.
5,000 RBCs per mm^3 is considered positive in a patient with low chest or high abdominal penetrating trauma where diaphragmatic perforation is a possibility.

❑❑ Define sensitivity and specificity.

Sensitivity is true positives divided by true positives plus false negatives. It represents how well a test identifies people who have a condition from among all the people who have the condition.

Specificity is true negatives divided by true negatives plus false positives. It is the percentage of people who do not have the disease correctly classified as negative by the test.

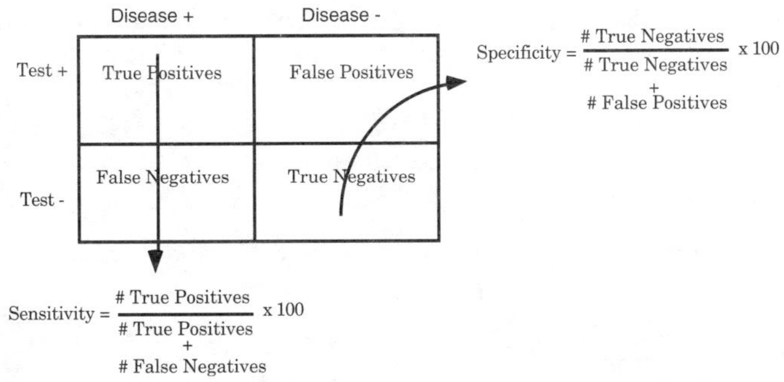

❑❑ Describe the zones of the neck and the appropriate treatment for injuries to each zone.

Zone 1 -- below the cricoid cartilage,
Zone 2 -- between the angle of the mandible and the cricoid cartilage,
Zone 3 -- above the angle of the mandible.

Treatment and evaluation:
Zones 1 and 3, angiography to evaluate major vessels.

Zone 2 requires surgical evaluation. ("2 surgery!!")

❑❑ What is the cause of death secondary to untreated tension pneumothorax?

Decreased cardiac output. The vena cava is compressed resulting in decreased right heart blood return and concomitant severe compromise in stroke volume, blood pressure and cardiac output.
[Editorial comment - 2° arrhythmias can also occur. V-tach in a young apparently healthy person is 2° to a tension pneumothorax until proven otherwise. JNA]

❑❑ How does a chronic pericardial effusion appear on chest x-ray?

Gradual pericardial sac distention results in a "water bottle" appearance of the heart.

❑❑ What are the symptoms and signs of adrenal insufficiency?

Fatigue, nausea, anorexia, abdominal pain, change in bowel habits and syncope are frequently reported symptoms. Hyperpigmentation, hypertension, vitiligo and weight loss may be noted.
Laboratory abnormalities can include hypoglycemia, <u>hyperkalemia</u>, <u>hyponatremia</u> and azotemia.

❑❑ Treatment for myxedema coma may include:

IV thyroid replacement with thyroxine, IV glucose, hydrocortisone and consideration of water restriction.

❑❑ What are the symptoms and signs of thyrotoxicosis?

Weight loss and weakness may be reported. Tachycardia and fever are common abnormal vital signs with hypotension and shock occurring less frequently. Mental status changes of decreased consciousness or psychosis may be present. Signs of CHF, thyromegaly, tremor, eye signs including lid lag and proptosis should also be sought.

❑❑ How do patients present with central retinal artery occlusion?

Patients present with a sudden, painless loss of vision in one eye.

❑❑ Describe a patient with acute narrow angle closure glaucoma.

Symptoms include nausea, vomiting and abdominal pain. Visual acuity is markedly diminished. The pupil is semi-dilated and nonreactive. There is usually a glassy haze over the cornea and the eye is red and very painful. Intraocular pressure may be as high as 50 or 60 mmHg.

❑❑ Describe the treatment of acute narrow angle glaucoma.

Mannitol to decrease intraocular pressure.
Miotics, such as pilocarpine, to open the angle.
Carbonic anhydrase inhibitor to minimize aqueous humor production. Iridectomy is eventually performed to provide aqueous outflow.

❑❑ What is the appropriate treatment for a hyphema?

Elevate the head.
Other treatment is controversial, however, most ophthalmologists believe patients should be hospitalized.
Treatment <u>may</u> include double eye patch, topical cortisone and cycloplegics. Visual acuity is often decreased.

❑❑ Describe the classic symptoms and signs of retinal detachment.

The patient is typically myopic and will complain of seeing a curtain coming down across his or her eye. This is usually accompanied by flashes of light but no discomfort. The patient may also see flashing lights, black dots, or sudden change in vision. On funduscopic exam, the detached areas will appear gray in comparison to the normal pink retina. Treatment includes bilateral eye patch, strict bedrest and consultation with an ophthalmologist for laser photocoagulation of the retinal detachment.

❑❑ What type of streptococci cause acute post-streptococcal glomerulonephritis?

Group A ß-hemolytic streptococci. Physical exam may reveal facial edema and decreased urinary output that are the most common presenting findings. Urine may be dark. Laboratory findings include normochromic anemia due to hemodilution, increased sedimentation rate, numerous RBCs and WBCs in the urine with casts, and hyperkalemia. Hospitalization is advised.

❑❑ Name the five major modified Jones criteria.

Dr. Jones, the EM Physician, is SNoring, she Can't Come.

Dr. Jones, the EM	Erythema Marginatum
Physician,	Polyarthritis
is SNoring,	Subcutaneous Nodules
she Can't	Carditis
Come.	Chorea

Other criteria include rheumatic fever or rheumatic heart disease, arthralgias, fever, prolonged PR interval on EKG, C reactive protein, elevated sedimentation rate, or antistreptolysin O titer.

❑❑ What disorder is present when the five major modified Jones criteria are met?

Rheumatic fever.

❑❑ Describe the symptoms and signs of varicella (chickenpox).

Varicella rash onset is one to two days after prodromal symptoms of slight malaise, anorexia and fever. The rash begins on the trunk and scalp. It first appears as faint macules, later becoming vesicles.

❑❑ Describe the signs of roseola infantum.

Roseola infantum usually affects children ages 6 months to 3 years. It is characterized by high fever that begins abruptly and lasts 3 to 5 days, possibly precipitating febrile seizures. A rash appears as the temperature drops to normal.

❑❑ Describe the symptoms and signs of rubella (German measles).

Rubella begins after a mild 1 - 5 day prodrome of upper respiratory infection symptoms. A rash begins on the face and spreads quickly. Suboccipital and posterior auricular adenopathy are associated findings.

❑❑ What is the standard dose of atropine in a child?

0.02 mg/kg is the standard atropine dose.

❑❑ What is the most common cause of bacterial meningitis in a child more than one month of age?

Hemophilus influenzae.
S. pneumoniae is second most common.
N. meningitis is third most common.
This is treated with ampicillin and chloramphenicol. Single agent treatment with a third generation cephalosporin may also be used.

❑❑ What is the initial dose of sodium bicarbonate in children during a cardiopulmonary arrest?

1 mEq/kg.

❐❐ How is the expected normal systolic blood pressure for a pediatric patient (toddlers and up) calculated?

Multiply the age by 2 and add 90 to the result to determine expected systolic BP.

Average SBP (mmHg) = (Age x 2) + 90

Low normal limit SBP (mmHg) = (Age x 2) + 70.

SBP for a term newborn is about 60 mmHg.

❐❐ How does sickle cell disease usually present in a patient older than 12 months?

Initial symptoms are often pain in the joints, bones and abdomen. The child may have abdominal tenderness and even rigidity. Mild icterus and anemia may be present.

❐❐ How does a child present with erythema infectiosum (fifth disease or slapcheek syndrome)?

Fifth disease typically does not infect infants or adults. There are no prodromal symptoms. The illness usually begins with sudden appearance of erythema of the cheeks followed by a maculopapular rash on the trunk and extremities that evolve into a lacy pattern.

❐❐ What is the correct dose of epinephrine and atropine during a pediatric code?

Epinephrine 0.01 mg/kg/dose.
Atropine 0.02 mg/kg/dose.

❐❐ What are the signs and symptoms of Kawasaki's disease?

Kawasaki's initial presentation is with a high spiking fever, conjunctivitis, morbilliform rash, strawberry tongue, and erythema of the distal extremities with cervical adenopathy. It is a disease of the mucocutaneous lymph nodes. Patients should be hospitalized to rule out myocarditis, pericarditis and coronary aneurysms. Aspirin is therapeutic.

❐❐ What is the initial antibiotic treatment for a child with epiglottitis?

The most likely cause is *H. influenzae*; the child should be treated with a second or third generation cephalosporin.

❐❐ What are the characteristics of a posterior hip dislocation?

Posterior hip dislocations are typically caused by posteriorly directed force applied to the flexed knee. The extremity is shortened, internally rotated and adducted. Acetabular fractures are associated with this injury. 90% of hip dislocations are posterior.

❐❐ Describe the key features of central cord syndrome.

Central cord syndrome typically occurs with hyperextension injuries in older patients with spondylosis, degenerative changes or stenosis in the cervical spine. Symptoms include weakness that is more pronounced in the arms than the legs.

❐❐ Key features of anterior spinal cord syndrome?

The anterior cord syndrome involves compression of the anterior cord causing complete motor paralysis and loss of pain and temperature sensation distal to the lesion. Posterior columns are spared - light touch and proprioception are preserved.

❐❐ **What is the typical organism of a paronychia?**

Staphylococcus aureus.

❐❐ **How does myasthenia gravis typically present?**

Weakness of voluntary muscles, usually the extraocular muscles. Diagnostic confirmation relies on the edrophonium (Tensilon) test that we don't do.
Treatment includes neurologic consultation, anticholinesterases, steroids and thymectomy.

❐❐ **What visual deficit is typically associated with lesions at the optic chiasm?**

Optic chiasm lesions typically produce bitemporal hemianopsia.

❐❐ **On CT scan of the brain of an immunocompromised patient, a ring lesion is noted. The patient also has lymphadenopathy, fever, headache and confusion. What diagnosis is suspected?**

Toxoplasmosis secondary to *Toxoplasma gondii* cyst. The disease is typically treated with pyrimethamine and sulfadiazine.

❐❐ **What are the signs and symptoms of posterior inferior cerebellar artery syndrome?**

Cerebellar dysfunction such as vertigo, ataxia and dizziness.

❐❐ **Describe the signs and symptoms of neuroleptic malignant syndrome.**

Patients present with muscle rigidity, autonomic disturbances and acute organic brain syndrome.
Blood pressure and pulse fluctuate wildly and temperature may reach as high as 42° C (108° F).
Muscle necrosis may occur with resultant myoglobinuria. Mortality ranges as high as 20%.

❐❐ **Describe the presentation of placenta previa.**

Placenta previa typically presents with painless bright red vaginal bleeding.

❐❐ **Describe the presentation of abruptio placentae.**

Dark red, painful, vaginal bleeding.

❐❐ **What is the most common growth plate (Salter class) injury?**

Salter II fracture.

❐❐ **Where is the most common site for esophageal foreign bodies to lodge?**

The cricopharyngeus muscle.

❐❐ **What is the most common organism causing a septic joint in a child?**

S. aureus.

❐❐ **What is the most common organism to cause a septic joint in an adolescent?**

Neisseria gonorrhoeae.

❐❐ **Signs of tension pneumothorax on physical exam include:**

Tachypnea, unilateral absent breath sounds, tachycardia, pallor, diaphoresis, cyanosis, tracheal deviation, hypotension and neck vein distention.

❑❑ **What is the most common cause of bacterial pneumonia, except for the first week of life?**

Streptococcus pneumoniae.

❑❑ **What is the most common cause of abdominal pain in children?**

Constipation.

❑❑ **What is the most common cause of an intestinal obstruction in a child under 2 years of age?**

Intussusception.

❑❑ **What is the most frequent carpal fracture.**

Navicular fracture.

❑❑ **What is the most frequently dislocated bone in the wrist?**

Lunate.
It is also the second most common fractured bone in the wrist.

❑❑ **What medications should be used to treat preeclampsia and eclampsia?**

Magnesium and hydralazine.

❑❑ **Do local anesthetics freely cross the blood brain barrier?**

Yes.
Most systemic toxic reactions to local anesthetics involve the CNS or cardiovascular system.

❑❑ **What is the most common cause of hemoptysis in the United States?**

Bronchitis and bronchiectasis.

❑❑ **What is the most common site of thrombophlebitis?**

The deep muscles of the calves, particularly the soleus muscle.

❑❑ **What is the most common cause of acute aortic regurgitation?**

Infectious endocarditis.

❑❑ **What are the most common causes of aortic stenosis (2)?**

Rheumatic fever and congenital bicuspid valve disease.

❑❑ **What is the most common cause of acute mitral regurgitation?**

Inferior wall infarcts.

❑❑ **What are the most common causes of pulsus paradoxus (2)?**

COPD and asthma.

❑❑ **What does Beck's triad consist of?**

Hypotension, elevated CVP (distended neck veins) and distant heart sounds.

❒❒ **What's it good for (Beck's triad that is)?**

Acute pericardial tamponade.

❒❒ **What is the <u>worst</u> way to confirm the diagnosis of a delayed pericardial injury after blunt trauma?**

Autopsy.

❒❒ **What is the <u>most</u> <u>common</u> conduction disturbance in acute myocardial infarction?**

First degree AV block.

❒❒ **How much fluid is needed in the pericardial sac to increase the cardiac silhouette on chest x-ray?**

About 250 mL.

❒❒ **What is the most common site of rupture in abdominal aortic aneurysms?**

Posterior lateral aorta.

❒❒ **What is the most common symptom in abdominal aortic aneurysm?**

Pain.

❒❒ **What is the most common dysrhythmia associated with Wolff-Parkinson-White syndrome?**

Paroxysmal atrial tachycardia.

❒❒ **What are the symptoms and signs of aortic stenosis?**

Exertional dyspnea, angina and syncope.
Narrowed pulse pressure with decreased SBP.
Slow carotid upstroke.
Prominent S_4.

❒❒ **What drugs are commonly associated with torsade de pointes?**

Type I-A antiarrhythmics - quinidine and procainamide.

These drugs lengthen the Q-T interval.

❒❒ **What common metabolic disorder is associated with hypercalcemia?**

Hypokalemia.

❒❒ **What does the urine dipstick show from a patient with myoglobinuria?**

The dipstick is "heme-positive" with few or no RBCs.

❒❒ **What is the <u>most</u> <u>common</u> cause of hepatitis transmitted through blood transfusions?**

Hepatitis C.

❒❒ **Are males or females more likely to get symptomatic gallstones?**

Females.

❒❒ What is the most common type of ulcers?

Duodenal ulcers are more commonly seen than gastric ulcers.

❒❒ What is the differential diagnosis of a red eye with decreased visual acuity?

Iritis, glaucoma and central corneal lesions.

❒❒ A patient has a non-red, painful eye with decreased visual acuity. What diagnosis do you suspect?

Optic neuritis.

❒❒ What disease is associated with retrobulbar optic neuritis?

MS.

❒❒ How could mydriasis caused by third cranial nerve compression be distinguished from mydriasis caused by anticholinergic drugs or mydriatics?

Mydriasis caused by third cranial nerve compression is reversible with pilocarpine, other causes are not.

❒❒ What is the best method to open an airway while maintaining C-spine precautions?

Jaw thrust.

❒❒ What is the only absolute contraindication to MAST?

Pulmonary edema.

❒❒ T/F: Increased blood pressure in hypovolemic patients associated with MAST application is primarily due to autotransfusion.

NOT! The primary mechanism of MAST appears to be due to increased peripheral vascular resistance. Autotransfusion of a few hundred mL of blood may occur but is not of great significance.

❒❒ What is the most common complication of using an EOA?

Tracheal intubation, 10%.

❒❒ At what child's age is a cuffed ET tube preferred?

6 years.

❒❒ What is the formula for appropriate ET tube size in children greater than 1 year-old?

ET size = (Age + 16) / 4.

❒❒ What is the correct ET tube size for a 1 - 2 year-old?

4.0 - 4.5 mm.

❒❒ What is the correct ET tube size for a 6 month-old?

3.5 - 4.5 mm. Hey, we didn't *make up* these answers!...

❐❐ **What is the correct ET tube size for a newborn?**

3.0 - 3.5 mm.
Premature - 2.5 - 3.0 mm.

❐❐ **What is the distance from the mouth to 2 cm above the carina in men and women?**

Men 23 cm; women 21 cm.

❐❐ **What is the treatment of hyperkalemia?**

Diurese with loop diuretic, e.g.., furosemide or ethacrynic acid.

Sodium polystyrene sulfonate ion exchange resin (Kayexalate) enema (associated Na^+ load can cause failure). Hours before effect is seen.

1 ampule of D_{50}, insulin 5 to 10 units IV for redistribution (follow by 50 g glucose and 20 U insulin over 1 hour). About 30 minutes for effect.

Sodium bicarbonate 50 - 100 mEq IV over 10 - 20 minutes. Five to ten minutes for effect.

Calcium. Calcium chloride has more Ca per ampule (13.4 mEq) than gluconate (4.6 mEq) and is faster acting. Give one ampule (10 mL of 10% solution) over 10 - 20 minutes. WATCH OUT if giving to a patient on digitalis, it will potentiate toxicity. Very rapid onset.

3% sodium chloride IV may serve as a temporary antagonist.

Peritoneal or hemodialysis.

Digoxin specific Fab (Digibind) if 2° to digitalis overdose.

❐❐ **How should hypercalcemia be treated?**

Furosemide and normal saline. Mithramycin may be used, especially in hypercalcemia secondary to bone cancer. Other treatments include calcitonin, hydrocortisone, and indomethacin.

❐❐ **What is the <u>most</u> <u>common</u> cause of multifocal atrial tachycardia?**

COPD.

❐❐ **What is the treatment for multifocal atrial tachycardia?**

Treat underlying disorder. Magnesium sulfate 2 grams over 60 seconds (with supplemental potassium to maintain serum K^+ above 4 mEq/l). A second treatment is verapamil 10 mg IV.

❐❐ **What is the treatment of ectopic SVT due to digitalis toxicity?**

Stop digitalis, correct hypokalemia, consider digoxin specific Fab, magnesium IV, lidocaine IV or phenytoin IV.

❐❐ **What is the treatment of ectopic SVT not due to digitalis toxicity?**

Digitalis, verapamil or ß-blocker to slow rate. Quinidine, procainamide or magnesium to decrease ectopy.

❐❐ **What is the treatment for verapamil-induced hypotension?**

Calcium gluconate 1 gram IV over several minutes.

❐❐ **What drugs are contraindicated for treatment of le torsade de pointes?**

A drug which prolongs repolarization (QT interval). For example, class Ia antiarrhythmics (quinidine, procainamide). Other drugs that share this effect include TCAs, disopyramide, and phenothiazines.

❑❑ **What is the treatment of torsade de pointes?**

Pacemaker cranked to 90 - 120 bpm to "overdrive" pace.
Isoproterenol is an other option. Magnesium is the agent of choice to treat drug-induced torsade de pointes. The initial dose of magnesium sulfate is 2 grams IV..
The goal is to accelerate the heart rate and shorten ventricular repolarization. (If it's me, start with the mag, SHP & JNA).

❑❑ **Discuss the treatment of digitalis toxicity.**

Charcoal.
Phenytoin (Dilantin) for ventricular arrhythmias (it increases AV node conduction) or lidocaine.
Atropine or pace for bradyarrhythmias.
Digoxin specific Fab (Digibind).

❑❑ **What hypos can lower the seizure threshold?**

Hypoglycemia, hyponatremia, and hypocarbia.

❑❑ **What are symptoms and signs of a vertebrobasilar artery lesion?**

Vertebral system supplies cerebellum and brain stem.
Vertigo, nausea, vomiting, ipsilateral 7th nerve deficit, contralateral hemiplegia.
Basilar artery occlusion leads to quadriplegia, coma or locked-in syndrome.

❑❑ **What motor function is spared in locked-in syndrome?**

Upward gaze.

❑❑ **What are signs and symptoms of a middle cerebral artery lesion?**

Hemiplegia or hemiparesthesia, homonymous hemianopsia and speech disturbance.

❑❑ **What is the most common cause of cerebral artery occlusion, embolic or thrombotic?**

Embolic.

❑❑ **What effects are likely to be present with an anterior cerebral artery lesion?**

Paralysis of contralateral leg with sensory loss in leg only and incontinence. No aphasia.

❑❑ **What deficits can result from ocular motor nerve paralysis?**

Ptosis as a result of levator palpebrae superioris/cranial nerve III injury. Lateral nerve gaze is controlled by cranial nerve VI, corneal reflex by cranial nerve V. The superior oblique muscle moves gaze downward and laterally; it is controlled by CN IV.

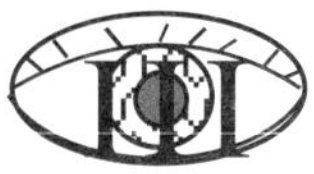

$(LR_6\ SO_4)_3$

❒❒ **Describe the symptoms and signs of pressure on the first sacral root (S1).**

Symptoms of S1 injury include pain radiating to the mid-gluteal region, posterior thigh, posterior calf and down to the heel and sole of the foot. Sensory signs are localized to the lateral toes. S1 root compression would typically involve the plantar flexor muscles of the foot and toes. The ankle reflex is decreased or absent.

❒❒ **In an infant, what is the most narrow segment of the airway?**

The cricoid cartilage ring. The glottic aperture is the most narrow part of the airway in the adult.

❒❒ **What is the ET tube size recommended for a term newborn infant?**

3 - 3.5 mm.
Premature infant requires a 2.5 mm tube.

❒❒ **What drug would you use to treat a patient in cardiac arrest secondary to hyperkalemia?**

Calcium chloride IV acts fastest.
Also provide $NaHCO_3$.

❒❒ **What are the potential complications of excess sodium bicarbonate?**

Cerebral acidosis, hypokalemia, hyperosmolality, and increased hemoglobin binding of oxygen.

❒❒ **What are the effects of dopamine at various doses?**

At 1 to 10 µg/kg, dopamine causes renal, mesenteric, coronary and cerebral vasodilation.
At 10 to 20 µg/kg, both α– and ß-adrenergic effects are present.
At 20 µg/kg, effects are primarily α–adrenergic.

❒❒ **What is the drug of choice for digitalis toxicity resulting in a ventricular arrhythmia?**

Phenytoin and digoxin specific Fab (Dilantin and Digibind).

❒❒ **What is the treatment for acute angle closure glaucoma?**

2% Pilocarpine drops every 15 minutes initially, acetazolamide (Diamox) 250 mg IV or 500 mg po, and po glycerol 1 g/kg with juice, or IV mannitol.

❒❒ **For each 100 increase in glucose, what is the effect on serum sodium?**

Each 100 increase in glucose decreases the serum sodium by 1.7 mEq/l.

❒❒ **What are common entities in the differential diagnosis of pinpoint pupils?**

Narcotic overdose, clonidine overdose, sedative hypnotic overdose including alcohol, cerebellar pontine angle infarct, and subarachnoid hemorrhage.

❒❒ **In a patient with tachycardia from cocaine abuse, what medications are appropriate?**

Sedation with benzodiazepines may calm the patient and decrease tachycardia. Nitroprusside may be used to treat hypertension. Caution must be used with ß-adrenergic antagonist agents alone as they may leave α–adrenergic stimulation unopposed, increasing the patient's risk for severe hypertension, intracranial hemorrhage, or aortic dissection.

❒❒ **What traditional anti-arrhythmic agents may be used to treat digitalis-induced ventricular arrhythmias in addition to phenytoin?**

Lidocaine and bretylium. Procainamide and quinidine are contraindicated in digitalis toxicity.

❑❑ **In a trauma patient receiving multiple units of transfused blood, when should the blood products be supplemented with fresh frozen plasma?**

For each five units of transfused blood, fresh frozen plasma is usually given.

❑❑ **What is a complication due to citrate present in stored blood?**

Citrate may bind calcium and result in hypocalcemia.

❑❑ **What is an anaphylactoid reaction?**

Anaphylactoid reactions are very similar to anaphylaxis, however, they do not require prior exposure to the reaction product. Cases may result from radiopaque contrast media or medications such as NSAIDs.

❑❑ **A child has a mild anaphylactic reaction. What is the correct route and dose of epinephrine?**

The correct dose is 0.01 mL/kg of a 1:1,000 solution, up to 0.3 mL, SQ.

❑❑ **What is universal donor blood?**

Type Rh negative blood with anti-A and anti-B titers of less than 1:200 in saline.

❑❑ **When would orthostatic hypotension typically develop in a 70 kg adult?**

Loss of over 1000 cc of blood would probably result in orthostatic hypotension. Class II hemorrhage (loss of 750-1500 mL) presents with tachycardia, normal BP and narrow pulse pressure. Class III hemorrhage (loss of 1500 to 2000 mL) presents with tachycardia > 120, hypotension and decreased urine output.

❑❑ **What are the common presentations of a transfusion reaction?**

Myalgia, dyspnea, fever associated with hypocalcemia, hemolysis, allergic reactions, hyperkalemia, citrate toxicity, hypothermia, coagulopathies and altered hemoglobin function.

❑❑ **What are the signs of the Cushing reflex?**

Increased systolic blood pressure and bradycardia.

❑❑ **In the Glasgow Coma Scale a dead person gets a 3. What number of points are possible measuring eye-opening response?**

4.
(I've an eye 4 U).

❑❑ **What number of points is the best verbal response worth in the Glasgow Coma Scale?**

5.

❑❑ **What number of points is the best motor response worth in the Glasgow Coma Scale?**

6.

❑❑ **What are normal findings in the oculocephalic reflex?**

Conjugate eye movement is opposite to the direction of head rotation.

❑❑ **In testing a patient's oculovestibular reflex, what is the direction of nystagmus anticipated in response to cold-water irrigation; toward or away from the irrigated ear?**

Recall that nystagmus is defined as the direction of the fast component of saccadic eye movement.
Emergency physicians commonly perform a crude but secure test of the oculovestibular reflex using ice water.
After irrigation, nystagmus should be away from the irrigated ear.
Try the mnemonic COWS - Cold Opposite, Warm Same.

❑❑ Signs and symptoms of an uncal herniation include:

Ipsilateral pupillary dilation and either ipsilateral or contralateral hemiparesis. Blunting of corneal reflex may occur. Oculovestibular response may be lost.

❑❑ Tonic eye movement toward irrigated ear in response to caloric testing in a comatose patient signifies.

Life.

❑❑ What effect do ß-blockers have on Prinzmetal's variant angina?

ß-blockers typically worsen the syndrome by allowing unopposed α–adrenergic stimulation of the coronary arteries.

❑❑ What are the symptoms and signs of an ophthalmoplegic migraine?

Typical duration is 3 to 5 days. Patient may complain of diplopia.
Mydriasis and exotropia may be noted.
Palsies of the muscles served by cranial nerves III, IV and VI may occur.

❑❑ Define strabismus.

A lack of parallelism of the visual axis of the eyes.
Esotropia = medially deviated,
Exotropia = laterally deviated.

❑❑ What common drugs cause bradycardia?

Agents such as ß-blockers, cardiac glycosides, pilocarpine and cholinesterase inhibitors such as organophosphates are responsible for bradycardia.

Sympathomimetics such as amphetamines and cocaine, and anticholinergics, such as atropine and cyclic antidepressants, commonly cause tachycardia.

❑❑ What drug commonly causes both horizontal and vertical nystagmus?

Phencyclidine (PCP).

❑❑ What life-threatening mnemonic may help you recall the signs of cholinergic poisoning?

DUELS. These fighters are wet.

D = diaphoresis,
U = urination,
E = eye changes (miosis),
L = lacrimation,
S = salivation.

❑❑ What is the antidote for organophosphates?

Atropine and pralidoxime (PAM).

❑❑ **How is an overdose of nitroprusside treated?**

Nitroprusside may induce methemoglobinemia. This is treated with 1% methylene blue solution.

❑❑ **For how long should sutures remain in the face, scalp or trunk, extremities and joints?**

Facial sutures	-3 to 5 days,
Scalp or Trunk	-7 to 10 days,
Extremities	-10 to 14 days,
Joints	-14 days.

❑❑ **What are the signs and symptoms of uncal herniation?**

Uncal herniation typically compresses the ipsilateral third cranial nerve resulting in ipsilateral pupil dilation. Contralateral weakness occurs because the pyramidal track decussates below this level. Occasionally, shift will be great enough to cause compression of both sides leading to a combination of ipsilateral or contralateral pupillary dilatation and weakness.

❑❑ **What is a common finding on sinus x-ray suggesting basilar skull fracture?**

Blood in the sphenoid sinus.

❑❑ **What bleeding sites are causes of subdural hemorrhages?**

Torn bridging veins.
Delayed hemorrhage from damaged parenchyma may also result in subdural hemorrhage.

❑❑ **In ordering x-rays of the face, what view gives the best view of the zygomatic arch?**

Modified basal view. This is also called jug-handle, submentaloccipital or submental-vertical view.

❑❑ **What x-ray view should be ordered to evaluate the maxilla, maxillary sinus, orbital floor, inferior orbital rim or zygomatic bones?**

The Water's view.

❑❑ **How long can an extracted tooth survive?**

One percentage point of likely survivability is lost for each minute the tooth is out.
A tooth may survive 4 to 6 h longer in a commercial solution.
If no commercial solution is available place in milk or under patient's tongue.

❑❑ **Name five drugs or conditions that cause hypertension.**

Sympathomimetics
Withdrawal
Anticholinergics
MAO Inhibitors
Phencyclidine (PCP). Mnemonic for this is SWAMP.

❑❑ **Name five drugs or conditions that cause tachycardia.**

Sympathomimetics
Withdrawal
Anticholinergics
MAO Inhibitors
Phencyclidine (PCP). SWAMP mnemonic.

❐❐ Name six common drugs that can cause hyperthermia.

Salicylates
Anticholinergics
Neuroleptics
Dinitrophenols
Sympathomimetics and PCP.

A psychotic friend of mine (on Stelazine) with bad allergies was on the beach smoking some Jimson weed laced with PCP. She took some antihistamine for the allergies and ASA for the sunburn. She was then stung by a beach-bee and required epi, but right about then the drugs were kicking in and it took 12 beach security guards to hold her down for her shot. Boy was she HOT!
The mnemonic is SANDS-PCP.

❐❐ What drugs/environmental exposures can induce bullous lesion formation?

Sedative hypnotics, carbon monoxide, snake bite, spider bite, caustic agents, and hydrocarbons.

❐❐ What drugs cause an odor of acetone on the breath?

Ethanol, isopropanol and salicylates. Ketosis often has the same odor.

❐❐ What substances induce an odor of almonds on the breath?

Cyanide, Laetrile, and apricot pits (latter two contain amygdalin).

❐❐ What drugs induce an odor of garlic on the breath?

DMSO, organophosphates, phosphorus, arsenic, arsine gas and thallium.

❐❐ What drug induces an odor of peanuts on the breath?

Vacor (RH-787).

❐❐ What drugs induce a pear-like odor on the breath?

Chloral hydrate and paraldehyde.

❐❐ What compounds induce an odor of rotten eggs on the breath?

Hydrogen sulfide, mercaptans and sewer-gas.

❐❐ What is the mnemonic for remembering what drugs or conditions commonly cause seizures?

SHAKE WITH eL SPOC!

S = salicylates,
H = hypoxia,
A = anticholinergics,
K = Karbon Monoxide (KO),
E = EtOH withdrawal,

W = withdrawal,
I = isoniazid,
T = theophylline and tricyclics,
H = hypoglycemia,

eL = lead, lithium and local anesthetics,
S = strychnine and sympathomimetics,
P = PCP, phenothiazines and propoxyphene,
O = organophosphates,
C = camphor, cholinergics, carbon monoxide and cyanide.

❒❒ What is a mnemonic for remembering the drugs that cause nystagmus?

MALES TIP

M = methanol,
A = alcohol,
L = lithium,
E = ethylene glycol,
S = sedative hypnotics and solvents,

T = thiamine depletion and Tegretol (carbamazepine),
I = isopropanol and
P = PCP and phenytoin.

❒❒ What is a mnemonic for remembering drugs that are radiopaque?

BAT CHIPS!

B = barium
A = antihistamines,
T = tricyclic antidepressants,

C = chloral hydrate, calcium, cocaine condoms,
H = heavy metals,
I = iodine,
P = phenothiazines, potassium,
S = slow-release (enteric coated).

❒❒ What is the antidote for Mercury, Arsenic and Gold (MAG) poisoning?

BAL & Dimercaptosuccinic acid (DMSA).

Play BAL with a DMSAl named MAG!

❒❒ What is the antidote for ß-blockers?

Glucagon.

❒❒ What are the antidotes for ethylene glycol?

Fomepizole, ethyl alcohol, and dialysis. Thiamine and pyridoxine are also important possibly to divert metabolism of EG to less toxic acids than oxalate.

❒❒ What three toxicologic emergencies require immediate dialysis?

Ethylene glycol, methyl alcohol and Amanita phalloides.

❒❒ What is the antidote for iron?

Deferoxamine.

❒❒ What are the antidotes for isoniazid?

Pyridoxine, diazepam, and sodium bicarbonate.

❑❑ **Antidote for reversing benzodiazepine overdose?**

Flumazenil.

❑❑ **What is the antidote for lead?**

EDTA. EDTA is ONLY used for treating lead poisoning.
Penicillamine.
BAL.

❑❑ **What is the antidote for mercury?**

Penicillamine and BAL.

❑❑ **What is the antidote for organophosphates?**

Atropine and 2-PAM.

❑❑ **What is the antidote for chronic bromide intoxication (bromism)?**

NaCl.

❑❑ **What is the antidote for tricyclic antidepressant overdose?**

Alkalinization.

❑❑ **Name some side effects of alkalization of the urine.**

Hypernatremia and hyperosmolality.

❑❑ **What drugs are commonly excreted using alkaline diuresis?**

BLIST

B = barbiturates (long-acting),
L = lithium (not so common),
I = INH,
T = TCAs,
S = salicylates.

❑❑ **What drugs require immediate dialysis?**

Ethylene glycol and methyl alcohol. Come on, you know it...yup, Amanita phalloides does too.

❑❑ **Can theophylline be dialyzed?**

Yes.

❑❑ **For what drugs may hemoperfusion be indicated?**

Salicylates, theophylline and long-acting barbiturates.

❑❑ **For what drugs may dialysis be indicated?**

Salicylates, theophylline and long-acting barbiturates.
Also - Methyl alcohol, ethylene glycol, amphetamine, lithium and thiocyanate.

❐❐ What are the four mechanisms by which tricyclics induce toxicity?

(1) Anticholinergic atropine-like effects 2° to competitive antagonism of acetylcholine.
(2) Block the reuptake of norepinephrine.
(3) A quinidine-like action on the myocardium.
(4) Alpha blocking action (promotes vasodilation, i.e., hypotension).

❐❐ What are the symptoms and signs of anticholinergic effects?

Peripheral effects include tachycardia, hyperpyrexia, mydriasis, vasodilatation, urinary retention, decreased GI motility, decreased secretions. Central effects include anxiety, disorientation, hallucinations, hyperactivity, delirium, seizures, coma and death. These patients are dry. In fact,
Dry as a bone,
Red as a beet,
Mad as a hatter,
Hot as a stone,
Blind as a bat.

❐❐ What are the four stages of acetaminophen toxicity?

I (within h)	- anorexia, nausea, vomiting and diaphoresis.
II (24-48 h)	- liver function test abnormalities and right upper quadrant pain.
III (72-96 h)	- jaundice, return of GI symptoms, peak of liver function abnormalities, coagulation defects.
IV (4 d-2 wk)	- Get better or die.

❐❐ When does acetaminophen become toxic?

When there is no glutathione to detoxify its toxic intermediate.

❐❐ How does N-acetylcysteine act to interrupt acetaminophen toxicity?

Exact mechanism unknown, however, likely that NAC enters cells, and is metabolized to cysteine which is a precursor for glutathione. Thus it may increase glutathione stores.

❐❐ Would you like to have FOUR ACEs.

Of course! So check ACEtaminophen level FOUR h after ingestion.

❐❐ What is the early acid base disturbance seen in salicylate overdose?

Respiratory alkalosis. Approximately 12 hours later, one might see an anion gap metabolic acidosis or mixed acid base picture.

❐❐ In salicylate overdose, is hyperglycemia or hypoglycemia expected?

This may present with either hyperglycemia or hypoglycemia.

❐❐ What are common symptoms and signs of chronic salicylism?

Fever, tachypnea, CNS alterations, acid base abnormalities, electrolyte abnormalities, chronic pain, ketonuria, and noncardiogenic pulmonary edema.

❐❐ A patient presents with an acute salicylate ingestion. What symptoms are expected with a mild, a moderate and a severe overdose?

Mild - Lethargy, vomiting, hyperventilation and hyperthermia.

Moderate - Severe hyperventilation and compensated metabolic acidosis.
Severe - Coma, seizures and uncompensated metabolic acidosis.

❑❑ What is the treatment of salicylate overdose?

Decontaminate, lavage and charcoal, fluid replacement, potassium supplementation, alkalize the urine with use of bicarbonate, cooling for hyperthermia, glucose for hypoglycemia, oxygen and PEEP for pulmonary edema, multiple dose activated charcoal, and dialysis.

❑❑ A patient presents with vomiting, hematemesis, diarrhea, lethargy, coma and shock. What cause is suspected?

Iron intoxication. Order a flat plate of the abdomen to look for concretions.

❑❑ What iron level is considered toxic?

Moderate overdose is considered to be 350 µg/dl, best measured 4 h after ingestion.
The amount of elemental iron ingested is used in calculations. 20-40 mg elemental iron/kg is toxic.
Symptomatic patients receive treatment without waiting for lab tests.

❑❑ Discuss the 4 stinking stages of iron toxicity.

I (h)..........................Abdominal pain, vomiting, diarrhea, possible GI bleeding and 2° lethargy and metabolic acidosis. Due to direct corrosive effect of iron.

II (3-12 h)..............GI symptoms resolve, physician falsely reassured.

III (>12 h)..............Iron makes it into cells, blocks oxidative phosphorylation, catalyzes formation of free radicals. Cellular and organ disruption ensue with edema and venous pooling. Hepatic dysfunction, renal and cardiac failure can occur. Stage III occurs earlier in severe poisoning.

IV (days-wk).........Small bowel and gastric outlet obstruction.

❑❑ What is the treatment of iron ingestion?

If patient has Ø symptoms ever for 6 h and is completely normal on exam, go home.

If patient has minimal symptoms and appears fine and has iron level close to maximum normal level (150 µg/dl) measured 4 h after ingestion, go home.

Cathartics for patients without diarrhea (controversial).
Hydration and treat GI hemorrhage.

Deferoxamine if:
- Moderate or severely symptomatic,
- Serum iron level > TIBC,
- Serum iron level > 350 µg/dl.

Deferoxamine is a specific agent for iron and will not chelate other metals. The IV dose of deferoxamine is 10 to 15 µg/kg/h.

❑❑ What are the symptoms and signs of cyanide overdose?

Dryness and burning in the throat, air hunger, and hyperventilation. If not removed from the toxic environment loss of consciousness, seizures, bradycardia and apnea follow prior to asystole.

❑❑ What is the treatment for cyanide overdose?

(0) Oxygen, CPR prn.
(1) Amyl nitrite perle inhaled.
(2) Sodium nitrite 10 cc of 3% solution in an adult which is 300 mg, or 0.2 - 0.33 mL/kg.
(3) Sodium thiosulfate 12.5 mg, in an adult which is 50 cc of a 25% solution or 1.0 - 1.5 mL/kg in a child (five times the volume of sodium nitrite).

Excess nitrites may require treatment with methylene blue for very, very rare case of dangerous methemoglobinemia.

❑❑ **What are the classic signs of PCP overdose?**

Hypertension, agitation, confusion, ataxia, vertical nystagmus, miosis, muscle rigidity, and catatonia.

❑❑ **What drugs can cause methemoglobinemia?**

Nitrites, local anesthetics, silver nitrate, amyl nitrite and nitrites, benzocaine, commercial marking crayons, aniline dyes, sulfonamides and phenacetin.

❑❑ **Atropine is used to treat:**

Organophosphate and carbamate overdose.

❑❑ **Pralidoxime (2-PAM) is used to treat:**

Organophosphate overdose.

❑❑ **Sodium chloride is used to treat:**

Chronic bromism.

❑❑ **Vitamin K is used to treat:**

Warfarin overdose.

❑❑ **Methylene blue is used to treat:**

Methemoglobinemia.

❑❑ **Pyridoxine is used to treat:**

Isoniazid and Gyromitra mushroom poisoning.

❑❑ **Name two selective cardioselective ß-blockers.**

Just remember the main cardioselective ß-blockers Metoprolol and Atenolol from the mnemonic "Look Ma!, I'm cardioselective!"

❑❑ **Overdose of ß-blockers may result in:**

Nausea, vomiting, bradycardia, hypotension, respiratory depression, seizure, CHF, bronchospasm, hypoglycemia and hyperkalemia.

❑❑ **Evaluating a pediatric cervical spine film, what are the normal values?**

Predental space < 5 mm or < 3 mm in an adult.
The posterior cervical line attaching the base of the spinous process of C1 to C3 should be considered. If the base of C2 spinous process lies greater than 2 mm behind the posterior cervical line, a hangman's fracture should be suspected. Anterior border of C2 to the posterior wall of the fornix distance < 7 mm.

Finally, anterior border of C6 to the posterior wall of the trachea distance would be 14 mm in children younger than 15 years of age, and less than 22 mm in an adult.

❒❒ Describe a hangman's fracture.

C2 bilateral pedicle fracture.

❒❒ What are key features of a vertical compression fracture?

Cervical and lumbar regions. Usually stable.

A Jefferson fracture of C1 may occur and is extremely unstable, although it is also very rare in occurrence.

❒❒ Injury to what cervical area results in Horner's syndrome (ptosis, miosis, and anhidrosis)?

Disruption of the cervical sympathetic chain at C7 to T2.

❒❒ What spinal level corresponds with dermatomal innervation of:

a. Perianal region,
b. Nipple line
c. Index finger
d. Knee
e. Lateral foot.

a. Perianal region	S2-S4
b. Nipple line	T4
c. Index finger	C7
d. Knee	L4
e. Lateral foot	S1

❒❒ Describe a patient with a central cord syndrome.

Injury to the ligamentum flavum and to the cord causing upper extremity neurologic deficit greater than lower extremity deficit.

❒❒ Describe a patient with Brown-Séquard syndrome.

Ipsilateral motor paralysis.
Ipsilateral loss of proprioception and vibratory sensation.
Contralateral loss of pain and temperature sensation.

❒❒ Describe a patient with anterior cord syndrome.

Complete motor paralysis and loss of pain and temperature sensation distal to the lesion.
Posterior column sparing results in intact proprioception and vibration sense.
Cause - occlusion of the anterior spinal artery or protrusion of fracture fragments into the anterior canal.

❒❒ Under water conditions, oops. Under what conditions does trench foot or immersion foot develop?

Trench foot occurs with exposure to wet or cold for days where the temperature is above freezing. The extremity develops superficial damage resembling partial thickness burns.

❒❒ What is pernio (chilblain)?

Chilblain refers to exposure of an extremity for a prolonged period of time to dry cold at temperatures above freezing. Patients develop superficial, small, painful ulcerations over chronically exposed areas. Sensitivity of the surrounding skin, erythema and pruritus may develop.

❒❒ What is frostnip?

Frostnip is the name for the condition preceding frostbite in which the skin becomes numb and blanched followed by cessation of discomfort. Sudden loss of cold sensation at the location of injury is a reliable sign of precipitant frostbite. Frostnip will proceed to frostbite if treatment is not initiated.

❒❒ How is frostnip treated?

Frostnip is the only form of frostbite which can be treated at the scene. It is treated by warming by hand, by breathing on the skin or by placing the frostnipped fingers or toes in the armpit (FUN!).
The affected part should not be rubbed. This may cause skin breakage, increases chances of infection, and does not thaw the tissues completely.

❒❒ What is appropriate treatment for frostbite?

The extremity in question should be rapidly rewarmed. Immerse in 42° C circulating water for 20 min or until flushing is observed. Dry heat should not be used. Refreezing thawed tissue greatly increases damage. Remember tetanus prophylaxis. Debride white or clear blisters as they contain toxic mediators (prostaglandin and thromboxanes). Hemorrhagic blisters should be left intact. Topical antibiotics such as silver sulfadiazine may be used. After admission, whirlpool treatments in warm antibiotic solution should be used twice per day.

❒❒ What are some common complications of frostbite?

Rhabdomyolysis, permanent depigmentation of the extremity, and increased likelihood of subsequent cold injury. X-ray approximately three to six months following frostbite injury reveals irregular, fine, punched out lytic lesions that may appear on the MTP, PIP and DIP joints, likely due to chronic subperiosteal inflammation.

❒❒ Where do endoscopic perforations of the esophagus typically occur?

They usually occur near the distal esophagus or at the site of pre-existing disease, such as a caustic burn.

❒❒ What are the three most common sites of foreign body perforation of the esophagus?

The levels of the cricopharyngeus muscle, the left mainstem bronchus, and the gastroesophageal junction.

❒❒ What laboratory abnormalities may be anticipated in acute cyanide poisoning?

An elevated anion gap - frequently 25 to 30 mEq/l, with lactic acidosis and decreased bicarbonate levels.

Venous PO_2 may be greater than 40 mmHg due to decreased tissue oxygen extraction.

❒❒ What is the most common site of penetrating ureteral injuries?

Penetrating ureteral injuries typically occur in the upper one-third of the ureter.

In pelvic fractures the most common site of injury is where the ureter crosses the pelvic brim.

❒❒ The most common cause of a coagulopathy in patients that require massive transfusions:

Thrombocytopenia.

❒❒ What percentage of ureteral injuries present without hematuria?

One-third of ureteral injuries present without hematuria.

❑❑ How may a posterior urethral tear be diagnosed in a male?

High riding, boggy prostate suggests this injury.

❑❑ Describe the mechanism of injury and signs & symptoms associated with an anterior urethral tear?

Straddle or crush injury mechanism.
Severe perineal pain with blood usually found at the meatus.
Good urinary stream is maintained.

❑❑ The best method of transporting an avulsed tooth?

Under the patient's tongue. If unable, transport in milk, saline or a wet handkerchief.

❑❑ What is the mechanism of a posterior urethral tear?

Associated with pelvic fracture.
Urethral stricture, impotence and incontinence.

❑❑ A patient has a pelvic fracture with suspected bladder or ureteral injury. What test should be performed first, a cystogram or an IVP?

When a pelvic fracture is present or suspected, the cystogram is usually performed first so that distal ureteral dye from the IVP will not mimic extravasation from the bladder.

❑❑ About what is the half-life of carboxyhemoglobin?

6.0 h in 21% F_IO_2,
1.5 h in 100% F_IO_2 and
0.5 h in 3 atmospheres of hyperbaric 100% F_IO_2.

❑❑ The most common cause of Ludwig's angina is:

Odontogenic abscess of a lower molar. Most common pathogen is hemolytic strep.

❑❑ The most common adverse effect of AZT:

Granulocytopenia and anemia. Less commonly a myopathy.

❑❑ Isopropyl alcohol, glycerol, or polyethylene glycol mixture is useful for treatment of what chemical burn?

Phenol (carbolic acid).

❑❑ The best means of transporting an amputated extremity:

Wrapped in sterile gauze moistened with saline, placed in waterproof plastic bag, immersed in ice water.

❑❑ What is the antidote for phosphorus poisoning?

Copper sulfate 1% solution. Remove within 30 minutes. Phosphorus may be identified by formation of insoluble black precipitate when swabbing with copper sulfate.

❑❑ What is the dose of SQ/intradermal 10% calcium gluconate used to treat hydrofluoric acid skin burn.

0.5 cc per cm^2 burned.

❐❐ Explain the significant features of each "axis" in the DSM-III official diagnostic criteria and nomenclature for psychiatric illnesses.

Axis I - organic brain syndromes caused by intoxication or physical illness, and major psychiatric disorders including psychosis, affective disorders and disorders of substance use.
Axis II - personality disorders including antisocial, schizoid and histrionic types.
Axis III - medical problems such as heart disease and infections.
Axis IV - life events that contribute to the patient's problems.
Axis V - patient adaptation to these problems.

❐❐ Which test is most reliable in predicting the severity of radiation exposure 48 h post exposure?

Absolute lymphocyte count. Presence or absence of GI symptoms following near-lethal doses is a good indicator of mortality.

❐❐ What local anesthetics may cause anaphylaxis?

The ester derivatives containing para-aminobenzoic acid (PABA) are known to stimulate IgE antibody formation and cause anaphylaxis.

These include procaine and tetracaine.

❐❐ What neighboring structures may be injured with a supracondylar distal humeral fracture?

The anterior interosseous nerve (which is a branch of the median nerve) and the brachial artery.

❐❐ Which test best discriminates between functional and organic blindness?

Optokinetic nystagmus.

❐❐ What is the most common carpal fracture?

Scaphoid (navicular); the more proximal the fracture, the more likely to develop avascular necrosis.

❐❐ How may a lunate dislocation be diagnosed?

Lateral view x-ray - the lunate appears dorsal or volar to its usual position within the radial fossa.

❐❐ The most common ligament injured after an inversion ankle sprain?

Anterior talo-fibular ligament.

❐❐ How may a perilunate dislocation be diagnosed?

AP and lateral x-ray - the lunate remains in alignment with the radial fossa and the other carpal bones appear displaced.

❐❐ What is the cause of lymphogranuloma venereum?

Chlamydia trachomatis.
Painful unilateral suppurative nodes may present with sinus tract.

Sx: Transient ULCER IS PAINLESS.
Dx: Compliment fixation.
Rx: Tetracycline, erythromycin, doxycycline.

❒❒ **What is the cause of granuloma inguinale?**

The bacterium Donovania granulomatis, recently renamed *Calymmatobacterium granulomatis.*

Dx: Bright, beefy-red, granulomatous lesions. Confirm diagnosis with finding of intracytoplasmic bacilli in macrophages (Donovan bodies).
Rx: Streptomycin, tetracycline, erythromycin, chloramphenicol, TMP/SMX.

❒❒ **The best diluent in solid lye ingestion is:**

Milk.

❒❒ **What is the cause of condylomata acuminata?**

Papova virus.

❒❒ **What is the mechanism of injury responsible for the greatest portion of injuries in the elderly?**

Falls. Most falls are caused by tripping but other medical causes underlying the initial fall should always be sought.

❒❒ **The organ most severely affected in a blast injury:**

The lungs.

❒❒ **The organ most commonly affected in a blast injury:**

The ears.

❒❒ **A patient has previous focal deficits from CVA's. Is it true that such a patient may present with confusion when having suffered a new focal lesion.**

Yes. The presentation of a new focal lesion may be with generalized or non-focal symptoms in the context of previous insults.

❒❒ **A patient with a dementia gets a wound infection. Is it true that such a patient may present with a severe decrease in mental status.**

Yes. Normally minor insults may cause drastic changes in neurologic functioning in those with pre-existing deficits.

❒❒ **The most common cause of extrauterine surgical emergencies in pregnancy:**

Appendicitis.

❒❒ **A patient had right arm and hand paralysis from a previous CVA. That deficit is mostly compensated with only residual weakness remaining. Should that patient subsequently have an episode of hyponatremia, can the presentation be with a right arm and hand paralysis?**

Sure. Formerly compensated deficits may return in response to a generalized neurological insult.

❒❒ **Red blood cell basophilic stippling is seen in what two disorders?**

Thalassemia and lead poisoning.

Zebe alert!

❒❒ **What triad is associated with Reiter's syndrome?**

Non-gonococcal urethritis, polyarthritis and conjunctivitis. The conjunctivitis is the least common and is seen in only 30 percent of patients. Acute attacks respond well to NSAIDs.

❒❒ **What is the most common cause of immediate postpartum hemorrhage?**

Uterine atony followed by vaginal/cervical lacerations, and retained placenta or placental fragments.

❒❒ **What complications of rheumatoid arthritis require emergency treatment?**

Vasculitis. This should be promptly treated with systemic steroids, otherwise irreversible neuropathy may occur.

❒❒ **What is Felty's syndrome?**

Rheumatoid arthritis with splenomegaly and neutropenia. It is a late complication of rheumatoid arthritis.

❒❒ **What drugs are commonly known to induce a lupus reaction?**

Procainamide, hydralazine, isoniazid and phenytoin.

❒❒ **What is the most serious complication of dental infections, aside from possible respiratory compromise in Ludwig's angina?**

Septic cavernous sinus thrombosis.

❒❒ **What joint is most commonly affected with pseudogout?**

The knee. The causative agent is calcium pyrophosphate crystals.

❒❒ **What joint is most commonly affected with gout?**

The great toe MCP joint.

❒❒ **What are the complications of impetigo?**

Streptococcal-induced impetigo can result in post-streptococcal glomerulonephritis.
It has not been shown to be associated with rheumatic fever.
Tx: erythromycin, dicloxacillin, cephalexin to help eliminate the skin lesions.
There is not clear proof that treatment prevents glomerulonephritis.

❒❒ **What are the clinical features of rubella (German measles)?**

Malaise, fever, headache, generalized lymphadenopathy, particularly the suboccipital and the posterior auricular nodes, with a pinkish maculopapular rash that first appears on the face.

❒❒ **How does measles (Rubeola) typically present?**

Fever, coryza and conjunctivitis. Pathognomonic Koplik's spots appear 2-4 d later on the buccal mucosa followed by the spreading maculopapular rash starting on the forehead and upper neck radiating to truck and extremities.

❒❒ **The most common early manifestation of a significant radiation exposure is:**

Nausea and vomiting.

❒❒ **How does roseola infantum appear?**

Roseola is typified by a high fever for three to four days, followed by a macular or maculopapular rash that is profuse on the chest and abdomen and mild on face and extremities. Patient feels well with rash.

❐❐ Describe the key features of the rash of Rocky Mountain Spotted Fever.

Rocky Mountain Spotted Fever is caused by *Rickettsia rickettsii* and is transmitted by Ixodidae ticks. Patients get sick, with high fever, headache, chills and muscular pain. On about the 4th d of fever, the rash begins on the wrists and ankles. The spread of rash is centripetal.

❐❐ The most effective dermal decontaminate following radiation exposure:

Wash with soap and water after removal of all clothes.

❐❐ Describe the rash of scarlet fever.

Sandpaper type texture rash beginning on the face, neck, chest, abdomen and spreads to extremities. Patients may have strawberry tongue.

❐❐ What is the most likely cause of unilateral transient loss of vision in a patient's eye (amaurosis fugax)?

Carotid artery disease. This is usually the result of platelet emboli from plaques in the arterial system.

❐❐ Syncope is a characteristic symptom of what valvular disease?

Aortic stenosis.

❐❐ What valvular lesion is most likely to cause syncope?

Aortic stenosis.

❐❐ The most common cause of a transudative pleural effusion?

Congestive heart failure.

❐❐ How does Landry-Guillain-Barré present?

Presentation in the third to fourth decade of a rapidly progressive ascending transverse myelitis. Weakness begins in lower extremities. Bulbar musculature may eventually be involved. Decrease or loss of DTRs is relatively specific for this disorder, though tick paralysis and Diphtheria neurotoxin can share this feature.

❐❐ How does a patient present with Eaton-Lambert Syndrome?

Proximal weakness with aching muscles especially in the lower extremities. Cranial nerve involvement is very rare. Patients often have a dry mouth. Unlike myasthenia gravis, which gets worse with activity, with E-L grip strength improves. There is no response to edrophonium test.

❐❐ How is an acute hemorrhagic overdose of Coumadin best treated?

Fresh frozen plasma, Vit K IM will help prevent subsequent hemorrhage.

❐❐ Where does botulism toxin exert its effects?

At the myoneural junction. It prevents the release of acetylcholine.

❐❐ How does botulism present?

Neurologic systems begin 24 - 48 hours after ingestion of contaminated foods. May start with nausea, vomiting or diarrhea. Most common early neurologic complaints are related to the eye and bulbar musculature. Symptoms involve all muscles of the trunk and extremities. Intestinal and bladder involvement may include ileus and acute urinary retention.

❒❒ Describe a patient with tick paralysis.

A rapid progressive ascending paralysis that develops over one to two days. First systems occur in the extremities and trunk and move to bulbar musculature. It is almost identical to Guillain-Barré Syndrome.

❒❒ Patient's with sickle cell trait most commonly present with:

Hematuria and decreased urine concentrating ability.

❒❒ Differentiate diphtheria with neurologic sequelae from toxicity due to botulism.

Diphtheria vs. botulism - Diphtheria is an acute febrile illness with pseudomembranous oropharyngitis and cardiac involvement.

❒❒ Differentiate neurologic sequela of botulism toxicity from neurologic deficits of Guillain-Barré syndrome.

G-B is an ascending transverse myelitis. It does not begin with bulbar musculature.

❒❒ How does infant botulism present?

The usual source is raw honey. (Honey abusers, huh! We know your type...)
Presentation with lethargy, failure to thrive, progresses to paralysis and death.

❒❒ What is the pathophysiology of myasthenia gravis?

Circulatory antibody against ACh receptor which binds at the motor end plate. In myasthenics, ACh receptors are in short supply resulting in fatigable weakness.

❒❒ What is the most serious transfusion reaction?

Hemolytic. Treat with aggressive fluid replacement and Lasix.

❒❒ What is the most common transfusion reaction?

Febrile.

❒❒ What diseases are associated with myasthenia gravis?

Rheumatoid arthritis, pernicious anemia, SLE, sarcoidosis and thyroiditis. 10 - 25% have associated thymoma.

❒❒ How does myasthenia gravis present?

Muscular weakness with fatigability. Strength improves after resting. First muscles involved are usually the extraocular muscles (other bulbar muscles *may* present earlier). The first symptom is either diplopia or eyelid ptosis. Bright light may increase ptosis and diplopia and heat may increase muscle weakness. Proximal muscles are typically weakest. Respiratory muscle involvement can be life-threatening.

❒❒ A patient presents with ocular, bulbar and limb weakness which gets worse during the day and decreases with resting - diagnosis?

Myasthenia gravis.

❑❑ **The best emergent treatment of an Ellis III dental fracture in an adult:**

Cover tooth with moist cotton then dry aluminum foil, and refer immediately to an orthodontist.

❑❑ **What are some factors commonly associated with meningitis?**

Age less than 5 years or greater than 60 years, low socioeconomic status, male sex, crowding, black race, sickle cell disease, splenectomy, alcoholism, diabetes and cirrhosis, immunologic defects, dural defect from congenital, surgical or traumatic source, contiguous infections such as sinusitis, household contacts, malignancy, bacterial endocarditis, intravenous drug abuse and thalassemia major.

❑❑ **A patient has xanthochromic CSF with a low protein count. What is the most likely cause?**

Subarachnoid hemorrhage.

❑❑ **A patient has xanthochromic CSF with a high protein count (greater than 150 mg/dl). What is the most likely cause?**

Traumatic tap.

❑❑ **What disease is associated with periaqueductal petechial hemorrhages?**

Wernicke's disease.

❑❑ **What disorders are associated with cerebrocortical neuronal degeneration?**

Anoxic, hypoglycemic and hepatic encephalopathies.

❑❑ **What is the most commonly abused volatile substance?**

Toluene.

❑❑ **A patient presents with hypokalemia of 2.0, hyperchloremia and acidosis. What is the most likely toxicologic cause?**

Chronic toluene abuse.

❑❑ **A patient has been abusing nitrous oxide for a long time. What symptoms might be expected?**

Paresthesias and motor weakness may be present in chronic abusers. Such symptoms are often mistaken for symptoms of multiple sclerosis.

❑❑ **Describe the features of each of the three stages of PCP intoxication.**

Stage I - agitated or violent, normal vital signs.
Stage II - tachycardia, hypertension and unresponsive to pain.
Stage III - unresponsive, depressed respirations, seizures and death.

❑❑ **Should the urine be acidified in the treatment of PCP intoxication?**

Although acidification of the urine is theoretically advantageous, clinical experience has not shown this to be efficacious. Let's call that a "no."

❑❑ **Explain how methylene blue functions as an antidote for methemoglobinemia.**

A normal level of 3% methemoglobin is usually maintained by a NADPH - dependent enzyme. This enzyme capacity can be exceeded with oxidant poisoning. Methylene blue enhances NADPH - dependent hemoglobin reduction by acting as a cofactor. Methylene blue is usually only needed for metHb levels > 30%; its dose is 1-2 mg/kg IV over 5 min.

❑❑ **A patient presents with belladonna alkaloid poisoning resulting in anticholinergic effects. Explain the dangers of treating this patient with physostigmine.**

Physostigmine acts to increase the acetylcholine levels. Doing so, it can precipitate a cholinergic crisis resulting in heart block and asystole. As a result, it is recommended to reserve physostigmine for life threatening anticholinergic complications.

Heart block and asystole.

❑❑ **Does botulism produce fever?**

No. This can be important in differentiating neurologic symptoms in a sick patient who could have diphtheria.

❑❑ **Describe a patient with Chlamydial pneumonia.**

Chlamydial pneumonia is usually seen in children 2 to 6 wk of age. The patient is afebrile. Patients do not appear toxic.

❑❑ **A patient has had three days of diarrhea which was abrupt in onset. The patient reports slimy green, malodorous stools that contain blood. In addition, the patient is febrile. What is the most likely cause?**

Salmonella.

❑❑ **Drug treatment for** Campylobacter**?**

Erythromycin or tetracycline.

❑❑ **In a child, does coarctation of the aorta typically cause cyanosis?**

No.

❑❑ **How much elemental iron will 100 mg of deferoxamine bind?**

About 8.5 mg of elemental iron is bound by 100 mg of deferoxamine.

❑❑ **Drug treatment for persistent** Escherichia coli**?**

Trimethoprim with sulfamethoxazole (TMP/SMX).

❑❑ **Drug treatment for** Giardia lamblia**?**

Quinacrine or metronidazole or furazolidone.

❑❑ **Drug treatment for persistent** Salmonella**?**

Ampicillin.
TMP/SMX.
Chloramphenicol.

❑❑ **Drug treatment for** Shigella**?**

TMP/SMX or Ciprofloxacin (if resistant).

❑❑ **Drug treatment for** Yersinia?

TMP/SMX.
Tetracycline.
3rd generation cephalosporin.

❑❑ **What are the 8 common clinical presentations of pediatric heart disease?**

Cyanosis, pathologic murmur, abnormal pulses, CHF, HTN, cardiogenic shock, syncope and tachyarrhythmias.

❑❑ **Complications of the use of sodium bicarbonate in severe metabolic acidosis include:**

Hypernatremia, paradoxical CSF acidosis, decreased oxygen unloading at the tissue level, hyperosmolality, dysrhythmias and hypokalemia.

❑❑ **What is the function of aldosterone?**

Aldosterone causes sodium conservation and K^+ excretion. As a result, it causes increased resorption of sodium and fluid.

❑❑ **What drug will most rapidly decrease K^+?**

Calcium chloride IV (1 - 3 minutes).

❑❑ **What is a potential side effect of the use of Kayexalate?**

Kayexalate exchanges sodium for K^+. As a result, sodium overload and CHF may occur.

❑❑ **What is Addison's disease?**

Deficiency or absence of mineralocorticoid (aldosterone). This results in increased sodium excretion. Potassium is retained. The urine cannot concentrate.

This can lead to severe dehydration, hypotension and circulatory collapse.

Deficiency of cortisol (also produced in the adrenal cortex) leads to metabolic disturbances, weakness, hypoglycemia and deceased resistance to infection.

❑❑ **What metabolic conditions will potentiate the toxic cardiac effects of digoxin?**

Hypokalemia and hypercalcemia.

❑❑ **What is the initial treatment for hypercalcemia?**

Saline and furosemide.

❑❑ **What conditions lead to hypocalcemia?**

Shock, impaired production, pancreatitis, hypomagnesemia, alkalosis, decreased serum albumin, hypoparathyroidism, osteoblastic mets, and fat embolism syndrome.

❑❑ **What vital sign might be affected with hypermagnesemia?**

Hypermagnesemia causes hypotension because it relaxes vascular smooth muscle. Deep tendon reflexes may disappear.

❑❑ What is the immediate treatment of thyroid storm?

1st -Draw blood for Free T4 index and free T3 and cortisol levels.
2nd -Supportive care (avoid aspirin - it may increase free T3 and T4).
3rd -IV glucocorticoids - 300 mg hydrocortisone per day.
4th -Inhibit thyroid hormone synthesis - propylthiouracil 900-1200 mg or methimazole 90 - 120 mg.
5th -Retard thyroid hormone release (iodine 1g q 8 hours IV).
6th -Block peripheral thyroid hormone effects (propranolol 1 mg q 1 min. to total of 10 mg.

❑❑ How is myxedema coma treated?

IV thyroxine 400 - 500 mg infused slowly, then 50 - 100 mg every day. Caution, lower dose of thyroxine if cardiac ischemia or arrhythmias are present.

❑❑ Common causes of hypercalcemia:

PAM P SCHMIDT.

P = Parathormone
A = Addison's
M = Multiple Myeloma

P = Paget's

S = Sarcoidosis
C = Cancer
H = Hyperthyroidism
M = Milk - alkali Syndrome
I = Immobilization
D = Vitamin D Excess
T = Thiazides

❑❑ What is the treatment for adrenal crisis?

100 mg hydrocortisone (Solu-Cortef) IV bolus and 100 mg hydrocortisone added to IV solution. Then, 200 mg hydrocortisone q 6 h for 24 hours.

(Refer to your preferred text for discussion of simultaneous testing and treatment with dexamethasone and corticotropin instead).

❑❑ What are the signs and symptoms of Wernicke's encephalopathy?

Oculomotor disturbances are common, usually with nystagmus and ocular palsies. Abnormal mentation and ataxia may be present. Ophthalmoplegias and nystagmus usually respond to thiamine, however, mental changes are often irreversible.

❑❑ When does alcoholic ketoacidosis commonly occur?

It usually occurs in chronic alcoholics after an interval of binge drinking followed by one to three days of protracted vomiting, abstinence and decreased food intake.

❑❑ ECG changes associated with tricyclic antidepressant overdose?

Prolongation of the PR, QRS and QT interval, as well as conduction defects such as bundle branch block, typically on the right.

❑❑ What is the treatment for TCA overdose?

Seizures
- Alkalinization.
- Diazepam.
- Phenytoin.
- Phenobarbital.

Tachycardia
- Alkalinization by hyperventilation.

Blocks and Ventricular Arrhythmias
- Alkalinization by hyperventilation.
- Sodium bicarbonate.
- Phenytoin (unproved).
- Lidocaine (unstudied).

Hypotension
- Alkalinization by hyperventilation.
- Fluids.
- Sodium bicarbonate.
- Pressors: epi, NE, dopamine.
- Digitalis (unstudied).
- Physostigmine (in extremis).
- Charcoal hemoperfusion.
- Cardiopulmonary bypass.

❒❒ **What drugs should be avoided in treatment of TCA overdose?**

Absolute - Procainamide. Also quinidine, disopyramide, and ß-blockers.

Relative - Corticosteroids, dopamine, isoproterenol, low dose dobutamine, bretylium, amiodarone, encainide and flecainide.

❒❒ **What dose of ASA will cause mild to moderate toxicity?**

200 - 300 mg/kg. Greater than 500 mg/kg is potentially lethal.

❒❒ **What is the ferric chloride test and what toxic ingestion does it detect?**

Add a few drops of 10% ferric chloride solution to a few drops of urine. Violet purple color indicates presence of salicylic acid. Ketones or phenothiazines can lead to false positive results.

❒❒ **What is the treatment of lithium overdose?**

Saline diuresis and hemodialysis.

❒❒ **What is the treatment for chloral hydrate overdose?**

Hemodialysis and/or charcoal hemoperfusion will clear the active metabolite, trichloroethanol.

❒❒ **What are the common effects of barbiturate overdose?**

Hypothermia, hyperventilation, venodilation with hypotension and negative inotropic effect on the myocardium. Clear vesicles and bullae may also be seen.

❒❒ **What is the pediatric dose of naloxone?**

0.01 mg/kg to a dose of 0.8 mg, may repeat.

❑❑ **What electrolyte abnormality is commonly seen in salicylate toxicity?**

Hypokalemia.

❑❑ **What is the treatment for acetaminophen overdose?**

Charcoal, cathartics and N-acetylcysteine.

❑❑ **What electrolyte abnormality may mimic the signs and symptoms of hypocalcemia?**

Hypomagnesemia.

❑❑ **What are some key signs and symptoms of Thrombotic Thrombocytopenic Purpura (TTP).**

Thrombocytopenia, purpura, microangiopathic hemolytic anemia. Presents with fever, fluctuating neurologic signs and renal complications. Untreated, the disease is almost uniformly fatal. Therapy includes steroids, splenectomy, plasmapheresis and exchange, and antiplatelet agents such as dipyridamole and aspirin.

❑❑ **How does a patient present with Boerhaave's syndrome?**

Boerhaave's syndrome is spontaneous esophageal perforation. It usually occurs after forceful vomiting. The patient suffers an acute collapse, chest and abdominal pain. A left pleural effusion is seen in 90 percent of patients on chest x-ray and most have mediastinal emphysema.

❑❑ **In what type of a patient is Staphylococcal pneumonia likely?**

Hospitalized, debilitated and drug abusing patients.

❑❑ **How low does the platelet count drop before spontaneous bleeding occurs.**

Below 50,000 per cubic millimeter spontaneous bleeding may occur. CNS bleeds usually do not occur until counts drop below 10,000 per cubic millimeter.

❑❑ **What factors affect the prothrombin time (PT)? Which pathway is this?**

I, II, V, VII, and X. 125710.
Extrinsic and common pathways.
PT is normal in hemophilia.
A normal PTT and increased PT suggests warfarin therapy, vitamin K deficiency, or liver disease.

❑❑ **What factors affect the partial thromboplastin time (PTT)? Which pathway is affected?**

VIII, IX, or XI. 8911.
Intrinsic pathway.
Heparin increases PTT.

❑❑ **What affect will heparin or warfarin overdose have on the PT and PTT?**

Both cause increases in PT and PTT in excessive doses.

❑❑ **What are the five key lab findings in DIC?**

Increased PT, PTT, and fibrin degradation products.
Decreased fibrinogen and platelet levels.

❑❑ In the thrombocytopenic patient, one unit of platelets will raise the platelet count by about how much?

One unit raises the platelet count by ≈10,000 / mm^3.

❑❑ What are the classic findings of shaken baby syndrome?

Failure to thrive, lethargy.
Seizures.
Retinal hemorrhages.
CT may show subarachnoid hemorrhage or subdural hematoma from torn bridging veins. (Bleeding in various stages, i.e., acute and chronic hemorrhages)

❑❑ Define spondylolysis.

Spondylolysis is a defect in the pars interarticularis.

❑❑ Define spondylolisthesis.

Spondylolisthesis is forward movement of one vertebral body on the vertebra below it.

❑❑ Define spondylosis.

Spondylosis is degenerative change in the vertebrae which may also include osteophyte formation at the disk spaces.

❑❑ T/F: High fever in neonates with bacterial pneumonia usually <u>follows</u> a period of general fussiness and decreased feeding.

True.

❑❑ Chlamydia pneumonia is more likely to occur in the neonate after how many weeks of age?

Three weeks.

❑❑ Conjunctivitis is an associated finding in about what percentage of neonates with Chlamydia pneumonia?

About 50%.

❑❑ Neonates with Chlamydia pneumonia are usually tachypneic with a bad cough; are they febrile?

Usually not.

❑❑ What is the immediate treatment for cord prolapse?

Displace the head cephalad.

❑❑ What is the most common bacterium causing septic arthritis of the hip?

Staphylococcus aureus.

❑❑ What nerve may be injured in a distal femoral fracture?

Peroneal nerve.

❑❑ Newborns should stop losing weight by how many days after birth?

About 6 days.

❑❑ **T/F: Stool color of neonates can be an important sign.**

False; with the exception of presence of blood, stool color is insignificant.

❑❑ **What is the difference between vomiting and regurgitation?**

Very little once it's on you!
Vomiting follows from forceful diaphragmatic and abdominal muscle contraction. Regurgitation occurs without effort.

❑❑ **Is regurgitation dangerous in an otherwise thriving neonate?**

No. It can be dangerous for newborns with failure to thrive or respiratory problems and it may be associated with chronic aspiration.

❑❑ **Projectile vomiting in the neonate is often associated with pyloric stenosis. When this is the case, such vomiting becomes a prominent sign after how many weeks of age?**

About two to three weeks.

❑❑ **What is the name for diarrhea associated with sepsis, otitis media, UTI or other systemic disease?**

Parenteral diarrhea.

❑❑ **Infectious diarrhea is most commonly viral. What are the two <u>most common</u> viruses?**

Rotavirus and Norwalk virus.

❑❑ **T/F: Bacterial and parasitic etiologies of diarrhea in the neonate are rare.**

True.

❑❑ **What are some entities in the differential diagnosis of bloody diarrhea in the neonate?**

Necrotizing enterocolitis, bacterial enteritis, iatrogenic causes secondary to antibiotics, milk allergy.

❑❑ **Neonates with necrotizing enterocolitis are sick; what are some of the signs of sepsis to look for?**

Poor feeding, lethargy, fever, jaundice, abdominal distention, and poor color.

❑❑ **What should be considered in the case of a neonate who has never passed stool?**

Meconium ileus or plug, Hirschsprung's disease, intestinal stenosis or atresia.

❑❑ **Anal stenosis, hypothyroidism and Hirschsprung's disease can all present with what clinical sign?**

Constipation that was not initially present but which had onset prior to one month of age.

❑❑ **Describe the signs and symptoms, and x-ray tests, for diagnosing a slipped capital femoral epiphysis.**

Gradual onset of hip pain and stiffness with restriction of internal rotation; patient may walk with a limp. X-ray analysis should include both the anterior-posterior and lateral views of both hips. The slip of the epiphyseal plate posteriorly is best seen on the lateral view.

❒❒ Describe the signs and symptoms of a patient with chondromalacia patellae.

Chondromalacia patellae typically occurs in young, active females.
The pain is localized to the knee. There is no effusion and no history of trauma. Patella compression test is usually positive.

❒❒ Describe the signs and symptoms of tarsal tunnel syndrome.

Insidious onset of paresthesia, burning pain and numbness on the plantar surface of the foot. Pain radiates superiorly along the medial side of the calf. Rest decreases pain.

❒❒ What is the cause of swimmer's itch (Schistosome dermatitis)?

An invading cercariae.

❒❒ Vector of malaria?

Anopheles mosquito.

❒❒ Insect vector of trypanosomiasis?

Tsetse fly.

❒❒ Infectious agent of elephantiasis?

Nematode microfilaria.

❒❒ What is the vector that transmits Chagas' disease (Trypanosoma Cruzi)?

Reduviid (Assassin or kissing bug).

❒❒ Cysticercosis is associated with:

New onset seizure.

❒❒ Hookworm is associated with what sort of anemia?

Iron deficiency anemia.

❒❒ Fish tapeworm (Diphyllobothrium latum**) is associated with:**

Pernicious anemia.

❒❒ Onchocerciasis (from Onchocerca volvalas**) is associated with what visual deficit?**

Blindness.

❒❒ Chagas' disease is associated with:

Acute myocarditis. Trypanosoma Cruzi invades the myocardium resulting in myocarditis. Conduction defects may occur.

❒❒ Roundworm is associated with:

Small bowel obstruction.

❒❒ **Describe the presentation of a patient with post-extraction alveolitis:**

Pain of "dry socket" occurs on the 2nd or 3rd day after extraction.

❒❒ **Ludwig's angina typically involves what spaces in the head?**

The submental, the sublingual and submandibular spaces.

❒❒ **What are the signs and symptoms of a peritonsillar abscess?**

Sore throat, dysarthria (hot potato voice), odynophagia, ipsilateral otalgia, low grade fever, trismus, and uvular displacement.

❒❒ **What is the presentation of a patient with diphtheria?**

Sore throat, dysphagia, fever and tachycardia. A dirty tough gray fibrinous membrane that may be so firmly adherent that removal causes bleeding may be present in the oropharynx. *Corynebacterium diphtheriae* exotoxin acts directly on cardiac, renal and nervous systems. Sure, it can cause ocular bulbar paralysis that may suggest botulism or, perhaps, myasthenia gravis. The exotoxin may also cause flaccid limb weakness. Of note, such weakness may also include decreased or absent DTRs, a finding usually suggestive of Guillain-Barré or of tick paralysis (*Dermacentor andersoni* neurotoxin).

❒❒ **How does a patient present with a retropharyngeal abscess?**

Patients typically prefer a supine position. Retropharyngeal abscesses are common under 3 years of age. On examination, the uvula and tonsil are displaced away from the abscess. Soft tissue swelling and forward displacement of the larynx are present. Soft tissue x-ray films of the neck may assist in the diagnosis.

❒❒ **How does an adult with epiglottitis present?**

Pharyngitis and dysphagia are prominent symptoms. Adenopathy is uncommon. The patient may have a muffled voice and speak softly; hoarseness is rare. Pharyngitis is present and pain is out of proportion to objective findings.

❒❒ **What are the two most common pathogens in adult acute sinusitis?**

Streptococcus pneumoniae and *Hemophilus influenzae.*

❒❒ **What is rhinocerebral phycomycosis?**

Rhinocerebral phycomycosis, also known as mucormycosis, is a fungal infection typically seen in diabetic patients while in ketoacidosis, and in immunocompromised patients. The disease is rapidly fatal if not recognized and treated quickly. Treatment includes antifungal drugs and surgical debridement.

❒❒ **Where is the typical location of a Mallory-Weiss tear?**

The laceration typically occurs in the cardioesophageal region in the stomach, below the gastroesophageal junction. The bleeding usually stops spontaneously and does not typically require surgery. It can be diagnosed by endoscopy. It is associated with hiatal hernia.

❒❒ **Magnesium containing antacids may cause:**

Diarrhea.

❒❒ **Aluminum containing antacids may cause:**

Constipation.

❑❑ **What is the treatment for hepatic encephalopathy?**

Lactulose and po. or per rectum neomycin.

❑❑ **When does an elevation of HBsAg occur in relation to symptoms of Hepatitis B?**

HBsAg always rises before clinical symptoms of hepatitis B.

❑❑ **Is hepatitis A associated with jaundice?**

Typically not, as more than 50 percent of the population have serologic evidence for hepatitis and do not recall being symptomatic.

❑❑ **Describe a patient with intussusception.**

Patients with intussusception are most likely very young. 70 percent occur within the first year of life. In children, the cause is thought to be secondary to lymphoid tissue at the ileocecal valve, whereas in adults, it is thought to be caused by local lesions, Meckel's diverticulum, or tumor. On exam, bowel sounds are usually normal. Intussusception typically involves the terminal ileum. Meckel's diverticulum is the single most common intrinsic bowel lesion involved.

❑❑ **Are adhesions a common cause of bowel obstruction in the large bowel?**

No. They are very common in the small bowel, but do not be fooled; they are extremely uncommon in large bowel obstructions.

❑❑ **Should salmonella be treated?**

Only if symptomatic infection persists. Treat with ampicillin, TMP/SMX, or chloramphenicol.

❑❑ **What is the most common cause of acute food-borne disease?**

Staph aureus and the enterotoxins it produces.

❑❑ **What are the common features of** Vibrio parahaemolyticus**?**

Organism associated with oysters, clams and crabs. Symptoms include cramps, vomiting, dysentery and explosive diarrhea. Severe infections are treated with tetracycline and chloramphenicol.

❑❑ **What types of anorectal abscesses can be drained in the emergency department?**

Perianal, submucosal, and pilonidal abscesses can be drained in the emergency department. Ischiorectal and supralevator abscesses need to be drained in the operating room.

❑❑ **Painful, bright red rectal bleeding is most often due to:**

Anal fissure. External hemorrhoids present with acute painful thrombosis and are not typically associated with constant, bright red bleeding. Internal hemorrhoids present with painless bright red bleeding, usually with defecation.

❑❑ **Where is the narrowest part of the ureter?**

The ureterovesical junction.

❑❑ **What percentage of kidney stones are radiopaque?**

90 percent. Most are made of calcium oxalate.

❑❑ In a patient with acute testicular pain, relief of pain with elevation of the scrotum (Prehn's sign) is classically associated with:

Epididymitis.

❑❑ Drug of choice for treating urinary tract infection due to Proteus mirabilis?

Ampicillin. This is common in young boys.

❑❑ Most common organism causing epididymitis in a 20 year-old?

Chlamydia trachomatis.

❑❑ How should hydralazine be dosed for a preeclamptic patient?

Hydralazine is given in 5 mg boluses every 20 minutes until adequate BP control is achieved or a total of 20 mg is reached.

❑❑ What is the antidote of overdose of magnesium sulfate?

Calcium gluconate infusion.

❑❑ In an ectopic pregnancy, is an adnexal mass a common finding?

No. An adnexal mass is actually found in less than 50 percent of cases. Abdominal pain is the most frequent sign. Amenorrhea is the second most common sign.

❑❑ As pCO_2 increases, pH will decrease. By how much is the pH expected to decrease for every 10 mmHg increase in pCO_2?

pH decreases by 0.08 units for each increase of 10 mm of pCO_2.

❑❑ How much protamine is required to neutralize 100 units of heparin?

1 mg of protamine will neutralize ≈ 100 units of heparin. The maximum dose of protamine is 100 mg.

❑❑ What is the <u>most common</u> symptom of a PE?

Chest Pain (88%)
Dyspnea (84%)

❑❑ What is the <u>most common</u> sign of a PE?

Tachypnea (92%)
Rales (58%)

❑❑ What is the <u>most common</u> radiographic finding of a PE?

An elevated hemidiaphragm (41%).

❑❑ What is the <u>most common</u> ECG finding of a PE?

T-wave inversion (42%)

❑❑ Of patients with a PE, what percentage have a normal ECG?

Normal (13%).

❑❑ Of patients with a PE, what percentage of ECGs show the classic S_1 Q_3 T_3 pattern?

S_1 Q_3 T_3 (12%), incidence is 18% with massive PE

❑❑ What test is most sensitive for evaluating a PE?

Perfusion scan is the most sensitive test, even more so than a pulmonary angiogram. Unfortunately, it is not a specific test, as 5 percent of normal volunteers will have an abnormal scan, and virtually any pulmonary pathology will produce an abnormal scan.

❑❑ What organisms are most commonly present in a pulmonary abscess?

Mixed anaerobes.

❑❑ What are some causes of thoracic outlet syndrome?

Compression of the subclavian artery by an anomalous cervical rib, compression of the neurovascular bundle as it passes through the interscalene triangle, and compression of the neurovascular bundle in the retroclavicular space anterior to the first rib when the arms are hyperabducted. Symptoms are typically produced when the shoulders are moved backward and downward.

The most common cause is a cervical rib.

❑❑ What is the most common cause of endocarditis in IV drug abusers?

Staphylococcus aureus, most commonly involving the tricuspid valve.

❑❑ What are the classic signs and symptoms of aortic stenosis?

Left heart failure, angina and exertional syncope.

❑❑ What patient position will enhance the murmur of mitral stenosis?

Left lateral decubitus.

❑❑ What is optimal patient position and maneuver for auscultation of aortic insufficiency?

Have the patient sit up and lean forward with the hands tightly clasped. During exhalation, listen at the left sternal border.

❑❑ What murmurs will the Valsalva maneuver increase?

Only IHSS. All other murmurs are diminished.

❑❑ What is the most common valvular disorder in the United States?

Mitral valve prolapse.

❑❑ What is the most common cause of endocarditis in late onset prosthetic valve endocarditis?

Streptococcus viridans.

❑❑ Symptoms of endocarditis?

Fever, chills, malaise, anorexia, weight loss, back pain, myalgia, arthralgia, chest pain, dyspnea, edema, headache, stiff neck, mental status changes, focal neurologic complaints, extremity pain, paresthesia, hematuria and abdominal pain.

❒❒ **Key physical finding of "malignant" hypertension?**

Papilledema.

❒❒ **Key diagnostic features of coarctation of the aorta?**

Rib notching seen on x-ray. Significant differences in the blood pressure between the upper and lower extremities.

❒❒ **What is an interesting diagnostic feature of aortic regurgitation?**

Head bobbing.

❒❒ **What is the most common arrhythmia associated with digitalis?**

PVC (60%).
Ectopic SVT (25%).
AV Block (20%).

❒❒ **What effect does furosemide have on calcium excretion?**

Furosemide causes increased calcium excretion in the urine.

❒❒ **What is the most common arrhythmia in mitral stenosis?**

Atrial fibrillation.

❒❒ **The most common cause of CHF in an adult is:**

Hypertension.

❒❒ **What is the differential diagnosis of pulmonary edema with a normal size heart?**

Constrictive pericarditis, massive MI, non-cardiogenic pulmonary edema, and mitral stenosis (not mitral regurgitation).

❒❒ **How does dobutamine differ from dopamine?**

Dobutamine decreases afterload with less tendency to cause tachycardia.

❒❒ **Describe Kerley A and Kerley B lines.**

Kerley A lines are straight, non-branching lines in the upper lung fields.

Kerley B lines are horizontal, non-branching lines at the periphery of the lower lung fields.

❒❒ **Does nifedipine typically effect preload or afterload?**

Nifedipine is a vasodilator whose primary effects are on afterload reduction.

❒❒ **What effect does the Valsalva maneuver have on the heart?**

Valsalva decreases blood return to both the right and left ventricles. All murmurs decrease in intensity except IHSS.

❒❒ **Does prednisone cross the placenta?**

No. Prednisone is metabolized through prednisolone which does not cross the placenta.

❑❑ You see a patient with a severe high concentration burn of hydrofluoric acid burn. How do you treat this patient?

In addition to topical jelly and cutaneous injections of calcium gluconate, provide IV treatment with 10 cc. of 10% Calcium Gluconate (not calcium chloride) diluted in 50 cc. of D_5W. This is given via a pump over 4 h.

❑❑ How should an ocular burn secondary to hydrofluoric acid be treated?

Use calcium gluconate in a 1% solution mixed with saline and irrigate the eyes with this solution. The solution is made by diluting one part of standard 10% calcium gluconate solution with ten parts of saline which produces a 1% solution.

❑❑ What electrolyte is depleted in a victim of a hydrofluoric acid burn?

Hydrofluoric acid results in hypocalcemia. Patients may require calcium replacement. Keep in mind that normal signs and symptoms of hypocalcemia such as Chvostek's sign do not typically appear with hypocalcemia secondary to HF.

❑❑ A 35 year-old female presents with altered mental status and a temperature of 105 °F. The patient's muscles are rigid and she feels very hot in the trunk but her extremities are cool. What diagnosis is likely?

Neuroleptic malignant syndrome. High fever and muscle rigidity should make you suspect a diagnosis of neuroleptic malignant syndrome. Check the CPK.

❑❑ How should a patient with neuroleptic malignant syndrome be treated?

1) Ice packs to the groin and axilla.
2) Cooling blankets.
3) Fan.
4) Alcohol evaporation.
5) Dantrolene at an IV rate of 0.8 to 3 mg/kg IV q 6 hours to a total of 10 mg/kg.

❑❑ How should a patient with a black widow spider bite be treated?

1) Antivenin.
2) IV calcium gluconate.
3) IV opiates plus IV benzodiazepines.

❑❑ T/F: Centruroides scorpion antivenin should be considered for all Centruroides **envenomations.**

NOT. False. Scorpion antivenin is rarely necessary and is only typically used in children who have a severe (Grade IV) envenomation with peripheral motor and cranial nerve involvement. It is most important to use *Centruroides* antivenin only in severe cases as serum sickness or rash after administration is very common. In fact, as many as 60% of patients develop a rash or serum sickness secondary to this antivenin.

❑❑ What is a significant complication of scorpion envenomation?

Rhabdomyolysis.

❑❑ In what states could a scorpion bite be deadly?

Centruroides, which is the most toxic of scorpion stings, is only found in Arizona, California, Texas and New Mexico.

❒❒ An elderly patient presents with the complaint of seeing halos around lights. What diagnosis is suspected?

Glaucoma. Another presenting complaint of glaucoma is blurred vision. Also, consider digitalis toxicity.

❒❒ A patient presents with back pain and complaints of incontinence. On exam, loss of anal reflex, and decreased sphincter tone is noted. What is your diagnosis?

Cauda equina syndrome. The most consistent finding with cauda equina syndrome is urinary retention. On physical exam, expect saddle anesthesia, that is, numbness over the posterior superior thighs as well as numbness of the buttocks and perineum.

❒❒ What is the most common site of lumbar disc herniations?

98% of clinically important lumbar disc herniations are at the L4-5 or L5-S1 intervertebral levels.

Evaluate by checking for weakness of ankle and great toe dorsiflexors (L5). Also check pinprick sensation over the medial aspect of the foot (L5) and the lateral portion of the feet (S1).

❒❒ What WBC count is expected during pregnancy?

WBC counts of 15,000 to 20,000 are considered normal in pregnancy.

❒❒ A trauma patient has a closed head injury with suspected elevated intracranial pressure. What treatments should be considered?

1) Paralyze the patient and hyperventilate.
2) Maintain hypovolemia (fluid restrict).
3) Elevate the head of the bed to 30 degrees after the C-spine has been cleared.
4) Consider mannitol 500 mL. of a 20% solution over 20 minutes for a 70 kilogram adult.

Use of diuretics like furosemide is controversial. Steroids are no longer recommended. Barbiturate use is also not recommended. Mannitol use is also losing favor.

❒❒ When monitoring a pregnant female trauma victim, which vital signs are more appropriate to follow - the mother's or those of the fetus?

It is probably best to consider monitoring the fetal heart rate since it is more sensitive to inadequate resuscitation. Remember that the mother may lose 10 to 20% of her blood volume without change in vital signs whereas the baby's heart rate may increase or decrease above 160 or below 120 indicating significant fetal distress.

❒❒ What two findings on physical exam are indicative of uterine rupture?

Loss of uterine contour and palpable fetal part.

❒❒ What physical exam findings may be discovered in abruptio placenta?

Rapidly increasing fundal height secondary to bleeding into the uterus or a higher than expected fundal height.

❒❒ What is the number one risk factor for uterine rupture?

Previous cesarean section.

❒❒ How should a diagnostic peritoneal lavage be performed for a pregnant patient?

Use an open supraumbilical approach. Always make sure an NG tube and Foley are in place.

❒❒ A gravid woman is sent to the OB floor for cardiotocography after a motor vehicle accident. What findings will suggest problems with the fetus.

On the OB floor, they will look for uterine contractions at a rate of greater than 8 per minute. They will also watch for late decelerations. Late deceleration are a slowing of the fetal heart rate near the end of a contraction.

❒❒ An unconscious, 60 year-old patient presents to the ED with a head injury. An ECG shows significant ST segment elevation. What is your concern?

Although MI should be considered, don't forget the possibility of an intracerebral hemorrhage. This may also cause significant ST segment elevation.

❒❒ Why should the use of atropine be considered in a pediatric patient prior to intubation?

Many pediatric patients develop bradycardia associated with intubation. This can be prevented by pre-treatment with atropine (dose is 0.01 mg/kg).

❒❒ What size tracheotomy tube is appropriate for an adult female and for an adult male?

An adult female generally requires #4 tracheostomy tube and an adult male requires a #5.

❒❒ After use of ketamine in a pediatric patient, what effects are expected?

The child will have eyes wide open with a glassy stare, nystagmus, hyperemic flush and hypersalivation. There will also be a slight rise in the heart rate. A very rare complication of ketamine use is laryngospasm. Hallucinations are a common side-effect in children over the age of 10; as a consequence, ketamine should be restricted to use only in patients under the age of 10.

Ketamine may also cause sympathetic stimulation which increases intracranial pressure, and may cause random movements of the head and extremities. It is thus not a good sedative for children going to CT scan.

❒❒ Contraindications to TAC?

Mucus membranes, burns, and large abrasions. TAC used on the tongue and mucus membranes has led to status epilepticus and patient death.

❒❒ Why are quinolones contraindicated in children?

Quinolones impair cartilage growth.

❒❒ A patient presents with a symmetric weakness which has been progressive over several days to weeks and has associated paresthesia. Diminished reflexes are noted. Diagnosis?

Guillain-Barré syndrome. Other signs and symptoms are diminished reflexes, minimal loss of sensation, paresthesias, and leg weakness.

❒❒ How is Guillain-Barré syndrome diagnosed in the ED?

Suspect the diagnosis based on signs and symptoms, but confirmation requires nerve conduction studies performed as an inpatient.

❒❒ What is the dose of acyclovir (Zovirax) used to treat herpes zoster infections in an immunocompetent adult?

800 mg. po. five times per day for 7 to 10 days.
For herpes simplex genitalis, the dose is much lower, 200 mg. po. five times a day for ten days!

❒❒ A patient is brought to the ED after exposure to ammonia gas. What are your chief concerns?

Ammonia gas affects the upper respiratory tract and may cause significant laryngeal and tracheal edema. Administer warm humidified O_2 to soothe the bronchial tract. Bronchodilators may also be given by nebulization for bronchospasm. Be ready to intubate if severe upper airway edema occurs.

❒❒ What signs and symptoms would lead to consideration of hyperbaric oxygen treatment for a patient with CO poisoning?

History of, or current, unconsciousness, arrhythmia or ischemia, neurologic impairment greater than a mild headache, and/or a carboxyhemoglobin level over 40%.

❒❒ What are the indications for giving digitalis specific Fab?

Ventricular arrhythmias.
$K^+ > 5.5$ mEq/L.
Unresponsive bradyarrhythmias.

Some authors refer to an ingestion of more than 0.3 mg/kg as requiring Fab (Digibind).
The dose of Fab is:

vials required = 1.33 x mg ingested,

or use formula to determine dose based on serum digoxin level,
or give 10 vials (40 mg Fab each) if amount ingested is not known.

Adolescents and children have an even higher sensitivity to the serious complications of digoxin overdose and may need Fab therapy with ingestion of less than the recommended level of 0.3 mg. per kilogram.

Remember - in an acute overdose situation, the serum level of digitalis is unreliable in evaluating toxicity. Digitalis levels typically only become accurate after 4 to 6 hours; this is too long to wait for treatment.

❒❒ You give digoxin specific antibody (Fab) to a digoxin-toxic patient with an elevated digoxin level. A repeat digoxin level is obtained after this treatment and it is much <u>higher</u> than the previous level! What gives? Didn't the Fab work?

Digoxin assay measures free <u>and</u> bound digoxin, the latter increases ≈ 15 x via binding to Fab.

❒❒ What electrolyte change is expected with a serious digoxin ingestion?

Expect hyperkalemia. After Fab, potassium level may drop quickly and the patient may become hypokalemic. Monitor carefully.

❒❒ A near drowning victim is comatose and intubated with a diagnosis of severe pulmonary edema. What specific pulmonary treatment should be provided in the Eme[illegible]nent?

It is important to give these patients PEEP early. PEEP will decrease int[illegible]shunting and prevent terminal airway closure.

❒❒ There are four types of hypersensitivity reactions. Name them in order:

Hypersensitivity Reaction	Mediator	Example
Type 1 - Immediate	IgE binds allergen, includes mast cells and basophils	Food allergy. Asthma in children.
Type 2 - Cytotoxic	IgG & IgM antibody reactions to antigen on cell surface activates complement and killers	Blood transfusion rxn. ITP, hemolytic anemia. The least common rxn.
Type 3 - Immune complex, Arthus	Complexes activate complement	Tetanus toxoid in sensitized persons. Poststreptococcal glomerulonephritis.
Type 4 - Cell mediated, delayed hypersensitivity	Activated T-lymphocytes	Skin tests

❑❑ What distinguishes heat stroke from heat exhaustion?

Heat exhaustion is progressive loss of electrolytes and body fluid depletion. Therapy is rehydration.

Heat stroke occurs when temperatures are above 42° C and enzyme systems cease to function normally. As a result, there is necrosis, denaturing, and organ failure. Heat stroke requires much more aggressive treatment than simple fluid rehydration.

Remember - in patients with an altered sensorium and a core temperature above 42° C, always suspect heat stroke. Half of patients will be diaphoretic.

❑❑ What lab abnormalities may be found with heat stroke?

High elevations in SGOT, SGPT and LDH.

❑❑ How should a patient with heat stroke be treated?

1) Cool the patient with lukewarm water and fans.
2) Pack the axillae, neck and groin with ice.
3) Give fluids cautiously as large boluses of fluids may precipitate pulmonary edema.
4) Treat shivering with chlorpromazine (Thorazine) 25 to 50 mg IV.

❑❑ What complications can result from heat stroke?

Renal failure, rhabdomyolysis, DIC, and seizures. Remember antipyretics will not help.

❑❑ You ... orking locum tenens in Arizona, California, Texa ... As these states will have t ... uroides scorpion, you are particularly concerned ... ting treatment. How shou ... ng be treated?

A scorpion sting should be treated with local ice compresses, analgesics, and perhaps antidote.
Patients who have extremity jerking, blurred vision, slurred speech, or hypersalivation probably will require antivenin as this represents a Grade IV envenomation with peripheral motor and cranial nerve involvement.

❑❑ Describe the appearance of a black widow spider bite?

Two tiny red marks with surrounding erythematous patch. The initial bite may be painless. If a "pinprick" type bite is followed by abdominal cramps, think of a black widow spider. Exam reveals abdominal rigidity without true tenderness. Patients are restless and move about the gurney. Antivenin should probably be given to patients who are pregnant, younger than 16 and older than 65, and symptomatic. It also should be given to patients with underlying cardiac disease. Other treatments include calcium, diazepam (Valium), or methocarbamol (Robaxin). Traditional treatment also includes calcium gluconate.

❑❑ What conditions may make the end tidal $C0_2$ monitor inaccurate?

Monitor may be falsely yellow due to contamination from acidic drugs such as lidocaine-HCl and epinephrine-HCl. Contamination with vomitus may produce false readings.

❑❑ You are having a hard time remembering which anesthetics are amides and which anesthetics are esters. What is a fairly easy way of telling these two classifications of anesthetics apart?

The word amide has an "i" in it and so do the am"i"des (in the syllable(s) before "caine").

Lidocaine (Xylocaine).
Bupivacaine (Marcaine).
Mepivacaine (Carbocaine).

Esters on the other hand have no "i",
Procaine (Novocain)
Cocaine
Tetracaine (Pontocaine)
Benzocaine.

So remember - those with i's are amides. (In the first syllable only, the caines don't count!)

❑❑ An elderly patient presents with sudden onset of severe abdominal pain followed by a forceful bowel movement. Diagnosis?

Acute mesenteric ischemia. Keep in mind that abdominal series may be normal early in acute mesenteric ischemia. Possible late x-ray findings include:

Absent bowel gas, ileus, gas in the intestinal wall and thumb-printing of the intestinal mucosa.
In most cases, films are normal or not specifically suggestive. Expect heme-positive stools. Patients especially prone to mesenteric ischemia include those with CHF and chronic heart disease.

❑❑ Under what conditions does neurogenic pulmonary edema occur?

Neurogenic pulmonary edema is commonly associated with increased intracranial pressure. It is commonly seen with head trauma, subarachnoid hemorrhage, and even with seizures.

❑❑ A patient had a very severe headache two days ago. The headache is now subsiding and physical exam is normal. Should the possibility of a subarachnoid hemorrhage be evaluated, and if so, how?

Yes. CT.
However, a significant percentage of scans will be negative 48 hours after intracranial hemorrhage.
LP done 2 to 3 days after a bleed should still be positive and xanthochromia typically persists for 7 to 10 days.

❑❑ What are the classic signs and symptoms of adrenal insufficiency?

Fatigue, weakness, GI symptoms, anorexia, hypotension, and dehydration. May also have the classic clue - history of chronic steroid use. Order plasma cortisol level. Remember - cortisol level should be drawn prior to giving steroid therapy.

❑❑ What is the initial treatment for adrenal insufficiency (don't worry about Rx while Dx)?

Fluids and hydrocortisone IV in a typical dose of 100 to 200 mg.

❑❑ An elderly patient presents with altered mental status, a history of IDDM and is hypoglycemic. Core temperature is 32° C. What endocrinologic condition is likely?

Myxedema coma.
Other clues to look for are history of thyroid surgery, hypothyroidism, and use of anti-thyroid medications.

❑❑ What three conditions may cause a falsely low sodium concentration?

Pseudohyponatremia may be caused by:

Hyperglycemia.
Hyperlipidemia.
Hyperproteinemia.

❑❑ A patient presents with very low sodium and you suspect SIADH. What lab findings would confirm the diagnosis?

Serum osmolality should be low and urine sodium and osmolality should both be high. Remember - treatment of severe symptomatic hyponatremia includes a loop diuretic such as furosemide and simultaneous infusion of small boluses of 3% saline over 4 hours or 0.9 normal saline. Too rapid a correction of hyponatremia may result in neurologic sequelae.

❑❑ A young competitive figure skater presents with a complaint of generalized weakness following practice. What might be the cause of this profound weakness?

Hypokalemic "paralysis" is a cause of acute weakness.

❑❑ How may hyperglycemic, hyperosmolar, non-ketotic coma be differentiated from DKA?

Serum osmolality is higher in NKHC.
$NaHCO_3$ is normal in NKHC and depleted in DKA.
pH is usually maintained at >7.2 in NKHC.

❑❑ How should non-ketotic hyperosmolar coma be treated?

Fluids, fluids and more fluids. Such patients can be as much as 12 liters deficient. Give normal saline until adequate blood pressure and urinary output are established. Follow with half normal saline. When blood glucose falls to 250 to 300 mg, the solution should be changed to saline and glucose to avoid cerebral edema.
It is important to note that these patient's require very little insulin. Give as little as 5 to 10 units of insulin IV. These patients are commonly deficient in potassium and will need 10 to 15 mEq per hour once urine flow has been established. This disorder has a grave prognosis with up to a 50% mortality for severe cases.

❑❑ T/F: Phenytoin is the drug of choice for a patient with non-ketotic hyperosmolar coma who experiences a seizure.

False. Phenytoin is contraindicated in patients with hyperglycemic, hyperosmolar, non-ketotic coma.
Drugs of choice for treating this seizure disorder are lorazepam (Ativan) or diazepam (Valium). Phenobarbital use is also appropriate.

❑❑ For what types of overdoses is activated charcoal <u>not</u> indicated?

Alcohol ingestion, electrolytes, heavy metals, lithium, hydrocarbons and caustic ingestions.

❒❒ **A young patient has a threatened abortion in the first trimester. Laboratory studies reveal she is Rh negative and her husband is Rh positive. Treatment?**

The patient will need 50 µg of Rh immunoglobulin (RhoGAM) IM. After the first trimester, the dose is increased to 300 µg IM. After 15-16 weeks gestation, the mother may require more RhoGAM based on the results of a ICB assay.

❒❒ **What type of blood test is used to determine if a patient needs RhoGAM therapy?**

A Kleihauer-Betke (KB) checks for fetomaternal bleeding.

❒❒ **What are the signs and symptoms of preeclampsia?**

Upper abdominal pain, headache, visual complaints, cardiac decompensation, creatinine greater than 2, proteinuria greater than 100 mg per deciliter, and a blood pressure of greater than 160 mmHg systolic or 110 mmHg diastolic.

Preeclampsia is most common in nulliparous women late in pregnancy, typically after 20 weeks gestation. Look for edema, hypertension, and proteinuria to diagnose these patients.

The ED treatment for preeclampsia is IV hydralazine titrated to a blood pressure of 90 to 110 diastolic using 5 mg boluses q 20 to 30 minutes. Blood pressure must be lowered slowly to avoid compromising the uteroplacental blood flow. Patients with moderate to severe preeclampsia need IV magnesium (though its true utility is not well demonstrated).

❒❒ **What is the most commonly missed hip fracture?**

Femoral neck fracture.

❒❒ **Which is more common - a medial or a lateral tibial plateau fracture?**

The lateral tibial plateau is most commonly fractured. If AP and lateral films are negative, follow-up with oblique views if suspicious of a tibial plateau fracture.

❒❒ **What is the most commonly missed fracture in the elbow region?**

A radial head fracture. Like the navicular fracture, radiographic signs of a radial head fracture may not show up for days after the injury. A positive fat pad sign may be the only finding suggestive of this injury.

❒❒ **What are the two most common errors made in the intubation of a neonate?**

1) Placing the neck in hyperextension - this moves the cords even more anteriorly.
2) Inserting the laryngoscope too far.

❒❒ **What is the most common cause of food-borne <u>viral</u> gastroenteritis?**

Norwalk virus commonly found in shell fish.

❒❒ **What are the symptoms of "Chinese Restaurant" syndrome?**

Headache, dizziness, abdominal discomfort, facial flushing, and chest or facial burning. Symptoms typically start within an h of eating Chinese food.

❒❒ **A patient is in anaphylactic shock. She happens to be taking ß-blockers. She is not responding to epinephrine. What alternative agents might you consider?**

Norepinephrine, diphenhydramine, and glucagon.

❒❒ A young boy is presented for evaluation after suffering a coral snake bite. He appears to be fine. What is appropriate management?

Admit to the Intensive Care Unit and be ready for respiratory arrest. Coral snake bites appear minor at first. When symptoms begin, the patient may quickly progress to respiratory arrest. Coral snake venom is neurotoxic.

❒❒ Describe the appearance of a coral snake.

The snake is red, yellow and black. There is a black spot on the head. It is a round snake.

Coral snake bites typically do not cause immediate local pain whereas viper bites do.
(Red on yellow, kill a fellow!)

❒❒ What type of rattlesnake bite leads to most deaths?

Diamond back rattlesnake is the cause of nearly all lethal snake bites in the United States. The Diamond Back accounts for only 3% of snake bites seen. Treat with 10 to 20 vials of antivenin.

❒❒ How does a stupid idiot recognize a pit viper?

If he gets close enough, he will observe an elliptical pupil that looks like a football stood on end.

❒❒ What are some more common entities in the differential diagnosis of a limp or gait abnormality in a child?

Legg-Calvé-Perthes disease (avascular necrosis of the femoral head), Osgood-Schlatter disease, avulsion of the tibial tubercle, infection, toxic transient tenosynovitis, patellofemoral subluxation, chondromalacia patella, slipped capital femoral epiphysis, septic arthritis, metatarsal fracture, proximal stress fracture, and toddler fracture (spiral tibia fracture).

❒❒ What are the treatment recommendations for a patient with cluster headache?

Treat similarly to migraine except skip ß-blockers, add O_2, try lidocaine 4% in the ipsilateral nostril.

❒❒ What is the treatment for trigeminal neuralgia?

Carbamazepine (Tegretol) 100 to 200 mg. tid. Obtain baseline CBC and platelet count before starting carbamazepine.

❒❒ What is the only absolute contraindication to IVP?

Profound hypotension - the kidneys won't be perfused. Two relative contraindications are renal insufficiency with a creatinine greater than 1.6 and a history of allergic reactions.

❒❒ What markers indicate that an HIV positive patient is at increased risk for opportunistic infections like PCP?

An absolute CD-4 count of less than 200.

CD-4 lymphocytic percentage less than 20%.

❒❒ What are the National Institutes of Health treatment recommendations for spinal cord injury?

Give high dose methylprednisolone (Solu-Medrol) 30 mg/kg bolus over 15 minutes followed by 45 minutes normal saline drip. Over the subsequent 23 hours the patient should receive an infusion of 5.4 mg/kg/h of methylprednisolone.

❑❑ **What is the most common cause of small bowel obstruction in the surgically virgin abdomen?**

Incarcerated hernia.

❑❑ **A patient with a temperature of 29° C develops V-fib. Is defibrillation likely to be successful?**

Defibrillation should be attempted but is unlikely to be successful at temperatures less than 29° C.

❑❑ **T/F: The presentation of infectious endocarditis in an IV drug abusing patient does not usually include a murmur.**

TRUE. Less than 1/2 present with a murmur.

❑❑ **How is a retropharyngeal abscess diagnosed on plain films of a one year-old child?**

Look for prevertebral thickening of the soft tissues. More than 3 mm suggests the possibility of a retropharyngeal abscess. Air/fluid level may be present.

If still unsure, order a CT of the neck. On CT scan retropharyngeal abscesses are just anterior to the vertebral column, will appear in only a few cuts, and appear as a gray area of about the same density as the spinal canal on CT.

❑❑ **In what age child is use of an uncuffed tube most appropriate?**

Children under 6 should receive an uncuffed tube.

❑❑ **A straight (Miller) blade is preferred for intubating children of less than what age?**

4 years.

❑❑ **What is the Parkland formula for treating a pediatric burn victim?**

Ringer's lactate 4 mL/ %BSA/ kg over 24 h with 1/2 given in first 8 h.

❑❑ **Large burns in children less than 5 years of age may require:**

Colloid (5% Albumin or FFP) at 1 mL/ %BSA/ kg/ d

❑❑ **A burned pediatric patient is receiving fluids per the Parkland formula. How much** additional **fluid should be given for maintenance requirements?**

100 mL/kg/d for each kg up to 10 kg
\+ 50 mL/kg/d for each kg from 10-20 kg
\+ 20 mL/kg/d for each kg thereafter.

❑❑ **When examining a lateral adult C-spine film, the predental space, that is the area between the dens and the anterior arch of C1, looks particularly wide. What width space is normal for an adult?**

Normal is 2.5 to 3 mm.

If this width is greater than 3 mm, consider that the transverse ligament has ruptured or is at least lax.

❑❑ **What is the upper limit of normal of prevertebral soft tissue at C3?**

Anything greater than 5 mm suggests hematoma or fracture.

❑❑ What disease is commonly associated with central retinal vein occlusion?

Hypertension.

❑❑ What are common eye findings in patients with AIDS?

Cotton wool spots and CMV retinitis.

❑❑ What is Purtscher's retinopathy?

Purtscher's retinopathy is associated with thoracic injuries and broken bones. Findings include retinal hemorrhage and cotton wool spots.

❑❑ What are the common features of central vertigo?

1) Symptoms are gradual and continuous.
2) Focal signs may be present.
3) Hearing loss is rare.
4) Nausea and vomiting.

❑❑ What are the signs and symptoms of peripheral vertigo?

1) Symptoms are usually acute and intermittent.
2) Hearing loss is common, nausea and vomiting are severe.

❑❑ In the evaluation of retropharyngeal abscess, what is the most common age of the patient, how do they present, what diagnostic tests are used in the evaluation, and what treatment modalities are recommended?

Retropharyngeal abscess is most commonly seen in children less than 4 years of age.

Usual presentation is with dysphagia, muffled voice, stridor, sensation of a lump in the throat. Patients usually prefer to lie supine.

Diagnosis is made with a soft tissue lateral neck film which may demonstrate edema and air/fluid levels. CT may be useful.

Treatment includes airway, IV antibiotics and admission to the ICU. Intubation may rupture the abscess.

❑❑ The causes of epiglottitis include:

Hemophilus influenzae is by far most common.
Pneumococcus, Staphylococcus, and *Branhamella* may also be causes.
Presentation is most common among children within a few years of age 5.
Dogma to never attempt direct visualization of epiglottis is being questioned.

❑❑ What is the most common cause of Ludwig's angina?

Ludwig's angina is often associated with dental infections. Hemolytic streptococcus or mixed anaerobic infections are most common.

It is commonly seen in elderly and debilitated patients. It often presents with sublingual pain, protruding tongue, dysphonia, brawny induration, and stridor.

❑❑ A set of perennial favorites from our friend, René Le Fort! What is a Le Fort I fracture?

A maxilla fracture extending to the nasal aperture often missed on x-ray.

❑❑ What is a Le Fort II fracture?

A "pyramidal" fracture extends vertically through the maxilla, through maxillary sinuses and infraorbital rims and across nasal bridge. Usually confirmed with Waters' view.

❑❑ What is a Le Fort III fracture?

Craniofacial dysfunction includes fracture through the frontozygomatic suture lines, across the orbits and through the base of the nose. Le Fort I or II may also be present.

❑❑ What is the usual cause of facial cellulitis in children less than 3 years of age?

H. influenzae.
In adults- *Staph* or *Strep*.

❑❑ A trauma patient presents with a complaint of severe burning pain in the upper extremities and associated neck pain. On physical exam, the patient has good strength in his upper extremities and no obvious neurologic deficits in the lower extremities. Although the C-spine series is negative, what problem is still suspected?

Central cord syndrome. This injury is due to hyperextension of the spinal cord.
Diagnostic findings include upper extremity neurologic symptoms and minimal or no lower extremity symptoms.
Tingling, paresthesias, burning pain, and severe weakness or paralysis in the upper extremities with little or no symptoms in the lower extremities.

❑❑ An asthmatic patient suddenly develops a supraventricular tachycardia. Blood pressure is normal and the QRS complex is also narrow. What therapy is most appropriate?

Verapamil.

Avoid the use of adenosine as it is relatively contraindicated and may exacerbate bronchospasm in asthmatic patients. Also avoid ß-blockers.

❑❑ How is a laryngeal fracture diagnosed on plain films?

On a lateral soft tissue x-ray of the C-spine, check for retropharyngeal air, and elevation of the hyoid bone.
The hyoid bone is usually at the level of C3 if there is no evidence of a laryngeal fracture.

Elevation of the hyoid bone above C3 suggests a laryngeal fracture.

❑❑ Differentiate between a hypertensive emergency and a hypertensive urgency.

Elevated BP + end organ damage = hypertensive emergency.
Elevated BP + no symptoms or signs of end organ damage = hypertensive urgency; usually DBP > 115 mmHg. Requires acute treatment.

❑❑ A patient presents with a history of forehead contusion. She cannot move her arms; lower extremity strength is intact. X-rays of the neck are normal. What is the suspected diagnosis?

Central cord syndrome. We just did this!
Management includes maintaining C-spine precautions, CT or MRI of the C-spine and neurosurgical consultation.

❑❑ What are the antibiotics of choice in a wound resulting from a skin diving incident?

Ciprofloxacin or TMP/SMX.

❑❑ How should a jelly fish sting be treated?

Rinse with saline.
Apply 5% acetic acid (vinegar) locally to the wound for approximately 30 minutes. In addition, corticosteroid agents may be applied topically. No antibiotics are necessary.
Tetanus prophylaxis.
Chironex flexneri antivenin only for this coelenterate.

❑❑ A young man was found on the street by police and is brought to the ED. He has a temperature of 105 °F, altered mental status and muscle rigidity. You find a bottle of thioridazine (Mellaril) in his pocket. What conditions should be considered?

Meningitis, encephalitis, hyperthyroidism, anticholinergic or strychnine poisoning and heat stroke come to mind. Another disease that should be considered is neuroleptic malignant syndrome .

Patients may also have hypotension, hypertension, and tachycardia.

❑❑ When does dysbaric air embolism typically occur?

DAE always develops within minutes of surfacing after a dive. Symptoms are sudden and dramatic and include loss of consciousness, focal neurologic symptoms such as monoplegia, convulsions, blindness, confusion, and sensory disturbances.

Sudden loss of consciousness or other acute neurologic deficits immediately after surfacing is due to DAE unless proven otherwise. Treatment includes high flow oxygen and rapid transport for hyperbaric oxygen treatment.

❑❑ A patient's blood gases reflect a mixed metabolic acidosis and respiratory alkalosis; what cause immediately comes to mind?

Salicylate intoxication.

❑❑ A two year-old has jammed a pencil into her lateral soft palate. What complication might develop?

Ischemic stroke is a complication of soft palate pencil injuries that results in contralateral hemiparesis.

❑❑ What is the appropriate paralyzing agent to use when intubation is required in a seizing patient?

Use pancuronium (Pavulon) as succinylcholine has greater tendency to increase serum potassium and to increase ICP.

❑❑ Distinguish the key differences between strychnine and tetanus poisoning:

Tetanus poisoning produces constant muscle tension whereas strychnine produces tetany and convulsions with episodes of relaxation between muscle contractions.

❑❑ What is the common name for Dermacentor andersoni**?**

Wood tick.

❑❑ What neurologic disorder presents similarly to symptoms caused by Dermacentor andersoni **(Wood Tick) bite?**

Guillain-Barré. Recall that tick paralysis may have decreased or absent DTRs as a clinical finding. Such DTRs may also be found associated with diphtheria exotoxin.

❑❑ **What nerve supplies taste to the anterior two thirds of the tongue, the lacrimal and salivary glands?**

Cranial nerve VII.

❑❑ **What disease is associated with anti-acetylcholine receptor antibodies that affect the post-synaptic neuromuscular site and is seen more commonly in females with a peak incidence in the third decade of life?**

Myasthenia gravis. 50% of myasthenia gravis patients have thymomas and 75% have lymphoid hyperplasia.

❑❑ **What antibiotics should be avoided in myasthenia gravis patients?**

Polymyxin and aminoglycosides have curare-like properties and may cause paralysis in these patients.

❑❑ **A baby presents to your emergency department with no facial movement, the lids sag and the child has a poor suck. She does not seem to move much and seems very weak. What causes do you consider?**

Myasthenia gravis or baby botulism.

❑❑ **A patient complains of pronounced weakness when attempting to climb stairs and even becomes tired when they do such simple tasks as brushing their teeth. Diagnosis?**

Myasthenia gravis.

❑❑ **What is the treatment for myasthenia gravis?**

Steroids, thymectomy, immunosuppressive drugs, plasmapheresis, and cholinergic agents such as pyridostigmine.

❑❑ **What disease is tick paralysis very similar to?**

It is very Guillain-Barré like.

❑❑ **Eaton-Lambert syndrome is associated with what class of diseases?**

Malignancies, particularly oat-cell carcinoma. Symptoms include aching muscle pain and weakness (the latter usually less than associated with MG); cranial nerves are not usually involved. Muscle strength may increase with repeated action in contradistinction to greater weakness with use encountered in MG.

❑❑ **What is a chalazion?**

This is a Meibomian gland granuloma.

❑❑ **How should a chalazion be treated?**

Surgical curettage.

❑❑ **Patient presents with eye pain. She has a constricted pupil, ciliary flush, and red injected sclera at the limbus. Diagnosis?**

Acute iritis.

❑❑ **A patient presents with <u>loss of central vision</u>. Likely diagnosis?**

A retrobulbar neuritis is likely. <u>MS is associated with about 25% of cases of retrobulbar neuritis</u>. Macular degeneration and central retinal vein occlusion can also lead to loss of central vision.

❐❐ I am used to treat acute angle closure glaucoma (and occasionally in vain attempts to treat retinal artery occlusion). I also play a role in treatment and prevention of acute mountain sickness. I decrease aqueous humor production via my mechanism of being a carbonic anhydrase inhibitor. What is my name?

Acetazolamide (Diamox).

❐❐ A patient presents with fever, neck pain or neck stiffness and trismus. Exam reveals pharyngeal edema with tonsil displacement and edema of the parotid area. Diagnosis?

PARAPHARYNGEAL Abscess.

❐❐ A patient presents with hearing loss, nystagmus, complaint of facial weakness, and diplopia. Vertigo is provoked with sudden movement. A lumbar puncture reveals elevated CNS protein. What diagnosis is suspected?

An acoustic neuroma.

❐❐ Can a parapharyngeal abscess present with an associated finding of edema in the area of the parotid gland?

Yes.

❐❐ In a trauma patient, facial dimpling of the cheek is associated with:

Zygomatic arch fracture.

❐❐ What x-rays should be ordered to diagnose a fracture of the zygoma?

A jug handle, Water's view or submental view.

❐❐ What are the key features of Stevens-Johnson Syndrome?

It is a bullous form of erythema multiforme with involvement of mucous membranes. It may cause corneal ulcerations, anterior uveitis and blindness.

❐❐ Blood is originating from a tooth after trauma. What Ellis classification?

Ellis class III.

❐❐ What are the most common drugs causing TEN?

Phenylbutazone, barbiturates, sulfa drugs, anti-epileptics and antibiotics.

❐❐ Rhomboid shaped crystals from a joint aspiration are associated with:

Pseudogout.

❐❐ Needle shaped crystals are associated with:

Gout.

❐❐ What is the most common site of aseptic necrosis?

The hip.

❑❑ **Acute treatment for gout?**

Colchicine, indomethacin and other NSAIDs.

❑❑ **Most common presentation of a Charcot's joint?**

A swollen ankle and a" bag of bones" appearance on x-ray.

❑❑ **On x-ray you see Charcot's joints. Diagnosis?**

Diabetes.

❑❑ **What is the most common cause of Charcot's joint?**

Diabetic peripheral neuropathy.

❑❑ **What is the most common tendon affected in calcified tendonitis?**

The supraspinatus.

❑❑ **Which epicondyle is involved in tennis elbow?**

The lateral epicondyle.

❑❑ **What is the <u>most</u> <u>common</u> and second most common site of infectious arthritis?**

The knee is the most common and the hip is the second most common.
Staphylococcus is the <u>most</u> <u>common</u> cause.

❑❑ **At what cervical level is the hyoid bone normally found?**

The third cervical vertebra.
If the hyoid is above this level a laryngeal fracture should be suspected.

❑❑ **At what cervical level is the thyroid located?**

Level of the fourth cervical vertebra.

❑❑ **What is the most common site of cervical disc herniation?**

C5-C6. Patient will complain of bilateral shoulder pain.

❑❑ **What nerve is located in the tarsal tunnel?**

The tibial nerve.

❑❑ **A patient has difficulty squa[illegible]ising. Likely spinal pathology?**

L4 root compression with involvement of quadriceps.
(Don't even *think about* X-linked Duchenne's muscular dystrophy!)

❑❑ **What STD pathogens cause** painful **ulcers?**

Type II Genital Herpes and chancroid.

STD	Ulcer	Node
Genital Herpes	**Painful**	Painful
Chancroid	**Painful**	Painful
Syphilis	Painless	Less Painful
Lymphogranuloma Venereum	Painless	Moderately

❑❑ A patient presents with a complaint of pain at the site of the deltoid insertion with radiation into the back of the arm (C5 distribution). On exam, there is increased pain with active abduction from 70° - 120°. X-rays reveal calcification at the tendinous insertion of the greater tuberosity. Diagnosis?

Supraspinatus tendonitis.

❑❑ Absent knee jerk. What level?

L4.

❑❑ Absent Achilles reflex. What level?

S1.

❑❑ Paresthesia of the great toe. Level?

L5.

❑❑ Paresthesia of the little toe. Level?

S1.

❑❑ What is the most common site of compartment syndrome?

Anterior compartment of the leg.

❑❑ Describe the leg position associated with an anterosuperior hip dislocation.

Anterosuperior - External rotation and slight abduction. In the pubic type, the hip is extended and in the iliac type, it is slightly flexed.

❑❑ Describe the leg position associated with an obturator hip dislocation.

In an obturator dislocation there is external rotation, flexion and abduction.

❑❑ Posterior hip dislocation - leg position?

Internal rotation, flexion and adducted. Most co

❑❑ A patient in the ED cannot recall ever having a tetanus shot. The nurse gives him a tetanus shot. Later, he develops a hypersensitivity reaction and recalls that he recently had a tetanus shot. What type of reaction does he have?

Type 3 - Arthus reaction. Type 3 reactions are caused by immune complexes or antigen-antibody complexes that activate complement and platelets forming aggregates and complexes with IgE.

❑❑ A positive TB test is what type of reaction?

Type 4 - cell mediated, delayed hypersensitivity.

Type 4 reactions do not involve complement or antibodies.

❒❒ What drugs commonly cause erythema multiforme?

Carbamazepine, penicillin, sulfa, pyrazolone, phenytoin, barbiturates.

❒❒ What aerobe is most commonly found in cutaneous abscesses?

Staphylococcus aureus.

❒❒ What is the most common gram negative aerobe found in cutaneous abscesses?

Proteus mirabilis.

❒❒ Describe the Gram stain appearance of Staphylococcus aureus.

Gram positive cocci in grape-like clusters.

❒❒ What is the most common cause of cellulitis in children less than 3 years of age?

Hemophilus influenzae.

❒❒ What is the most common cause of cellulitis in the adult?

Staphylococcus aureus.

❒❒ What is the cause of erysipelas?

Group A , ß-hemolytic *streptococci.*

❒❒ How is erysipelas treated?

Penicillin (or clarithromycin).

Erythromycin for penicillin allergic patients.

❒❒ What is the most common cause of toxic shock syndrome?

Staphylococci. Toxins C and F are the proteins that mediate toxic shock syndrome.

❒❒ A child presents to the ED with a history of fever, conjunctival hyperemia, and erythema of the mucus membranes with desquamation. Diagnosis?

Kawasaki's Disease. Remember - Kawasaki's Disease may have lesions resembling erythema multiforme.

❒❒ Clostridium tetanus, a Gram and anaerobe, produces a neurotoxin. Is it an endotoxin or an exotoxin?

Tetanospasmin is an exotoxin. Its major effect is prevention of transmission of inhibitory neurons in anterior horn cells resulting in motor system disinhibition.

❒❒ What are some of the common causes of prerenal acute renal failure?

Volume depletion and decreased effective volume (CHF, sepsis, cirrhosis).

❒❒ What are the causes of acute renal failure which are renal in nature?

Acute Tubular Necrosis, acute interstitial nephritis, acute glomerulonephritis and vascular disease.

❑❑ What are the causes of post-renal failure?

Ureteral and urethral obstruction.

❑❑ What findings mark the presentation of a patient with rapidly progressive glomerulonephritis?

Most common - hematuria.
Also edema (periorbital), HTN, ascites, pleural effusion, rales, and anuria.

❑❑ What arrhythmia is frequently encountered during renal dialysis.

Hypokalemia induced ventricular fibrillation.

❑❑ In which trimester of pregnancy is UTI and pyelonephritis most common?

Third.

❑❑ What is inflammation of the foreskin called?

Balanitis or balanoposthitis.

❑❑ What is phimosis?

A condition in which the foreskin cannot be retracted posterior to the glans. The preliminary treatment is a dorsal slit.

❑❑ What is paraphimosis?

A condition in which the foreskin is retracted posterior to the glands and cannot be advanced over the glans.

❑❑ What are causes of priapism?

Prolonged sex (I *hate* it when...), leukemia, sickle cell trait and disease, blood dyscrasias, pelvic hematoma or neoplasm, syphilis, and urethritis. Drugs - Phenothiazines, prazosin, tolbutamide, anticoagulants, corticosteroids.

❑❑ What causes a green to gray frothy vaginal discharge with mild itching.

Trichomonas vaginitis. On physical exam, the cervix may have a strawberry appearance (20%).

❑❑ Describe the presentation of a patient with Gardnerella vaginitis?

On physical exam, note a frothy, gray-white, fishy smelling vaginal discharge. Wet mount may show clue cells (clusters of bacilli on the surface of epithelial cells).

Sherlock Holmes always uses his magnifying lens to look for *Clues* in the *Garden*.

❑❑ Do you know why I hate **it when my foot falls asleep during the day?**

It'll be up <u>all night</u>!

❑❑ Sulfamethoxazole may lead to hemolysis in a patient with:

G6PD deficiency.

❒❒ **What disease is associated with painless bright red bleeding per vagina in the third trimester?**

Placenta previa.

❒❒ **Painful third trimester vaginal bleeding likely represents?**

Abruptio placenta.

❒❒ **What affect does pregnancy have on BUN and creatinine?**

Both the creatinine and BUN are decreased. This is as the result of increased renal blood flow and increased glomerular filtration rate.

❒❒ **When can one auscultate the fetal heart?**

Ultrasound- 6 weeks.

Doppler- 10 - 12 weeks.

Stethoscope- 18 - 20 weeks.

❒❒ **Describe a Brudzinski sign.**

Flexion of the neck produces flexion of the knees.

❒❒ **Describe Kernig's sign.**

Extension of the knees from the flexed thigh position results in strong passive resistance.

❒❒ **What is the normal opening pressure in a spinal tap?**

15 cm H_2O.

❒❒ **What is the normal CSF protein level?**

40 mg/dl

❒❒ **What opening pressure and protein level are expected in bacterial meningitis?**

Opening pressure of near 30 cm H_2O and protein level of greater than 150 mg/dl. Glucose level will drop with bacterial meningitis, with TB and with fungal infections.

❒❒ **What does the India ink test show?**

Cryptococcus neoformans.

❒❒ **What is the most significant pathophysiologic mechanism of death from cyclic antidepressants?**

Myocardial depression, including hypotension and conduction blocks.

❒❒ **Of patients who die from CA overdose, what percentage are awake and alert at the time of first prehospital contact?**

25%.

❒❒ **What are some common side effects of phenothiazine use?**

Malaise, hyperthermia, tachycardia, anticholinergic effects, and quinidine-like membrane stabilization. The most dangerous side effect is neuroleptic malignant syndrome.

❒❒ How should stable ventricular tachyarrhythmias associated with phenothiazine overdose be treated?

Lidocaine and phenytoin.

❒❒ Which antibiotic may either increase or decrease lithium secretion?

Tetracycline.

❒❒ How is lithium overdose treated?

Lavage, saline diuresis, furosemide, and hemodialysis. Alkalinization *may* be appropriate.

❒❒ Is phenobarbital more quickly metabolized by children or by adults?

Adults. Neonates are especially slow at metabolizing phenobarbital.

❒❒ How should barbiturate poisoning be treated?

Supportive, charcoal, alkalinization of the urine, charcoal hemoperfusion or hemodialysis.

❒❒ What drugs increase the half-life of phenytoin?

Sulfonamides, isoniazid, dicumarol, and chloramphenicol.

❒❒ What hypersensitivity skin rashes are noted with phenytoin use?

Lupus-like and Stevens-Johnson syndrome.

❒❒ What are the cardiac effects of phenytoin?

Inhibits sodium channels, decreases the effective refractory period and automaticity in the Purkinje fibers. Little effect on QRS width or action potential duration.

❒❒ What symptoms are expected with a phenytoin level of > 20, of > 30, and of > 40 μg/mL?

> 20 - lateral gaze nystagmus.
> 30 - lateral gaze nystagmus plus increased vertical nystagmus with upward gaze.
> 40 - lethargy, confusion, dysarthrias, and psychosis.

❒❒ In endocarditis (all comers), what is the most commonly involved cardiac valve?

Mitral > Aortic > Tricuspid > Pulmonic.

❒❒ Infectious endocarditis in an IV drug abuser most commonly affects which valve?

#1 - Tricuspid.
#2 - Pulmonary.

❒❒ What is the <u>most common</u> causative bacterium associated with right-sided endocarditis in IV drug abusers?

S. aureus.
<u>Left- sided</u> endocarditis in IV drug abusers is likely due *to E. coli, streptococcus, Klebsiella, Pseudomonas* and *Candida.*

❒❒ **A heroin addict presents with pulmonary edema. What is the best treatment?**

Naloxone, O_2 and ventilatory support.
Don't bother using diuretics. This seems like a good test question.

❒❒ **What is the most common neurologic complication of IV drug abuse?**

Nontraumatic mononeuritis - painless weakness 2 -3 h after injection.

❒❒ **Name two frequently observed organisms causing septic arthritis in drug addicts.**

Serratiae and *Pseudomonas.*
These are rare causes in non-addicts.

❒❒ **An alcoholic patient presents with complaints of abdominal pain and blurred vision. The patient is very photophobic and blood gases reveal a metabolic acidosis. Diagnosis?**

Methanol poisoning. These patients may describe seeing something resembling a snow storm.

❒❒ **What is the mechanism of action of clonidine?**

Clonidine is a central acting α–agonist. It leads to decreased sympathetic outflow and lowers catecholamine levels.

❒❒ **What is the lethal dose of methanol?**

30 mL.
Formate levels in methanol poisoning are greatest in vitreous humor.

❒❒ **What alcohol poisoning is suggested by a plasma bicarbonate level of zero (cipher, null, empty set, zip, Ø)?**

Methanol.

It also produces a large osmolar gap and large anion gap. Methanol poisoning is treated with IV ethanol and hemodialysis.

❒❒ **Positive birefringent calcium oxalate crystals are pathognomonic for poisoning with what substance?**

Ethylene glycol.
The lethal dose of ethylene glycol is 100 mL.

❒❒ **What are the signs and symptoms of ethylene glycol poisoning?**

Hallucinations, nystagmus, ataxia, papilledema, and a large anion gap.

❒❒ **How should ethylene glycol poisoning be treated?**

Gastric lavage, sodium bicarbonate, thiamine and pyridoxine, IV ethanol and hemodialysis.

❒❒ **What are the major lab findings in a patient with isopropanol poisoning?**

Elevated osmolal gap.
Acetonemia and acetonuria. Acetone.
Ø acidosis.

❒❒ A patient presents to the ER with ataxia, altered mental status, and sixth nerve palsy. What is your diagnosis?

Wernicke's encephalopathy.

❒❒ What are the signs and symptoms of isopropanol poisoning?

Sweet odor of breath (acetone), hypotension and hemorrhagic gastritis, CNS depression from isopropanol and from its metabolite, acetone.

❒❒ What is the treatment of cocaine toxicity?

Sedate with benzodiazepine.
Treat unresponsive hypertension with nitroprusside or phentolamine.
Return to text book to re-read discussion of worsening symptoms with ß-adrenergic antagonists.

❒❒ Vertical nystagmus?

PCP.
(O.K., there *are* some other causes...brainstem disease, vestibular disease.)

❒❒ X-ray finding in a patient with salicylate toxicity:

Noncardiogenic pulmonary edema.

❒❒ Describe central nervous system affects of salicylate poisoning:

Lethargy, confusion, seizures, and respiratory arrest.

❒❒ Salicylate levels should ideally be checked how long after an ingestion?

6 hours.

❒❒ What is the minimum likely toxic dose of salicylates?

150 mg/kg.

❒❒ Salicylate level, measured at 6 h after ingestion, greater than _____ is associated with toxicity.

45 mg/dl.

❒❒ ACEtominophen level, measured 4 ACEs after ingestion, greater than _____ is associated with toxicity.

150 µg/mL.

❒❒ For what drugs will alkalinization of the urine increase excretion?

CA's, salicylates, and long-acting barbiturates.
May be of some use to enhance lithium excretion.

❒❒ What are the signs of salicylate poisoning?

Hyperventilation, hyperthermia, mental status changes, nausea, vomiting, abdominal pain, dehydration, diaphoresis, ketonuria, metabolic acidosis, and respiratory alkalosis.

❑❑ A child presents with lethargy, seizures, and hypoglycemia. A history of several days of preceding viral syndrome symptoms is elicited. Name two disorders that should be considered.

Reye's syndrome and salicylate intoxication.

❑❑ What laboratory test can aid in evaluation of a possible toxic iron ingestion?

Total iron binding capacity measured 3 to 5 hours after ingestion.
If serum iron level is significantly less than the total iron binding capacity, a toxic iron ingestion is less likely.

❑❑ What is the antidote for a toxic ingestion of iron?

Deferoxamine chelates only free iron.

❑❑ Deferoxamine should be given for a serum iron level greater than:

350 μg/dL.

❑❑ Deferoxamine should be given for what ratio of serum iron to total iron binding capacity?

Give deferoxamine if serum iron is > total iron binding capacity.

❑❑ How many hours after an iron ingestion should total iron binding capacity be measured. Feel the Force, Luke; we just did this.

3-5 hours.

❑❑ What type of hydrocarbons are most toxic?

"Oh no...not that reverse viscosity stuff!"

Kinematic viscosity (u), shear rates unrelated to apparent viscosity (∂) neglecting Fähraeus-Lindqvist effect.

O.K. - Thus, substances with <u>low</u> viscosities (measured in Saybolt Seconds Universal (SSU)) are <u>more</u> toxic than higher viscosity compounds. Your gasoline, kerosene and paint thinner (all aliphatic hydrocarbons with SSU's of < 60), are all more toxic than your motor oil, your tar and your petroleum jelly, which all have SSUs > 100.

Of the compounds with SSUs < 60, the most toxic are those that are not aliphatic, including your benzene, toluene, xylene and tetrachloroethylene.

❑❑ What is the most reliable site for detecting central cyanosis?

The tongue.

❑❑ You are taking boards and are presented with a patient with a history of placement of an aortic graft or of abdominal aortic aneurysm. The patient has been vomiting up some coffee ground emesis. What infrequent entity needs to be considered?

The dreaded aortoenteric fistula. These patients may present with a limited herald bleed before massive bleeding develops. A CT showing air in the periaortic area is indicative of need for immediate surgery.

❑❑ What is a common complication of pancuronium?

Tachycardia from its vagolytic action.

❒❒ What is the most common cause of hypermagnesemia in a patient with renal failure?

Patient use of compounds high in magnesium, such as antacids.
This can result in neuromuscular paralysis.
Consider IV calcium.
Saline and furosemide assisted diuresis may not help this patient with renal failure, so consider dialysis.

❒❒ How much energy should be used in cardioversion of an unstable infant with a wide complex tachycardia?

0.5 to 1.0 J/kg.

❒❒ How much energy should be used to cardiovert unstable VF in an infant?

2 J/kg.

❒❒ What is the most common malposition of the nasotracheal tube?

Into the piriform sinus. The second most common malposition is the esophagus.

❒❒ What is the <u>most</u> <u>common</u> physical sign of a PE?

Tachypnea.

❒❒ What are the three most common presenting signs of aortic stenosis?

Syncope, angina, and heart failure.

❒❒ When do CK levels first begin to rise and when do they peak in an MI?

CK - MB earliest rise 6-8 h.
Peak 24-30 h.
Normalizes 48 h.

❒❒ When does LDH first begin to rise and when does it peak in an MI?

LDH-I (from heart) earliest rise 12 to 24 h.
Peak 48 to 96 h.

❒❒ What is the effect of nitrates on preload and afterload?

Nitrates mostly dilate veins and venules to decrease preload.

❒❒ <u>Inferior</u> wall MIs commonly lead to what two types of heart block (via mechanism of damage to autonomic fibers in the atrial septum giving increased vagal tone impairing AV node conduction)?

First degree AV block.
Mobitz Type I (Wenckebach) second-degree AV block.
Sinus bradycardia can also occur.

Progression to complete AV block is <u>not</u> common.

❒❒ <u>Anterior</u> wall MIs may directly damage intracardiac conduction. This may lead to what type of arrhythmias?

The <u>dangerous</u> type! Mobitz II second-degree AV block that can suddenly progress to complete AV block.

❑❑ What are some of the potential, sometimes rare, complications of Mycoplasma pneumonia?

Non-pulmonary: Hemolytic anemia, aseptic meningitis, encephalitis, Guillain-Barré syndrome, pericarditis, and myocarditis.

Pulmonary: ARDS, atelectasis, mediastinal adenopathy, pneumothorax, pleural effusion and abscess.

❑❑ Under what conditions should Staphylococcal pneumonia be considered as a possible diagnosis?

Although it only accounts for 1% of bacterial pneumonias, it should be considered in patients with sudden chills, hectic fever, pleurisy and cough, especially following a viral illness such as measles or influenza.

❑❑ Of the following anesthetics, which has the shortest duration of action - lidocaine, procaine, bupivacaine or mepivacaine?

Procaine.

❑❑ Differential diagnosis of a ring lesion on CT scan:

Toxoplasmosis, lymphoma, fungal infection, TB, CMV, Kaposi's, and hemorrhage.

❑❑ Does erythema multiforme itch?

Not typically. It may be tender.

❑❑ A patient presents with granuloma inguinale. What does it look like?

Papular, nodular or vesicular painless lesions. These can progress to extensive destruction of local tissues. Cause is Calymmatobacterium granulomatis.

❑❑ What causes chancroid?

Hemophilus ducreyi.
Painful necrotic ulcerative lesions and painful nodes.

❑❑ Describe lesions associated with Chlamydia.

Painless shallow ulcerations, papular or nodular lesions or herpetiform vesicles wax and wane.

❑❑ What type of diarrhea causing disease may be transmitted by pets?

Yersinia.

❑❑ What state is associated with akinetic mutism?

N. Dakota is a bucolic state.
Akinetic mutism is an abulic state (which is like a coma vigil). Patients seem awake and may have eyes open. They respond to questions very slowly.
The cause is typically due to depressed frontal lobe function.

❑❑ What is normal blood pressure in a newborn?

60 mmHg.

❑❑ What is the initial drug of choice to treat SVT in a pediatric patient.

Adenosine 0.1 mg/kg is drug of choice.
Digoxin 0.02 mg/kg may take ≈ 4 h for conversion.

Verapamil may be used in children > 2 years of age. It is contraindicated in younger children due to several deaths.
Synchronized cardioversion at 0.5-1.0 J/kg.

❐❐ After the first mo of life, what is the number one cause of meningitis and of pneumonia in children?

Most common cause of meningitis after the first mo of life is *H. influenza.*

Most common cause of pneumonia after the first mo of life is *S. pneumoniae; H. influenza* is the second most common cause.

For bacteremia in children greater than one mo, the most common causes are *S. pneumoniae* (70%) and H. influenza (20%) of the time.

❐❐ Discuss infantile spasms.

Onset is by 3 to 9 months of age, typically lasts seconds, and may occur in single episodes or bursts. The EEG is most often abnormal.
85% of these patients go on to be mentally handicapped.

❐❐ Erythema multiforme can be associated with which anticonvulsants?

Phenobarbital, phenytoin and carbamazepine.

❐❐ Hepatic failure is commonly associated with what anticonvulsant?

Valproic acid.

❐❐ A patient presents with fever, neck pain and trismus. Exam reveals pharyngeal edema with tonsil displacement and edema of the parotid area. Diagnosis?

PARAPHARYNGEAL abscess.

❐❐ Does H. influenza typically cause abscesses?

No.

❐❐ What drugs, activities and cooking habits are associated with increasing clearance of theophylline (decreasing the theophylline level)?

Phenytoin, phenobarbital, cigarette smoking and charcoal Bar-B-Queing.

❐❐ Anaphylaxis is a common cause of what type of renal failure?

Prerenal.

❐❐ What are the end products of methanol, of ethylene glycol and of isopropyl alcohol metabolism?

Methanol - formate.
Ethylene glycol - oxalate and formate.
Isopropyl alcohol - acetone.

❐❐ What type of alcohol ingestion is associated with hypocalcemia?

Ethylene glycol.

❑❑ What type of alcohol ingestion is associated with hemorrhagic pancreatitis?

Methanol.

❑❑ Arsenic produces an odor on the breath similar to what?

Garlic.

❑❑ When does ECM show up in Lyme disease?

Stage I - 3 to 32 days after the bite.

❑❑ For what disorder is vigorous digital massage of the orbit indicated?

Central retinal artery occlusion.
DO NOT do this in central vein occlusion!

❑❑ What pathogen is suggested by a pneumonia with a single rigor?

Pneumococcus.

❑❑ What pathogen does a strawberry cervix suggest?

Trichomonas.

❑❑ What are the key features of Ellis Type I, II, and III?

Enamel, dentin, pulp.
Enamel, dentin, pulp. Pulp bleeds.

❑❑ What is the vector and causative organism of Lyme disease?

The vector is *Ixodes dammini* and the organism is *Borrelia burgdorferi*. It is the most frequently transmitted tick-borne disease.

❑❑ Q fever cause:

Coxiella burnetii, aka *Rickettsia burnetii.*
First found in *Dermacentor andersoni* tick.
Fever, headache, malaise, chest pain.

❑❑ A hordeolum is:

A Meibomian gland infection, usually of upper lid.

❑❑ Ludwig's angina pathology:

Hemolytic streptococci, staphylococcus, mixed aerobes and anaerobes.

❑❑ The three most common locations of malignant melanoma:

1) Skin.
2) Eye.
3) Anal canal.

❑❑ What is the initial dose of blood to be given in children?

10 mL/kg of packed RBCs.

❐❐ What is achalasia?

Disorder of esophageal motility and incomplete relaxation of the lower esophagus.

❐❐ Suspected mesenteric ischemia may be virtually confirmed by what invasive exam other than laparotomy?

Angiography.

❐❐ Enterotoxin producing organisms that can cause food poisoning:

Clostridium.
Staph aureus.
Vibrio cholerae.
E. coli.

❐❐ Antibiotics should be avoided in what infectious diarrhea?

Salmonella. Clear exceptions are in severe cases of diarrhea in immunocompromised patients and in children less than 6 months of age.

❐❐ Anal fissures:

Crohn's.

❐❐ Diphtheria - growth medium:

Loffler's medium or tellurite.
O.K.

❐❐ Three disorders that are associated with decreased DTRs:

Guillain-Barré.
Tic paralysis due to Dermacentor andersoni (Wood Tick) bite.
Diphtheria exotoxin.

❐❐ What is the most common cause of bacterial pneumonia in children greater than 4 weeks of age?

S. pneumoniae is the most common.
H. influenza is the second most common.

❐❐ Likely cause of CHF in a premature infant?

Premature infants = PDA.

❐❐ Likely cause of CHF presenting in the first 3 d of life?

First 3 d = transposition of the great vessels which will cause cyanosis and failure.

❐❐ Likely cause of CHF presenting in the first week of life?

First week = hypoplastic left ventricle.

❐❐ Likely cause of CHF presenting in the second week of life?

Second week = coarctation.

❑❑ Do you treat Shigella with antibiotics?

In general, yes.

❑❑ What is a pinguecula?

It is a yellowish nodule, particularly on the nasal aspect of the eye, but it may be lateral. Often caused by wind and dust.

❑❑ What is a pterygium?

It is a chronic growth over the medial or lateral aspect of the cornea approaching the pupil. It is much thicker than pingueculae.

❑❑ What is the most common cause of painless upper GI bleeding in an infant or child?

Varices from portal hypertension.

❑❑ What is the <u>most</u> <u>common</u> cause of major painless lower GI bleeding in an infant or child?

Meckel's diverticulum.

❑❑ Common cause of orbital cellulitis:

Staph aureus.

❑❑ Who should receive prophylaxis after exposure to Neisseria meningitidis**?**

People living with the patient or having close intimate contact.

❑❑ Name some common hydrocarbons that are considered to be most toxic and have SSU's of less than 60.

Aromatic hydrocarbons, halogenated hydrocarbons, mineral seal oil, kerosene, naphtha, turpentine, gasoline and lighter fluid.

Others considered less toxic have SSU's greater than 100, such as grease, diesel oil, mineral oil, petroleum jelly, paraffin wax, and tar.

❑❑ What drug is absolutely contraindicated in the treatment of hydrocarbon poisoning?

Epinephrine as it sensitizes the myocardium, potentially leading to arrest.

❑❑ What drug is contraindicated in a glue sniffing patient?

Epinephrine. Like solvent abusers, these patients may be scared to death.

❑❑ What is a delayed complication of acid ingestion?

Pyloric stricture.

❑❑ What is the difference between carbamates and organophosphates?

Carbamates produce similar symptoms as organophosphates, however, the bonds in carbamate toxicity are reversible.

❑❑ What are key signs and symptoms of organophosphate poisoning?

Ataxia, abdominal pain and cramping, blurred vision, seizures, ataxia and miosis.

❑❑ A patient presents with miotic pupils, muscle fasciculations, diaphoresis and diffuse oral and bronchial secretions. The patient has an odor of garlic on his breath. What is your diagnosis?

Organophosphate poisoning.

❑❑ What ECG changes may be associated with organophosphate poisoning?

Prolongation of the QT interval, and ST and T wave abnormalities.

❑❑ What is the key laboratory finding in the diagnosis of organophosphate poisoning?

An elevated red blood cell cholinesterase level.

❑❑ Treatment of organophosphate poisoning?

Decontaminate, charcoal, atropine and pralidoxime prn.

❑❑ What are the key features in the diagnosis of Trench foot?

Exposure must be for one to two days of wet, cold temperatures above freezing.
Trench foot represents a superficial partial burn with no deep tissue damage.

❑❑ What is chilblain?

Chilblain is prolonged exposure to dry cold.

❑❑ At about what core body temperature does shivering cease?

30 to 32° C.

❑❑ What is the sequence of arrhythmia development in a patient with hypothermia?

Bradycardia → Atrial fibrillation → Ventricular fibrillation → Asystole.

❑❑ What is the common pathogen in a cat bite?

Pasteurella multocida.

❑❑ What would you expect to find in the hippocampus of a patient with rabies?

Negri bodies. Incubation for rabies is 30 to 60 days. Treatment includes cleaning of the wound, rabies immune globulin, and Human Diploid Cell Vaccine. Remember, 1/2 the rabies immune globulin goes around the wound and the other half goes IM.

❑❑ How do you treat the bite of a Megalopyge opercularis caterpillar?

Calcium gluconate, 10 mL of a 10% solution IV.
Stings cause immediate rhythmic pain.

❑❑ What kind of tick transmits Rocky Mountain Spotted Fever?

The female andersoni tick. It transmits rickettsia rickettsii.

❑❑ What is the most common symptom in Rocky Mountain Spotted Fever?

Headache occurs in 90% of patients.

❑❑ **Describe the rash of Rocky Mountain Spotted Fever.**

It is a macular rash, 2 to 6 mm in diameter, and located on the wrists and palms, spreading to the soles and trunk.

❑❑ **What tick transmits Lyme disease?**

The *Ixodes dammini* tick.
Spirochete *Borrelia burgdorferi* is diagnosed by culture on Kelly's medium.

❑❑ **Describe skin lesion seen in Lyme disease.**

A large distinct circular skin lesion called erythema chronicum migrans. It is an annular erythematous lesion with central clearing.

❑❑ **Describe a patient with tick paralysis.**

Bulbar paralysis, ascending flaccid paralysis, paresthesias of hands and feet, symmetric loss of deep tendon reflexes and respiratory paralysis.

❑❑ **What drug is contraindicated in a Gila monster bite?**

Meperidine (Demerol).
(May be synergistic with venom!)

❑❑ **What is the causative organism of otitis externa?**

Pseudomonas.

❑❑ **Signs and symptoms of Lyme Disease, stages I-III:**

I. Erythema Chronicum Migrans.
Malaise, fatigue, headache, arthralgias, fever, chills.

II. Neurologic, cardiac.
Headache, meningoencephalitis, facial nerve palsy, radiculoneuropathy, ophthalmitis and 1°, 2° and 3° AV blocks.

III. Arthritis.
Knee > shoulder > elbow > TMJ > ankle > wrist > hip >hands > feet.

❑❑ **A diver levels off at 33 feet. How many atmospheres of pressure is he experiencing?**

Two. Sea level is one, 33 feet is two, 66 feet is three, etc.

❑❑ **After a diver surfaces, she immediately experiences aphasia, paralysis and blindness. Diagnosis?**

Dysbaric air embolism.

❑❑ **After a blast injury, the most life threatening injury is likely to have occurred where?**

In the lungs.

❑❑ **Describe the wound resulting from AC .**

AC produces an entrance and exit wound of similar size.
The damage from AC is usually worse than that from DC.

❐❐ **Describe a DC wound.**

Small entrance wound, large exit wound.

❐❐ **What type of arrhythmia does lightning produce?**

It is a DC and produces asystole.

❐❐ **What type of arrhythmia does AC tend to produce?**

Ventricular fibrillation.

❐❐ **A patient, who works in a plant that makes chemical deodorizers presents after exposure to phenol. Treatment?**

Clean the patient with olive oil and water.

❐❐ **What are the most common complaints in a patient with carbon monoxide poisoning?**

The most common is headache. Also dizziness, weakness, and nausea.

❐❐ **What signs and symptoms are expected after radiation exposures of 100 REM, 300 REM, 400 REM and 2000 REM, less than two hours post exposure?**

100 REM produces nausea and vomiting.
300 REM produces erythema.
400 REM produces diarrhea.
2000 REM produces seizures.

❐❐ **What drug blocks the uptake of radioactive iodine?**

Potassium iodine.

❐❐ **Psilocybin mushroom is associated with:**

Hallucinations.

❐❐ **In brain stem herniation is decorticate or decerebrate posturing expected?**

Decerebrate posturing (hyperextension)
Decorticate posturing is flexion of the upper extremities and extension of the lower extremities.

❐❐ **A patient presents after experiencing trauma to the head. The patient has an elevated systolic blood pressure and bradycardia. Diagnosis?**

Cushing reflex.

❐❐ **What are the three components to the Glasgow coma scale, and how many points is each worth?**

Eye opening (4).
Verbal response (5).
Motor response (6).

❐❐ **What is the name for a flexion mechanism fracture through the anterior aspect of a vertebral body that is associated with ligamentous damage and an anterior cord syndrome?**

A teardrop fracture.

❒❒ **Describe the corneal reflex.**

Conducted by the ophthalmic branch of the 5th nerve and the afferent branch of the facial (7th) nerve.

❒❒ **What is the most unstable cervical spine injury?**

Rupture of transverse atlantal ligament > dens fracture > burst fracture (flexion teardrop) > bilateral facet dislocation.

❒❒ **What is the eponym for a C1 burst fracture from vertical compression?**

Jefferson fracture.

❒❒ **A patient in a motor vehicle accident sustains a hyperextension injury of the neck. Plain films reveal a C2 bilateral facet fracture through the pedicles. You describe this fracture in consultation with the neurosurgeon. What type of fracture have you described?**

A Hangman's fracture.

❒❒ **A patient has an avulsion fracture of the spinous process of C7 with a history of a hyperflexion mechanism. Diagnosis?**

Clay shoveler's fracture - fracture involving the spinous process of C6, C7, or T1. The mechanism is usually flexion or a direct blow.

❒❒ **A patient suffers a bilateral interfacetal dislocation. What is your concern?**

Injury occurs as a result of flexion and is very unstable with ligament disruption.

❒❒ **What is the most unstable <u>fracture</u> of the cervical spine?**

A dens fracture with rupture of the atlantal ligament.

❒❒ **Stable or unstable: a Clay shoveler's fracture?**

Stable.

❒❒ **Stable or unstable: fracture of the posterior arch of C1?**

Stable.

❒❒ **Name the four stable cervical spine fractures.**

Simple wedge.
Clay shoveler's.
Pillar.
C1 posterior neural arch.
The rest are unstable or potentially unstable!

❒❒ **A patient presents with a history of a blow to the forehead. Her neck was hyperextended. Patient complains of weakness in the arms with minimal weakness in the lower extremities. Diagnosis?**

Central cord syndrome.

❒❒ **You see a patient with an obvious traumatic spinal cord lesion. On physical exam, he has motor paralysis, loss of gross proprioception and loss of vibratory sensation on one side, and loss of pain and temperature sensation on the opposite side. Diagnosis?**

Brown-Séquard's syndrome.

❑❑ What is the most common cause of shock in patients with blunt chest trauma?

Pelvic (or extremity) fracture.

❑❑ What is a frequent complication of ethmoid sinusitis?

Orbital cellulitis.

❑❑ What is the most common site of aspiration pneumonitis?

Right lower lobe.

❑❑ What is the most common ECG finding associated with a myocardial contusion?

ST-T wave abnormalities.

❑❑ What is the most common valvular injury associated with blunt cardiac injury?

A ruptured aortic valve.

❑❑ What is the most common site of a traumatic aortic laceration?

The vast majority occur just distal to the left subclavian artery.

❑❑ What is the most common x-ray finding in traumatic rupture of the aorta?

Widening of the superior mediastinum.

❑❑ What is the most accurate x-ray finding in traumatic rupture of the aorta?

Rightward deviation of the esophagus more than 1 - 2 cm.

❑❑ A patient presents with a history of high speed traumatic injury to the chest. On physical exam, a systolic murmur over the precordium is auscultated The patient has a slightly hoarse voice. The nurse tells you the pulse is also stronger in the upper extremities. Diagnosis?

Traumatic rupture of the aorta.

❑❑ A patient presents with a history of chest trauma, a systolic murmur and an infarct pattern on ECG. Diagnosis?

Traumatic ventricular septal defect.

❑❑ A person with a history of a motor vehicle accident has x-ray findings of retroperitoneal air seen on a flat plate of the abdomen. What is a likely diagnosis?

Duodenal injury. Tentative test is a contrast study. Extravasation confirms a duodenal injury.

❑❑ On an x-ray of the hand, the AP view shows a triangular shaped lunate. Diagnosis?

Lunate dislocation.
Lateral films will show a cup spilling out water.

❑❑ What x-ray view is required to diagnose a perilunate dislocation?

Lateral view.

❒❒ A patient presents describing a snapping sensation in the wrist and a click. Diagnosis:

Scaphoid dislocation.

❒❒ X-ray of the hand reveals a 3 mm space between the scaphoid and the lunate. Diagnosis?

Scaphoid dislocation.

❒❒ In a boxer's fracture, how much angulation of the 5th metacarpal neck is acceptable.

50 degrees.

❒❒ What ligament in the hand is commonly injured in a fall while skiing?

Thumb MCP joint ulnar collateral ligament rupture (Gamekeeper's thumb).

❒❒ Posterior dislocation of the shoulder is often missed with a standard radiographic shoulder series. What x-ray view aids in diagnosis?

The scapular "Y" view.

❒❒ Name the four muscles of the rotator cuff.

Supraspinatus, infraspinatus, teres minor and the subscapularis. Patients with a rotator cuff tear will not be able to fully abduct or to internally or externally rotate the arm normally.

❒❒ What is the usual mechanism of injury in a supracondylar fracture?

A fall on the outstretched arm.

❒❒ What artery is commonly injured with a supracondylar fracture?

Brachial artery.

❒❒ What nerve is commonly injured with a supracondylar fracture?

Injury to the anterior interosseous nerve, which is a branch of the median nerve.

❒❒ Elbow X-ray. Posterior fat pad sign! Diagnosis?

Occult fracture such as a supracondylar fracture of the humerus. Posterior fat pad seen on a lateral radiograph of the flexed elbow is usually due to hemarthrosis caused by a fracture.

❒❒ What nerve injury is associated with a medial epicondyle fracture?

Ulnar nerve.

❒❒ About how many liters of blood can a patient lose in the retroperitoneal space?

About 6 liters.

❒❒ Which type of pelvic fracture has the greatest amount of bleeding?

Vertical sheer.

❒❒ A patient presents to the emergency department with a history of a limp. Physical exam reveals pain with extension and abduction of the hip. Diagnosis?

Greater trochanteric fracture, the result of an avulsion at the insertion site of the gluteus medius.

❑❑ A patient presents with a history of hearing an audible pop in the knee and ankle as he fell. Diagnosis?

Tear of the anterior cruciate and Achilles tendon rupture.

❑❑ What nerve may be injured with a knee dislocation?

The peroneal nerve.

❑❑ What is the most common site of a stress fracture in the foot?

Second and third metatarsal.

❑❑ What is the most frequent cause of superior vena cava obstruction?

Bronchogenic carcinoma.

❑❑ What is the most common level of malignant spinal cord compression?

Thoracic.

❑❑ What is the most common site of bursitis?

Olecranon.

❑❑ What is the most common cause of subarachnoid hemorrhage in teenagers?

AV malformations.

❑❑ A patient presents with a painful, red eye and a decrease in visual acuity. What is the differential?

Central corneal lesions, glaucoma, and iritis.

❑❑ What is the most common symptom of acute mesenteric ischemia?

Abdominal pain.

❑❑ Where does pulmonary embolism rank in terms of lethality in the United States?

It is the third most common cause of death in the United States.
About 650,000 cases occur annually with overall mortality of 8%.

❑❑ What are the most common findings of osteomyelitis on x-ray?

Periosteal elevation and demineralization.

❑❑ For what conditions is hydralazine commonly used?

Treatment of preeclampsia and eclampsia.

❑❑ What is the most common cause of acute aortic regurgitation?

Infectious endocarditis.

❑❑ **What is the most common congenital valvular disease?**

Bicuspid aortic valve.

❑❑ **What infarct is most commonly associated with acute mitral regurgitation?**

Inferior wall.

❑❑ **What metabolic abnormality is commonly associated with hypercalcemia?**

Up to 1/3 will have hypokalemia.

❑❑ **What form of hepatitis is most commonly transmitted through blood transfusions?**

Hepatitis C.

❑❑ **On funduscopic exam, microaneurysms and soft exudates are typical of:**

Hypertension.

❑❑ **On funduscopic exam, macular microaneurysms and hard exudates are typical of:**

Diabetes.

❑❑ **In a patient with retrobulbar optic neuritis, what is the most likely cause?**

Multiple sclerosis.

❑❑ **How is pancuronium reversed?**

Atropine and neostigmine.

❑❑ **What paralyzing drug typically causes transient hyperkalemia?**

Succinylcholine.

❑❑ **What are the contraindications to succinylcholine use?**

Rhabdomyolysis, narrow angle glaucoma, neurologic disorders, renal failure, myopathies, muscle trauma and burns.

❑❑ **What are the initial symptoms of a patient with hypocalcemia?**

Paresthesias around the mouth and fingertips, irritability, hyperactive deep tendon reflexes and seizures.

❑❑ **What ECG change is associated with hypocalcemia?**

Prolonged T waves.

❑❑ **A patient is digitalis toxic. What electrolytes will need to be replaced?**

It is important to replace potassium and magnesium.

❑❑ **What EKG changes are expected in hypokalemia?**

Low voltage QRS.
Flattening of T waves.
Depressed ST segment.

Prominent P and U waves.
Prolonged QT and PR intervals

❑❑ **What ECG changes may be seen in hyperkalemia?**

Tall or peaked T waves.
Prolonged QT and PR intervals.
Diminished P wave amplitude.
Depressed ST segments.
QRS widening.

❑❑ **What ECG findings are anticipated with hypercalcemia?**

Depressed ST segments.
Widened T waves.
Decreased QT intervals.
Bradycardia.
BBBs leading to 2° and 3° heart blocks.

❑❑ **What ECG findings suggest hypomagnesemia?**

Prolonged QT and PR intervals.
Widened QRS.
Depressed ST segments.
Inverted T waves.

❑❑ **What is the most common complication of verapamil and how should it be treated?**

Hypotension, treated with calcium gluconate IV over several minutes.

❑❑ **Third degree heart block is often seen in what type of myocardial infarction?**

Acute anterior wall myocardial infarction.

❑❑ **What is the most common arrhythmia associated with Wolff-Parkinson-White syndrome?**

PAT. The patient presents with angina, syncope, and shortness of breath.

❑❑ **How may mydriasis caused by mydriatics and anticholinergic drugs be distinguished from those caused by third cranial nerve compression?**

Pilocarpine. Pilocarpine will reverse cranial nerve compression but will have no effect on anticholinergic drugs or mydriatics.

❑❑ **During CPR, the mean cardiac index is what percentage of normal?**

25%.

❑❑ **Outline treatment of atrial flutter.**

Cardioversion 25 to 50 joules, verapamil, digoxin, propranolol, procainamide, and quinidine.

❑❑ **How should atrial fibrillation be treated?**

Procainamide, digoxin, verapamil, and propranolol.
Cardioversion with 100 to 200 joules.

❑❑ **Why is verapamil a bad choice to treat ventricular tachycardia?**

Verapamil could increase heart rate and decrease blood pressure, without converting the rhythm.

❑❑ **What drugs should never be used in atrial fibrillation with Wolff-Parkinson-White?**

Digitalis, verapamil, and phenytoin.
Atrial fibrillation with Wolff-Parkinson-White should be treated with cardioversion or procainamide.

SVT with Wolff-Parkinson-White should be treated with verapamil or adenosine.

❑❑ **What does VVI mean?**

Ventricular pace, ventricular sense, and inhibited.

❑❑ **What complications can result from excessive lidocaine administration?**

Seizures and methemoglobinemia.

❑❑ **Name the drug of choice for Wolff-Parkinson-White with atrial flutter or fibrillation?**

Procainamide.

❑❑ **What makes the first heart sound?**

Closure of the mitral valve and left ventricular contraction.

❑❑ **What makes the second heart sound?**

Closure of the pulmonary and aortic valves.

❑❑ **What is the cause of the third heart sound.**

This is caused by the deceleration of blood flowing into the ventricle when the ventricle reaches its final stages of filling.

❑❑ **What is the cause of the fourth heart sound?**

It is caused by vibrations of the left ventricular muscle, the mitral valve and the left ventricular flow tract.

❑❑ **What is a common pathologic cause of an S3?**

Congestive heart failure.

❑❑ **What is the pathologic cause of an S4?**

Often decreased left ventricular compliance due to acute ischemia. Relevant circumstances include: aortic stenosis, subaortic stenosis, HTN, coronary artery disease, myocardiopathy, anemia and hyperthyroidism.

❑❑ **What is the chief effect of dopamine and what is the chief complication of dopamine?**

The chief effect is prompt elevation of blood pressure with ß-adrenergic effects at low doses and α–adrenergic effects at high doses. The primary complication is tachycardia which unfortunately, increases myocardial oxygen demand.

❑❑ **What is the chief effect of dobutamine?**

Dobutamine increases the cardiac contractility. It has only minor effects on peripheral α–receptors. It can increase cardiac output without increasing blood pressure.

❒❒ What effect does morphine have on preload and afterload?

Morphine decreases both preload and afterload.

❒❒ Does furosemide affect preload or afterload?

Furosemide decreases preload.

❒❒ What is the most common cause of post splenectomy sepsis?

Streptococcus pneumoniae.

❒❒ What laboratory findings are expected in a child with pyloric stenosis?

Hypokalemia, hypochloremia, and metabolic alkalosis.

❒❒ What is the most common cause of tricuspid regurgitation?

Right heart failure secondary to left heart failure, typically caused by mitral stenosis.

❒❒ What drug is preferred to treat hypertension in a patient with renal failure?

Labetalol (metabolized in the liver).

❒❒ Treatment for a propranolol overdose?

Glucagon.

❒❒ Preferred treatment for a patient with hypertensive encephalopathy?

Nitroprusside and labetalol.

❒❒ What are the x-ray findings in ischemic bowel disease?

"Thumb" printing on the plain film and a ground glass appearance with absence of bowel gas.

❒❒ A patient with currant jelly sputum is likely to have what type of pneumonia?

Klebsiella or type 3 *Pneumococcus*.

❒❒ What two diseases does the deer tick, Ixodes dammini**, transmit?**

Lyme disease and *Babesiosis*.

❒❒ How do patients present with Babesia infection?

Intermittent fever, splenomegaly, jaundice, and hemolysis. The disease may be fatal in patients without spleens. The disease can simulate rickettsial diseases like Rocky Mountain spotted fever. Treatment is with clindamycin and quinine.

❒❒ Time for a food question! There are 9 questions in this book that deal with either strawberry tongue, strawberry cervix, currant jelly sputum or currant jelly stool. Describe the pathology associated with each of these.

Strawberry tongue - Scarlet fever, Kawasaki's disease.
Strawberry cervix - Trichomonas.
Currant jelly sputum - *Klebsiella*, less commonly type 3 *Pneumococcus*.
Currant jelly stool - Intussusception.

❒❒ **What is the most frequently transmitted tick-borne disease?**

Lyme disease. Causative agent - spirochete *Borrelia burgdorferi.* Vector - *Ixodes dammini* (deer tick) also *I. pacificus*, *Amblyomma americanum,* and *Dermacentor variabilis.*

❒❒ **What is the second most common tick borne disease?**

Rocky Mountain spotted fever. Causative agent - *Rickettsia rickettsii.* Vector - Female Ixodid ticks *Dermacentor andersoni* (wood tick) and *D. variabilis* (American dog tick).

❒❒ **If you melt enough dry ice, can you swim without getting wet?**

Probably not!

❒❒ **What is a direct interview?**

An important source of information about a subject is the direct interview, which is a person-to-person interaction.

❒❒ **What are indirect surveys?**

Indirect surveys, are structured self-report forms that may be used for gathering research data. However, they lack the clinical judgment of an experienced practitioner that is necessary in some instances.

❒❒ **What is reliability?**

Reliability refers to whether or not the findings of the assessment instrument or diagnostic procedure are reproducible.

❒❒ **What is inter-rater reliability?**

Inter-rater reliability means the results of the survey can be replicated when the instrument is used by different examiners. It is measured using the kappa value.

❒❒ **What is test-retest reliability?**

Test-retest reliability means the results of the survey can be replicated when the instrument is used on different occasions.

❒❒ **What is validity?**

Validity refers to whether the test measures what it is supposed to measure.

❒❒ **What are sub-categories of validity?**

Criterion, face, content, and concurrent.

❒❒ **What is bias?**

Analytic studies can be flawed by bias, an error in construction that favors one outcome over another.

❒❒ **What does the double-blind method help with?**

The double-blind method helps to eliminate bias.

❑❑ What is randomization?

Randomization of a sample is a method in which each member of the total group studied has an equal chance of being selected. It also helps eliminate bias.

❑❑ What is sensitivity?

Sensitivity is the ability of an assessment instrument to detect the thing being evaluated.

❑❑ What is specificity?

Specificity refers to the ability of an assessment instrument to assess only the variable chosen for study.

❑❑ What is predictive value?

Assessment instruments should also have a good predictive value, which is the proportion of true-positive to true-negative results.

❑❑ What is analysis of variance (ANOVA)?

ANOVA is a set of statistical procedures designed to compare two or more groups of observations and determines whether the differences between groups are due to experimental influence or chance alone.

❑❑ What is factor analysis?

Factor analysis is a data reduction technique used to reduce a large number of variables to a smaller number of linear combinations of variables.

❑❑ What is multivariate analysis?

Multivariate analysis is a method for considering the relationship of three or more variables.

❑❑ What is a coefficient of correlation?

A coefficient of correlation shows the relationship between two sets of paired measurements, with a maximum value of 1 and a minimum value of 0 (indicating that no relationship exists between two variables).

❑❑ What is a Chi-square?

A Chi-square is a non-parametric statistic used to evaluate the relative frequency or proportion of events in a population that falls into well-defined categories.

❑❑ Name four multivariate methods.

Multiple regression, discriminant analysis, canonical correlation, and factor analysis are multivariate methods.

❑❑ What is the Null hypothesis?

The Null hypothesis is the assumption that there is no significant difference between two random samples of a population. When it is rejected, observed differences between groups are deemed to be improbable by chance alone.

❑❑ What does the "P value" mean?

A "P value" of 0.05 means that the result will occur more than 5 times out of every 100 times by chance alone.

❑❑ **What is a T-test?**

A statistical procedure designed to compare two sets of observations is the T-test.

❑❑ **What is a type-I error?**

The false claim of a true difference because the observed difference is due entirely to chance is a Type I error.

❑❑ **What is a type-II error?**

The false acceptance of the null hypothesis when, in fact, there is a true difference but the difference is so small that it falls within the acceptance region of the null hypothesis is a Type II error.

❑❑ **What are independent variables?**

Independent variables are those qualities that the experimenter systematically varies (for example, time, age, sex, type of drug).

❑❑ **What are Dependent variables?**

Dependent variables are those qualities that measure the influence of the independent variable or the outcome of the experiment (for example, the measurement of a person's specific physiological reactions to a drug).

❑❑ **What is the sensitivity of a test?**

Sensitivity is the proportion of patients with the condition in question that the test is able to detect.

❑❑ **What is the specificity of a test?**

Specificity is the proportion of patients who do not have the condition that the test calls negative.

❑❑ **What is the sensitivity in the following test?**

	Disease	No Disease
Test +	90	20
Test -	10	80
Totals	100	100

Sensitivity = $\frac{\text{True Positive}}{\text{True Positive + False Negative}}$

In the table shown in the question, it is clear that **90** people who were tested have the disease, which means they are **True Positive**. **Twenty** people tested positive but have no disease so they are **False Positive**. **Eighty** people tested negative and have no disease so they are **True Negative**. **Ten** people have the disease but tested negative (hence, they are **False Negative**). Know the formulas and fill in the numbers to get correct answers in % values.

❑❑ **What is the specificity in above test?**

Specificity = $\frac{\text{True Negative}}{\text{True Negative + False Positive}}$

❑❑ **What is the positive predictive value in above test?**

Positive Predictive Value = $\dfrac{\text{True Positive}}{\text{True Positive + False Positive}}$

❑❑ **What is the negative predictive value in above test?**

Negative Predictive Value = $\dfrac{\text{True Negative}}{\text{True Negative + False Negative}}$

❑❑ **A medical student had the following scores in the simulated examination he tried at home: 11, 9, 7, 6, 6, 4, and 6. What is the mode in this case?**

The mode is the number 6. The most important precaution is to ARRANGE the given numbers in an ascending pattern; otherwise answers will be wrong. Once arranged; find the middle number; and that is the median. Since there is a total of 7 numbers; the middle number is 6 in the series 4, 6, 6, 6, 7, 9, 11. Had there been 8 numbers (4, 6, 6, 6, 7, 8, 9, 11) we would have had to take average of the two middle numbers (6, 7) to get the median, which would then be 6.5. The mode is the number which occurs MOST frequently. (Remember Mode and Most start with MO) and the number 6 is the number occurring most frequently in the above series.

❑❑ **What is the median in the above case?**

Six.

❑❑ **The average duration of dementia is 4.5 years and its incidence is 3 per 1,000 each year. What is the prevalence of dementia?**

Prevalence = incidence X duration of a disease

Since incidence = 3 and duration of dementia = 4.5 years (in the given population), prevalence can be calculated by multiplying 4.5 by 3. The answer is 13.5.

❑❑ **What is the definition of the standard deviation?**

The standard deviation is the square root of the variance, which gives an estimate of the average deviation from the mean.

BIBLIOGRAPHY

BOOKS:

Adler, J.N., Plantz, S.H. & Collman, D.D. Emergency Medicine Pearls of Wisdom (4th. Ed.). 1997.

Adler, J.N., Brenner, B., Dronen, S., Feied, C., Mallon, W.K., O'Conner, R.E., Plantz, S.H., Pollack, C.V., Roberge, R.J. eMedicine: Emergency Medicine. St. Petersburg: eMedicine, 1999.

Advanced Cardiac Life Support. Dallas: American Heart Association, 1992.

Advanced Trauma Life Support. Chicago: American College of Surgeons, 1995.

Anderson, J.E. Grant's Atlas of Anatomy (8th Ed.). Baltimore: Williams & Wilkins, 1983.

Auerbach, P.S. Management of Wilderness and Environmental Emergencies 3rd Ed.). St. Louis: C.V. Mosby Company, 1995.

Berkow, R. The Merck Manual (17th Ed.). Rahway: Merck Sharp & Dohme Research Laboratories, 1999.

Bryson, P.D. Comprehensive Review in Toxicology for Emergency Clinicians (3rd Ed.) Aspen Publishers, Inc., 1996

Dambro, M.R. Griffith's 5 Minute Clinical Consult. Williams and Wilkins, 1999.

DeGowin, E.L. Bedside Diagnostic Examination (6th Ed.). New York: Macmillan Publishing Co. Inc., 1994.

Edwards, L., Dermatology in Emergency Care, Churchill Livingstone, 1997.

Fitzpatrick, T.B. Color Atlas and Synopsis of Clinical Dermatology (3rd Ed.). New York: McGraw-Hill Publishing Company, 1996.

Harris, J.H. The Radiology of Emergency Medicine (3rd Ed.). Baltimore: Williams and Wilkins, 1993.

Harrison, T.R. Principles of Internal Medicine (14th Ed.). New York: McGraw-Hill Book Company, 1997.

Harwood-Nuss, A. The Clinical Practice of Emergency Medicine. Philadelphia: J.B. Lippincott Company, 1996.

Lester, B.: The Acute Hand, Appleton & Long, 1998.

Marriott, H.J.L. Practical Electrocardiography (9th Ed.). Baltimore: Williams and Wilkins, 1994.

Moore, K.L. Clinically Oriented Anatomy. Baltimore: Williams & Wilkins, 1999.

Physicians' Desk Reference (53rd Ed.). Oradell: Medical Economics Company Inc., 1999.

Plantz, SH. Emergency Medicine PreTest, Self-Assessment and Review, McGraw- Hill, 1990.

Robbins, S.L. Pathologic Basis of Disease (6th Ed.). Philadelphia: W.B. Saunders Company, 1998.

Rosen, P. Emergency Medicine Concepts and Clinical Practice (4th Ed.). St. Louis: Mosby Year Book, 1997.

Rowe, R.C. The Harriet Lane Handbook (15th Ed.). Chicago: Year Book Medical Publishers, Inc., 1999.

Rudolph, A.M., Fondamentals of Pediatrics (2nd Ed.), 1998
Simon, R.R. Emergency Orthopedics The Extremities 3rd Ed.). Norwalk: Appleton & Lange, 1995.

The Hand Examination and Diagnosis (2nd Ed.). London: Churchill Livingstone, 1983.

The Hand Primary Care of Common Problems (2nd Ed.). London: Churchill Livingstone, 1990.

Tintinalli, J.E. Emergency Medicine A Comprehensive Study Guide (4th Ed.). New York: McGraw-Hill, Inc., 1995.

Weinberg, S. Color Atlas of Pediatric Dermatology (2nd Ed.). New York: McGraw-Hill, 1990.

Weiner, H.L. Neurology for the House Officer (4th Ed.). Baltimore: Williams & Wilkins, 1989.

Wilkins, E. W. Emergency Medicine (3rd Ed.). Baltimore: Williams & Wilkins, 1989.

APPENDIX

ECG 1

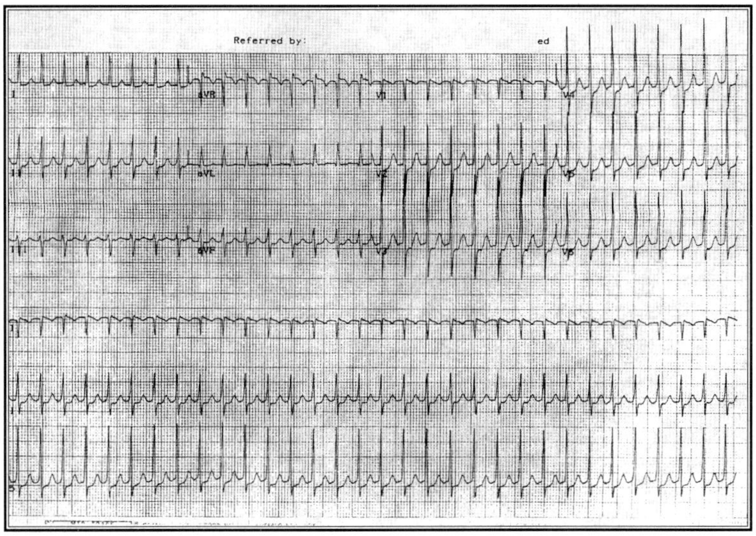

This tracing demonstrates a supraventricular tachycardia. It also displays a very tall R wave in the precordial V leads, in particular in lead V_2. This is consistent with a posterior wall myocardial infarction. Mild ST depression in leads V_2 and V_3 are the equivalent of ST elevation in AMI (ST elevation might be seen if the leads had been placed on the posterior thorax). The ST segment elevates in posterior wall infarction in V_2 because the posterior wall of the LV has infarcted (its "dead") and there is now unmasking of the normal anterior forces (of the anterior left ventricular wall) which have vectors directed primarily at V_2. These vectors produce the tall R wave in lead V_2. Subendocardial infarction can also cause ST segment depression in the precordial leads.

ECG 2 (3 simultaneous rhythm tracings)

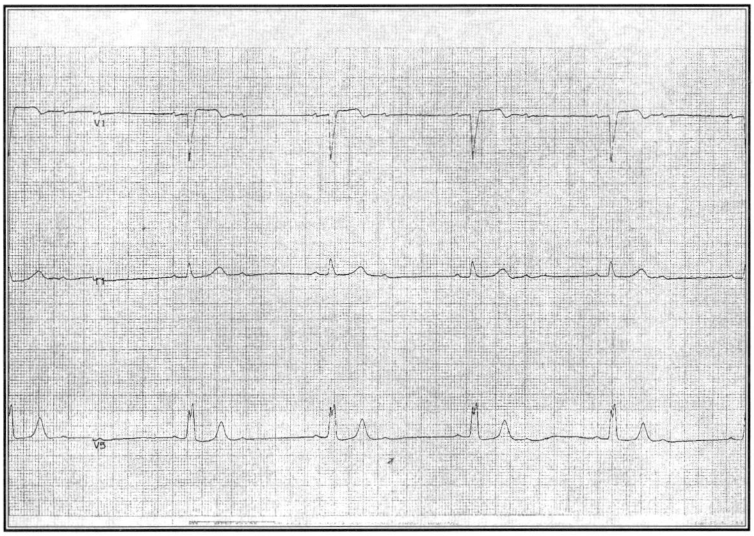

This tracing demonstrates three leads (V_1, II, V_5) recorded simultaneously. Both P waves and QRS complexes are seen. The P waves are not "related" to the QRS complexes (some are appearing after the QRS and several do not have a QRS complex which immediately follow the P wave). The QRS rate is very slow. Thus, the PR interval would be interpreted as variable. The QRS complexes are moderately widened. This patient is experiencing complete heart block with atrioventricular dissociation. The ventricles and atria are depolarizing in an independent fashion. This is an indication for immediate placement of a transcutaneous pacing device or transvenous pacemaker. This disturbance is associated with ischemia to the infranodal conduction pathways during an acute myocardial infarction. It may have been preceded by a Mobitz II AV block which has now progressed to complete heart block.

ECG 3a

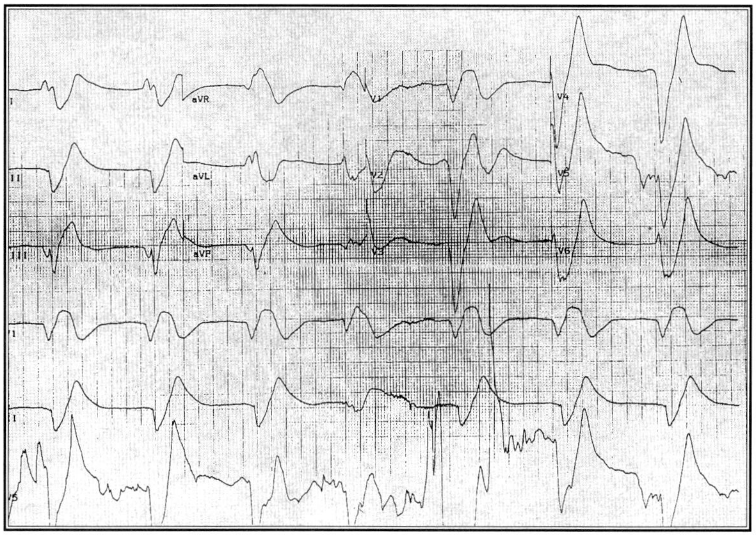

This tracing was recorded 19 minutes prior to ECG 3b from the same patient (see below). The first tracing demonstrates a very wide QRS complex in all leads depolarizing at a slow rate. The P waves are not visible and the T waves are tall. At very high serum potassium levels, e.g., above 7 mEq/L, impulses may still be conducted from the SA node to the ventricles. However conduction may be very impaired through the AV node and eventually result in an idioventricular rhythm. The tracing below was recorded after initial treatment for the hyperkalemia.

ECG 3b

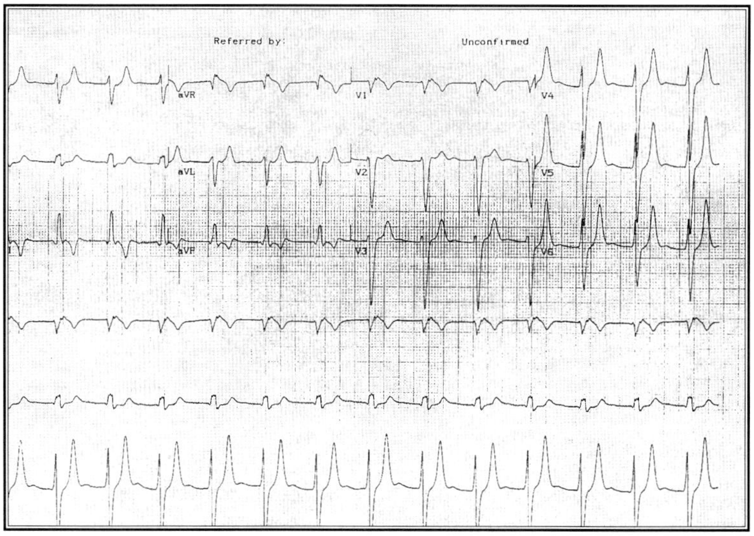

This tracing was recorded 19 minutes after ECG 3 from the same patient. It demonstrates loss of the P waves, some widening of the QRS complexes, sagging ST segments and narrow ("pinched waist"), peaked T waves. These findings are the primary electrocardiographic findings of hyperkalemia. Acute treatment might include various agents including parenteral calcium chloride (*or* gluconate), sodium bicarbonate, insulin and glucose (coadministered), ß-agonist inhalation, a loop diuretic (furosemide), and dialysis (hemodialysis or peritoneal dialysis). The cause of the hyperkalemia, e.g., postobstructive uropathy or digitalis toxicity, should be sought and corrected immediately. Oliguric renal failure is the most common cause of dangerous hyperkalemia. This tracing demonstrates the classic findings of hyperkalemia after improvement occurred from acute therapy for very severe hyperkalemia (ECG 3a).

ECG 4 (Rhythm strip)

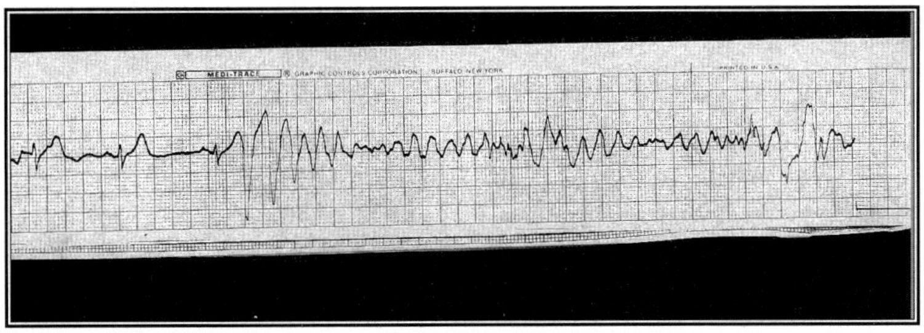

This tracing is a single lead (unspecified) rhythm tracing. It demonstrates three sinus beats with ST elevation followed by a wide complex tachyarrhythmia which has a gradually changing (rotating) QRS axis. This is consistent with Torsades de Pointes ("a twisting of the points"), a specfic type of atypical ventricular tachycardia which involves a single focus. It is associated with conditions that prolong the QT interval and results from a triggered arrhythmic mechanism after a period of prolonged, uneven ventricular repolarization. There are both acquired (administration of type Ia antiarrhythmic drugs [procainamide, disopyramide, quinidine], cyclic antidepressants, phenothiazines, electrolyte disturbances, hypothermia) and congenital (Jervell-Lange-Nielson syndrome, Romano-Ward syndrome) forms. Electrolyte disturbances especially hypomagnesemia, hypokalemia, and hypocalcemia should be considered and corrected. This rhythm may be seen in patients with any serious myocardial disease. Treatment with lidocaine is usually ineffective. Acceleration of the heart rate to shorten the QT interval using a pacemaker is the safest and most effective treatment. Intravenous bolus and infusion of magnesium sulfate is useful (especially with drug-induced torsades), but may be associated with recurrences during the infusion.

ECG 5

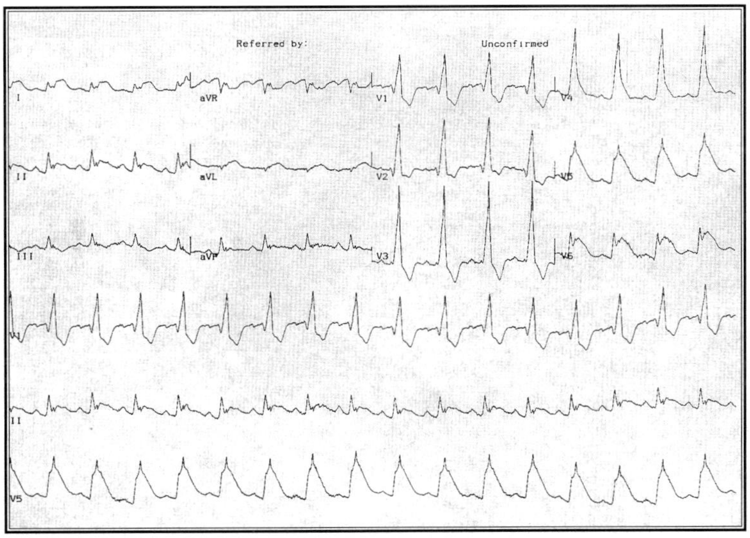

This tracing reveals a sinus rhythm with a wide complex QRS (180 msec) at approximately 100 beats per minute. The wide (and tall) QRS complexes in the right precordial leads may be consistent with right ventricular hypertrophy. The inferior lead (II, III, aVF) ST elevation, and lateral lead ST elevation (V_5, V_6, I, aVL), are consistent with inferior and anterolateral injury or acute infarction. Although no clinical information has been provided, keep in mind that any grouping of ECG findings can occur in the setting of acute pulmonary embolism. Poor cardiac output can contribute to myocardial hypoperfusion (with resulting left ventricular ischemia or injury) in the setting of right ventricular strain due to an obstructed pulmonary artery outflow tract.

ECG 6

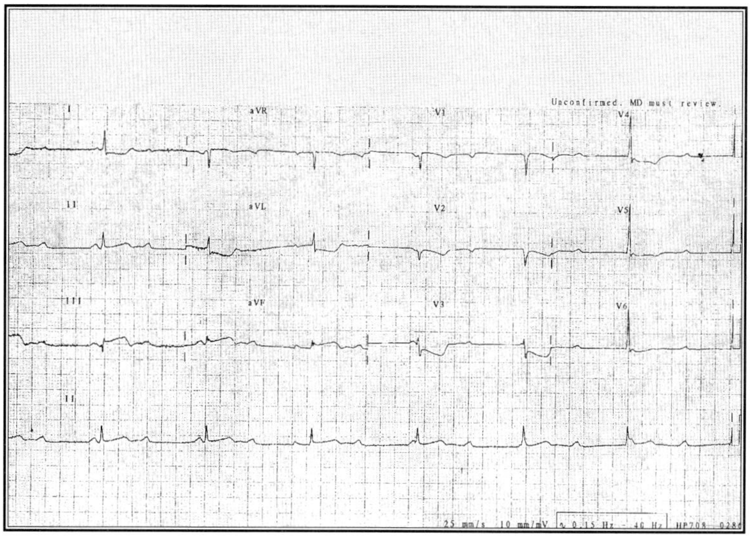

This tracing reveals a bradycardia at 42 beats per minute with both P waves and narrow QRS complexes visible. In the lead II rhythm strip the P waves are independent of the QRS complexes. This is most consistent with AV dissociation with an infranodal (His-Purkinje) pacemaker initiating ventricular depolarization (conduction is blocked through the AV node). Ventricular pacemaker sites always result in a wide QRS complex, so the pacemaker origin is eminating from a site higher in the conduction system in this patient. The inferior leads demonstrate ST elevation (reciprocal changes are seen in the anterolateral V leads); this is most consistent with inferior wall injury in the setting of acute myocardial infarction. Conduction through the AV node is impaired when the node is ischemic (as in the setting of inferior wall MI). The conduction block is usually transient in this situation and will spontaneously resolve or respond to atropine or pacing.

ECG 7

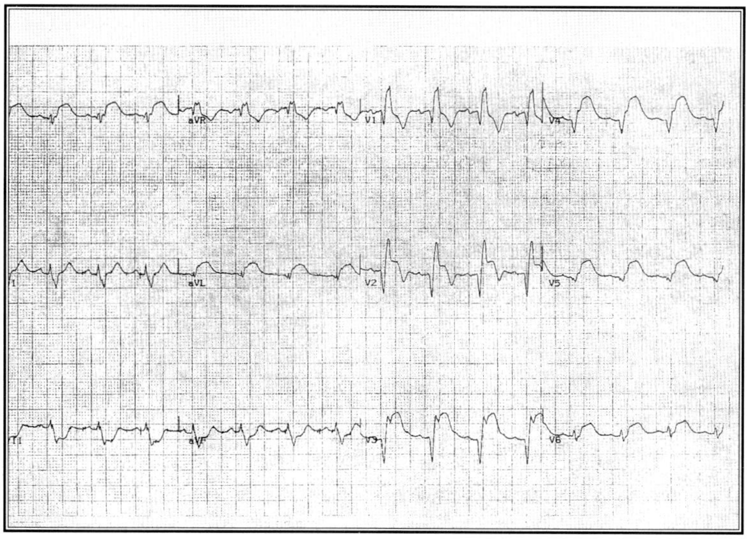

This tracing reveals a sinus rhythm at 91 beats per minute with normal P waves (look at lead II) and wide QRS complexes visible (QRS duration is 152 msec). The anterolateral V leads and leads I and aVL (lateral leads) demonstrate ST elevation consistent with acute anterolateral injury (infarction). Reciprocal ST-T wave changes (depressions) are seen in the inferior leads (II, III, aVF).

ECG 8

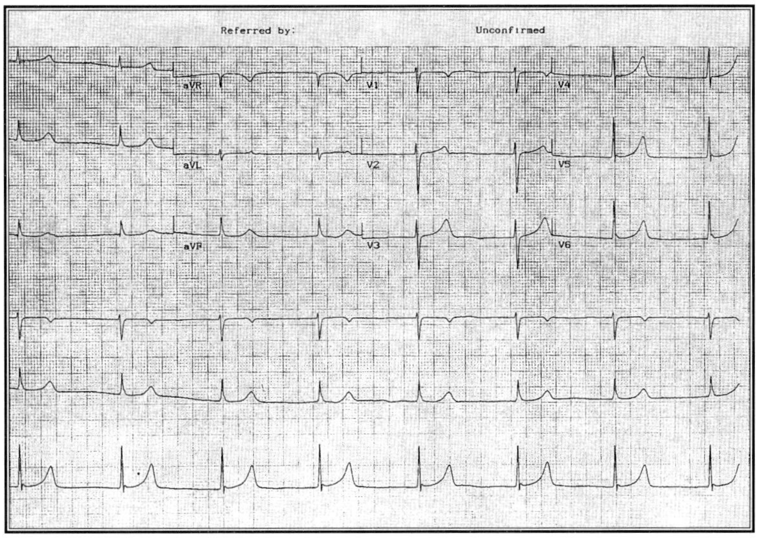

This tracing reveals a bradycardia at 45 beats per minute. An absence of P waves in the setting of a narrow QRS bradycardia is most consistent with a junctional rhythm. A junctional impulse is considered one that arises from the AV node or bundle of His proximal to the bifurcation of the main bundle branches. Atrial activation may not be seen if retrograde conduction is blocked or if atrial depolarization is occuring simultaneously with ventricular depolarization (P waves are obscured by the QRS complexes). AV junctional beats usually pace the ventricles at a rate of 40-60 beats per minute depending on the level of the pacemaker site. Junctional rhythms occur whenever there is a long enough delay in the impulses reaching the AV junction. This is seen in many conditions including congestive heart failure, hypokalemia, or digitalis toxicity. Myocarditis may also present with this rhythm disturbance. The primary treatment is to treat the underlying condition.

ECG 9

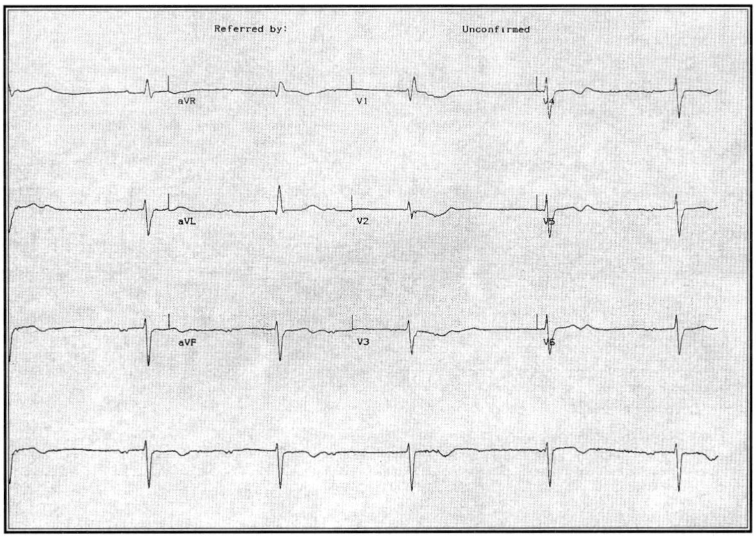

This tracing from a 78-year-old patient reveals a sinus rhythm with a prolonged PR interval of more than .2 msec (1° AV block), an rSR' configuration of lead V_1 (consistent with a right bundle branch block), and left axis deviation more negative than minus 45° (consistent with a left anterior superior fasicle block, i.e., the R wave in lead I is greater than the R waves in leads II and III, a qR wave is seen in lead aVL and deep S waves are seen in leads II, III and aVF). The primary concern in the setting of a "trifasicular block" is the sudden development of complete heart block; most patients with this type of tracing have advanced organic heart disease. However, placement of a ventricular (demand) pacemaker is indicated only when symptoms are due to documented bradyarrhythmias. Most patients still have a relatively low risk of sudden death from ventricular asystole in this setting.

ECG 10a

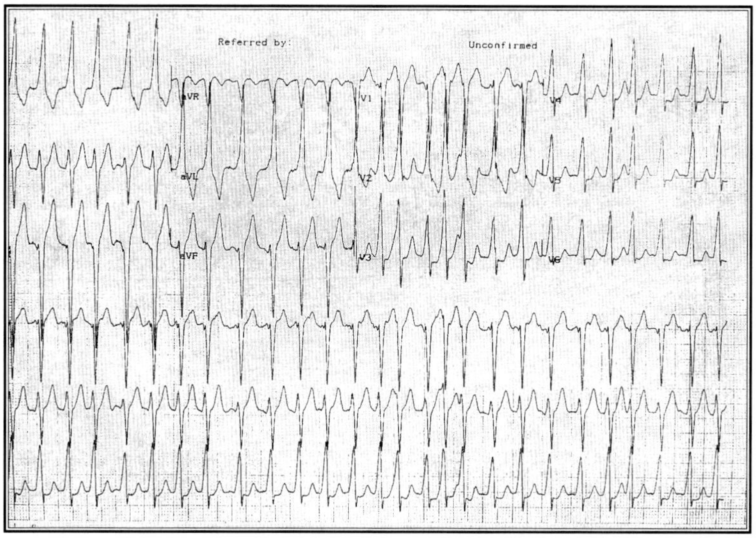

This tracing reveals a wide QRS complex tachyarrhythmia at approximately 163 beats per minute. Some irregularity of the rhythm is noted. Because it is irregular, one should suspect a supraventricular arrhythmia with abberant conduction. Ventricular tachycardia is always considered initially as the most important diagnosis (in the setting of a rapid wide complex), but the irregularity in this case is a clue in favor of SVT with aberrancy. However, note that P waves are not apparent. The same patient had a repeat ECG after an intervention (ECG 10b-see below) during the same visit to the emergency department. It reveals the underlying condition!

ECG 10b

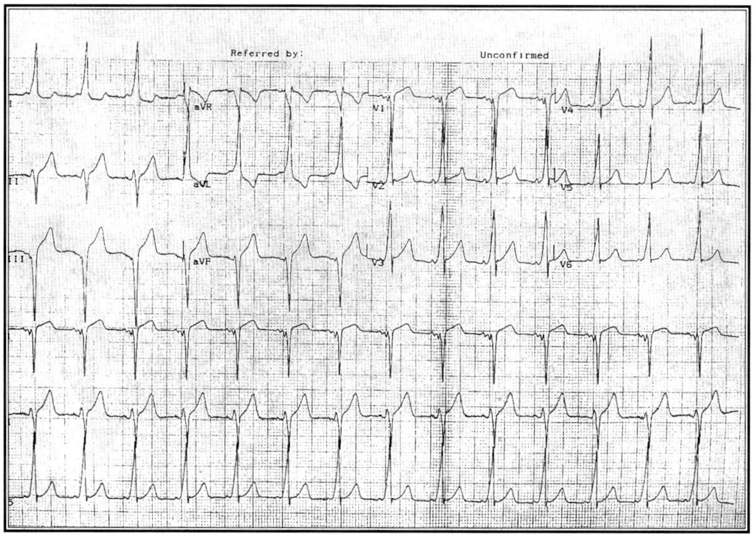

This tracing reveals a sinus rhythm with a short PR interval and a delta wave (slurred upstroke of the QRS complex-look at leads I, V_4, V_5, V_6). These findings are consistent with a particular type of preexcitation syndrome, i.e., Wolff-Parkinson-White (WPW) syndrome. In this case it is WPW type B (there are three subtypes, i.e., A, B, and C, based on the anatomic location of the bypass tract). The short PR is due to a bypass tract originating in the atrium and inserting into the ventricular muscle (conduction through these fibers bypasses the normal His-Purkinje network). The bypass tract allows for rapid conduction which is more rapid than the conduction through the normal AV node (the AV node is responsible for the normal length of the PR interval—its relatively slower conduction allows time for ventricular filling). Now that the patient who was previously in a circus movement, wide-complex tachyarrhythmia (ECG 10a), has been converted to sinus rhythm, the classic findings for Wolff-Parkinson-White syndrome are apparent.

ECG 11

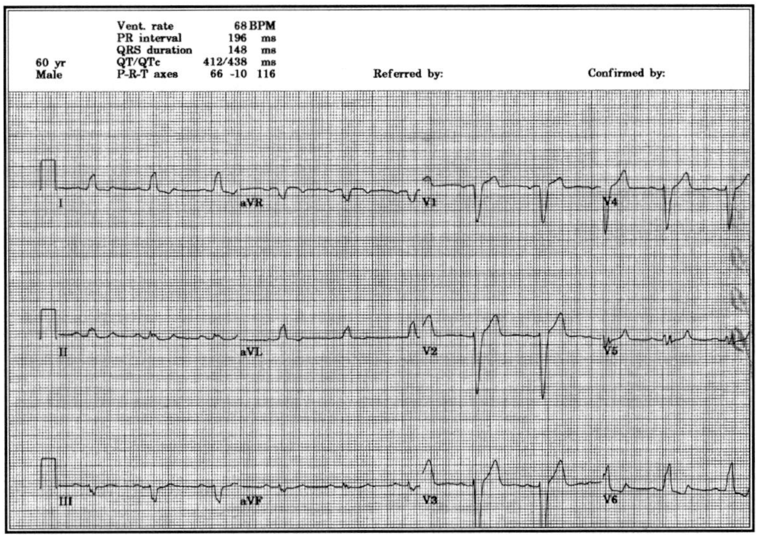

This tracing of a 60 year-old male demonstrates a sinus rhythm with a left bundle branch block pattern (LBBB). This patient was complaining of substernal chest pressure and was diaphoretic. The ECG criteria for LBBB include a QRS duration of more than 0.12 s plus large and broad R waves in leads I, aVL, V5, and V6, as well as a small r wave and an associated deep S wave in the inferior leads and in leads V1-V3. In LBBB the normal septal q wave is not seen in leads I, V5-V6 as well as in lead aVF. A new LBBB pattern in the clinical setting of an acute myocardial infarction can be an indication for thrombolysis even if the patient's ECG does not display the standard criteria for thrombolysis, i.e., new ST segment elevations in at least two adjacent limb (≥ 1 mV) or precordial (≥ 2 mV) leads.

ECG 12

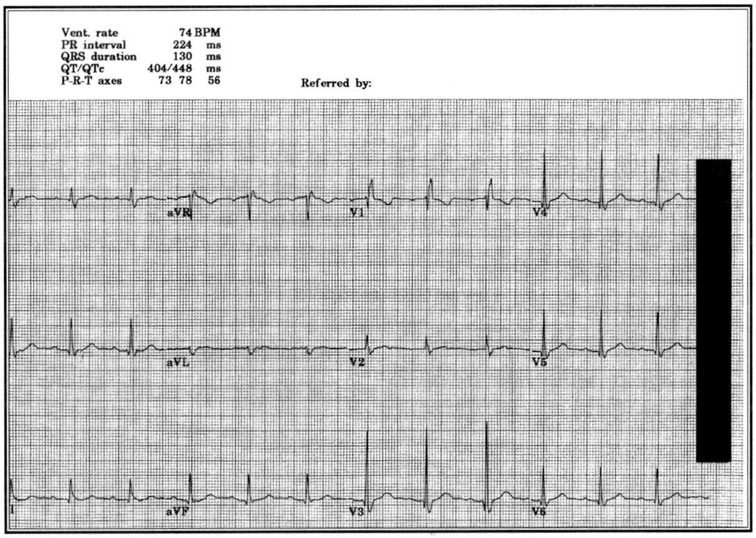

This tracing demonstrates a first degree AV block defined as a PR interval prolonged more than 0.20 s. It also displays a RBBB pattern (rSR' pattern in lead V1). Both P waves and QRS complexes are seen. Each P wave is related to the subsequent QRS complex. The QRS rate is normal. This patient is experiencing two blocks, one at the AV node (a slowing of conduction through the AV node which produces the PR interval lengthening, and one at the right main bundle branch. Neither conduction disturbance is an indication for immediate placement of a transcutaneous pacing device or transvenous pacemaker. A first-degree AV block does not usually require specific intervention and it is occasionally detected in a normal heart; it is also seen in association with increased vagal tone, digitalis toxicity and myocarditis. RBBB can be due to many causes including ischemia, myocarditis, cardiomyopathy, and degenerative change. Multiple conduction disturbances, as in this patient, can be associated with acute ischemia to portions of the conduction pathways during an AMI, e.g., acute inferior infarction. Again, they may also represent chronic changes; a prior ECG would be helpful to make this determination.

ECG 13

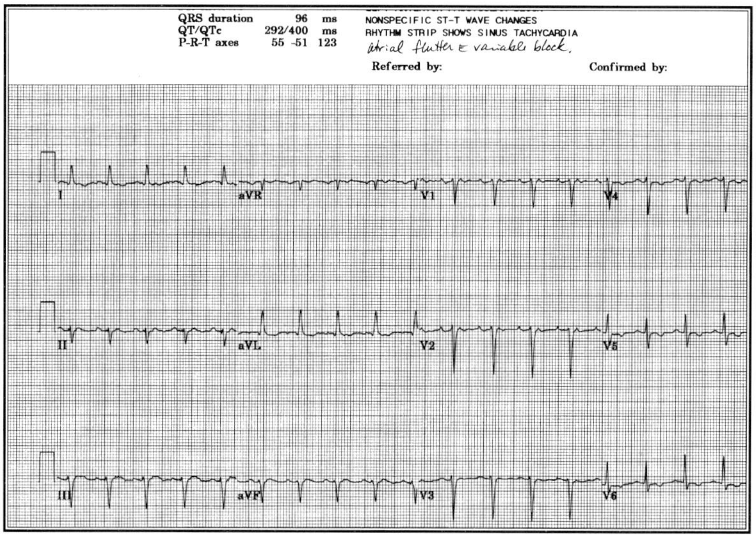

This tracing was demonstrates a pattern of P (flutter) waves with a slightly variable ventricular response of about 120 beats per minute (i.e., not an exact 2:1 block). The QRS complexes are slightly widened and there is left axis deviation. The latter two findings are the criteria for a left anterior fasicle block (LAFB). A helpful clue to diagnose atrial flutter is a ventricular rate of exactly 150 beats per minute on the tracing when there is a 2:1 conduction block. During a rapid supraventricular rhythm, such as atrial flutter, a conduction distubance in one fasicle may become apparent as in this case. The tracing also displays nonspecific ST-T wave changes. This latter finding and the conduction distubances are consistent with acute ischemia and/or a chronic underlying anatomic change, e.g., left atrial enlargement secondary to mitral stenosis or mitral regurgitation. Atrial flutter typically occurs only in patients with some form of heart disease. Conditions or circumstances that may be associated with the appearance of atrial flutter include hypertension, acute myocardial infarction, myocarditis or cardiomyopathy, thyroid disease, pulmonary embolism and the use of digitalis. Management of AF typically includes electrical or chemical cardioversion.

ECG 14

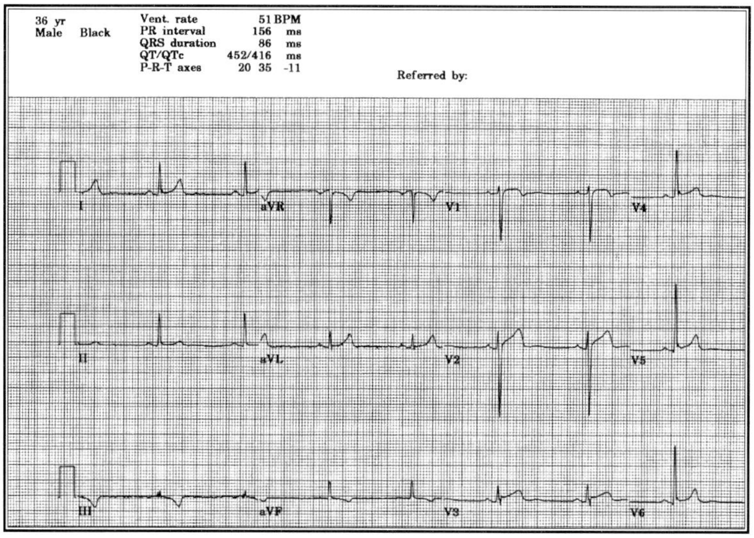

This tracing was recorded from a 36 year-old black, male patient who presented with nonspecific chest pain. It demonstrates a sinus bradycardia with multiple leads displaying ST elevation. The configuration of the ST elevation is most consistent with benign early repolarization (especially in leads I, II, aVL, V3-V6 in this patient). Two of the inferior leads, III and aVF, display T wave inversions; this finding could be consistent with acute ischemia. Diffuse T wave inversions can be associated with pericarditis after the ST segments have returned to the baseline (stage 4). Depression of the PR segment is also seen during acute pericarditis in the leads that display ST segment elevations. The T wave in lead II in this patient is flat and may invert on a subsequent tracing. Again, this could represent acute ischemia. The differential diagnosis for ST segment elevation includes benign early repolarization, acute current of injury (AMI), pericarditis, and ventricular aneurysm. An ST-to-T wave amplitude ratio (height at the onset of the ST segment compared to the peak of the T wave) of less than 25% is more consistent with benign early repolarization than with acute pericarditis. Clinical hallmarks of acute pericarditis include a friction rub and chest pain that improves when the patient sits up and leans forward.

ECG 15

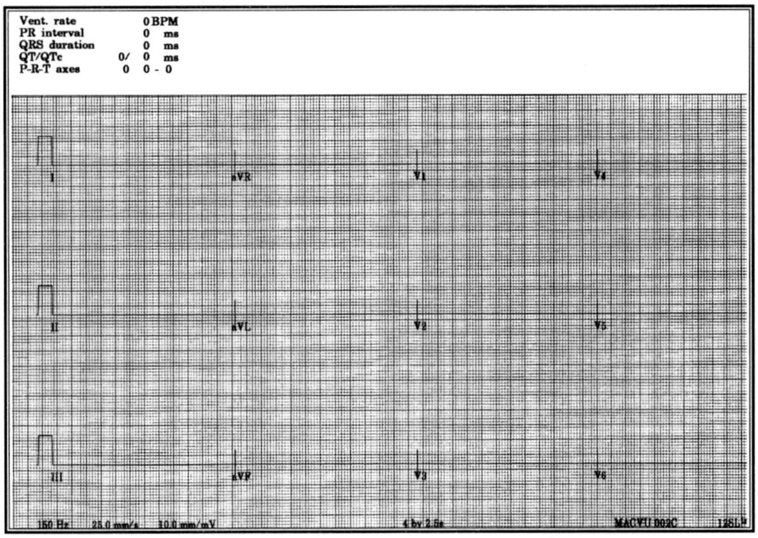

This tracing is from a victim of multiple stab wounds with penetrating thoracoabdominal injuries. The patient did not recover after aggressive attempts were made to rapidly diagnose and manage traumatic causes of cardiac asystole. The clinician should first look for the presence of tension pneumothorax (including bilateral tension pneumothorax), cardiac tamponade and profound hypovolemia. These are the most treatable injuries that will ultimately result in irreversible cardiac standstill if they are not rapidly identified and corrected. This patient had a brief period of electromechanical dissociation prior to the development of asystole. Alpha-adrenergic agents and ongoing cardiopulmonary resuscitation are used to initiate cardiac electrical activity in a patient with asystole secondary to a nontraumatic etiology. Although some form of ventricular pacing might also be attempted in that circumstance, it is generally not helpful if these measures are not effective in reestablishing effective cardiac contractions.

ECG 16

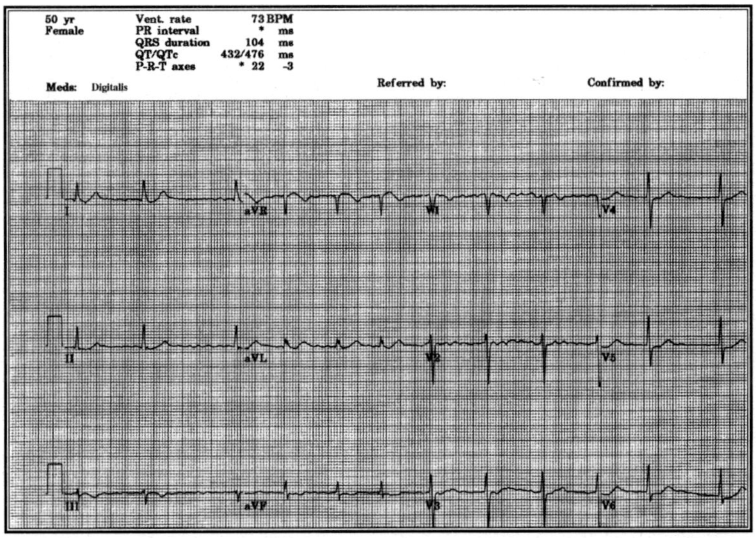

This tracing was obtained from a 50 year-old female complaining of severe abdominal pain that began suddenly two hours ago. She presented with mild hypotension and reported that she took digitalis on a chronic basis. Her abdominal examination was notable for mild diffuse direct tenderness and her stool was positive for occult blood. Abdominal films were nonspecific. This ECG tracing demonstrates atrial fibrillation with narrow QRS complexes and a relatively slow ventricular response at 73 beats per minute. The QT interval is prolonged. This presentation is most compatible with acute occlusive mesenteric ischemia, most likely from embolism of a cardiac mural thrombus to the superior mesenteric artery or one of its major tributaries. Acute myocardial infarction should be suspected when considering the etiology for a mural thrombus and/or the hypotension. Because of the history of digitalis use, she could also have nonocclusive mesenteric ischemia secondary to digitalis-induced mesenteric vasospasm. The correct diagnosis would be established by angiography. Other causes of mesenteric ischemia include a low-flow state (low cardiac output state), acute arterial thrombosis, and venous thrombosis secondary to a coagulopathy.

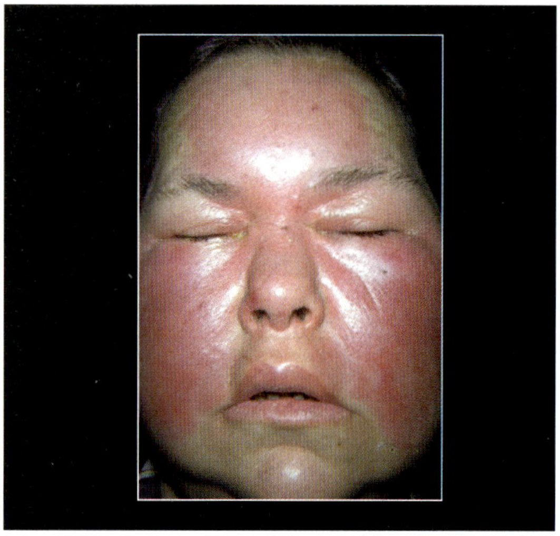

VISUAL PEARL

This adult female was toxic and febrile. She developed this facial rash with subsequent bulla formation, but rapidly improved with intravenous penicillin in twenty-four hours. What is your diagnosis? What is the causative organism? What antibiotic may be employed in a penicillin allergic patient?

ANSWER

The diagnosis is erysipelas–a superficial cellulitis with lymphatic involvement usually caused by group A *Streptococcus*. The physical findings are essentially diagnostic. The plaques are sharply demarcated, red, shiny, and painful. Local lymphadenopathy is common. Erysipelas is very sensitive to penicillin. A macrolide or a cephalosporin may be utilized in penicillin allergic patients.

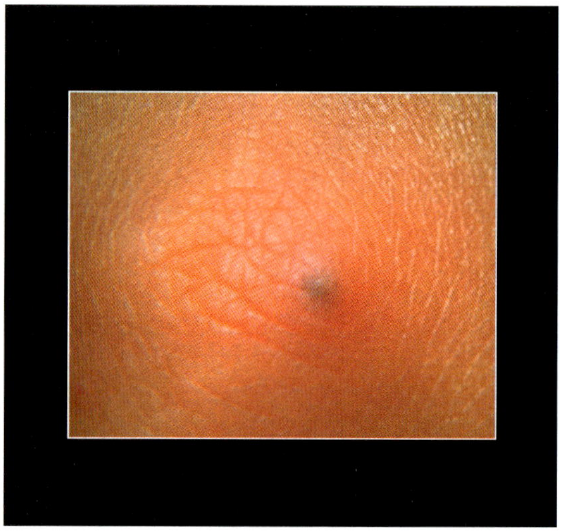

VISUAL PEARL

This teenage female patient presented with general malaise, arthralgias and a few of these sparsely distributed, tender lesions on her extremities. She denies any other symptoms. What is the most likely diagnosis?

ANSWER

The finding is a small pustule on an erythematous base. The primary clinical consideration is disseminated gonococcemia. The lesions in meningococcemia are generally larger and hemorrhagic. The diagnosis of disseminated gonococcemia is problematic because only 20 to 50% of skin lesion, blood, or joint cultures become positive. Pharyngeal, cervical, and rectal specimens are the most helpful in making a culture diagnosis.

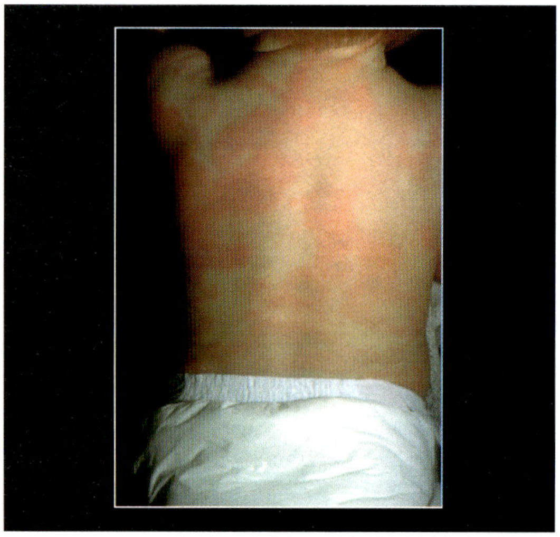

VISUAL PEARL

This toddler was brought to the emergency department with this rash. There was no history of a previous similar rash. The child is afebrile and feeding well. There is no other significant finding on physical examination. What is your diagnosis based on this clinical information?

ANSWER

Hives (urticaria). Hives are due to local capillary vasodilation and result in an erythematous or white nonpitting plaques. They may be confused with many conditions including erythema multiforme. Up to 20% of the general population will experience one episode. Both acute and chronic forms exist. Therapy includes eliminating potential causes, and treatment using one or several agents including antihistamines, steroids, and epinephrine in severe cases.

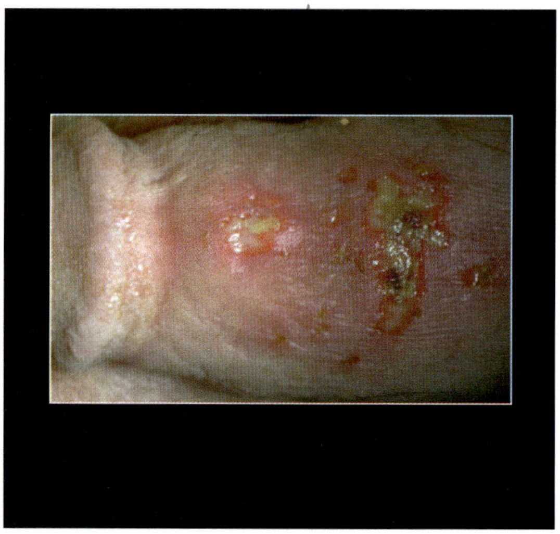

VISUAL PEARL

This adult male complained of painful blisters on his penis. Many of the blisters have coalesced and converted into ulcerations. The patient appeared mildly ill with inguinal discomfort, but no adenopathy. What is your diagnosis based on this appearance? What else should the physician consider when evaluating this patient?

ANSWER

Genital herpes (herpes simplex). This is a primary infection based on the patient's presentation. He denied any prior similar lesions. Orally administered acyclovir or other currently available antivirals are effective in treating primary genital herpes. Recurrences are usually less painful. Frequency of recurrence varies in different patients. Daily suppressive therapy is indicated in selected patients for up to one year. The patient should then be reassessed for additional recurrences. The physician should consider the possibility of another concomitant STD in this patient as well as the need for HIV testing.

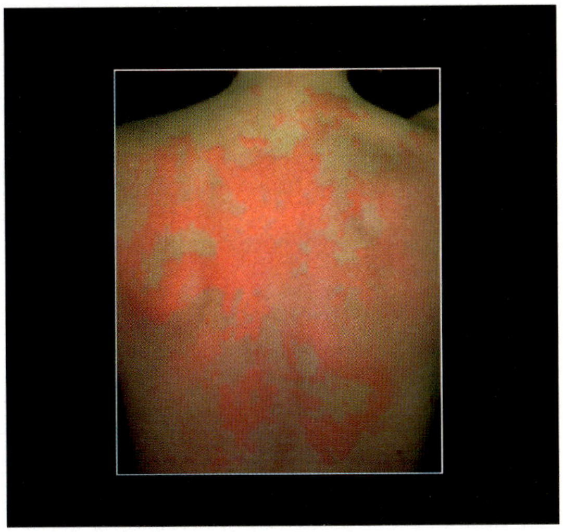

VISUAL PEARL

This 27-year-old female complained of repetitive episodes of swelling of her lips, abdominal pain and this very itchy rash. This is the appearance of the rash. What is your diagnosis based on this clinical information?

ANSWER

Angioedema is a well demarcated localized edema of the deeper skin layers and subcutaneous tissue. Classifications of urticaria with angioedema include IgE-dependent, complement mediated, nonimmunologic (mast cell-releasing agents: antibiotics, opiates, radiocontrast media), and idiopathic. Most chronic cases are idiopathic. Elimination of etiologic factor(s) is the best therapeutic approach. Topical steroids are of no benefit. H^1 antihistamines and sympathomimetics provide symptomatic relief. Hydroxyzine, and a combination of H^1 and H^2 antihistamines may be even more effective.

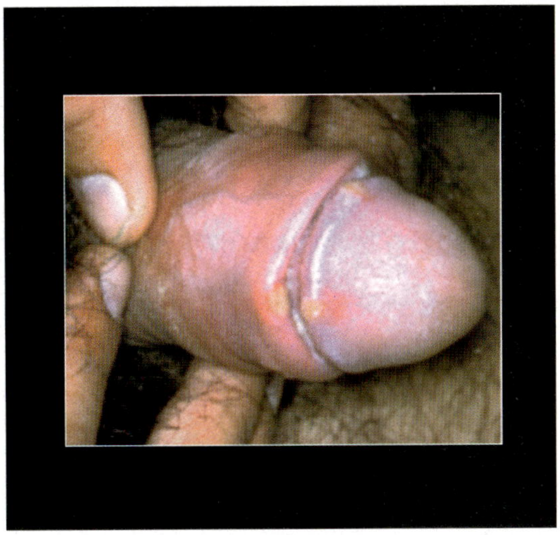

VISUAL PEARL

This male patient presented with a tender papule on his penis which ulcerated. Multiple lesions then developed; some of them coalesced. The patient complained of left inguinal pain, but had minimal constitutional symptoms and no skin rash. What is the most likely diagnosis and the treatment?

ANSWER

Chancroid is due to a pleomorphic gram-negative coccobacillus (*Haemophilus ducreyi*) that causes irregular-shaped, genital ulcers with red halo formation and lymphadenitis after the initial appearance of a painful, red papule. Ulcers are deeper than those in herpes and they spread laterally; autoinoculation produces multiple lesions. Painful inguinal adenopathy may be followed by bubo formation with spontaneous rupture. Diagnosis is made clinically, but syphilis should be considered. Azithromycin, ceftriaxone, or erythromycin base are all recommended treatments.

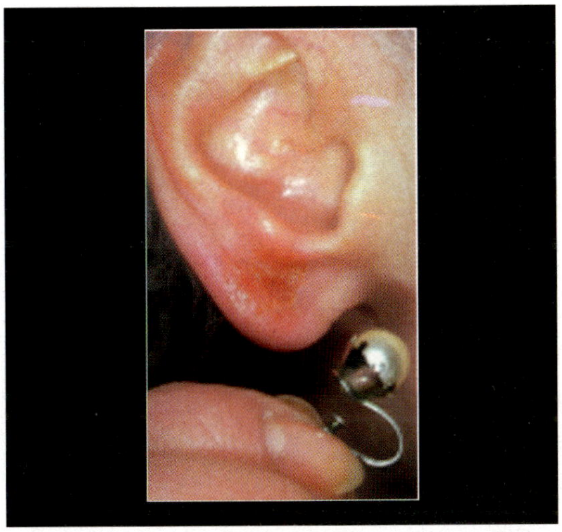

VISUAL PEARL

This female patient complained of a mildly tender, weeping, red tender area of her right earlobe after wearing a new pair of earings. Her ears are not pierced. What is your diagnosis?

ANSWER

This is nickel-induced contact dermatitis (one of the most common causes of allergic contact dermatitis). The acute problem will resolve, but the patient should be advised that it will reoccur upon repeat contact with earings made of nickel. Some gold earings contain nickel. Stainless steel or plastic earings are clinically safe for nickel sensitive patients.

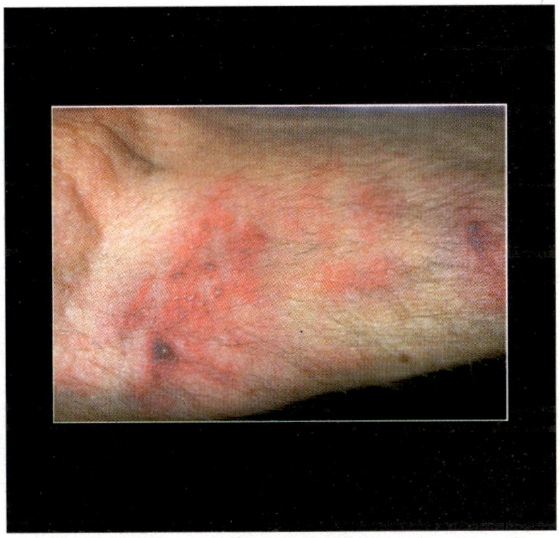

VISUAL PEARL

This adult male patient presents with an itchy blistering rash which began 2 days after hiking through a wooded area. He now has several regions of involvement with a linear distribution on skin surfaces that were previously protected by clothing during the hike.

ANSWER

Toxicodendron (*Rhus*) dermatitis. Principle causes include poison ivy and poison oak in North America, but it may also occur after exposure to poison sumac. Scratching disseminates the antigen contained in sap under a person's fingernails. Blister fluid contains no antigen. Treatment may include oral steroid therapy. Rebound dermatitis may occur if the steroid therapy is tapered too rapidly.

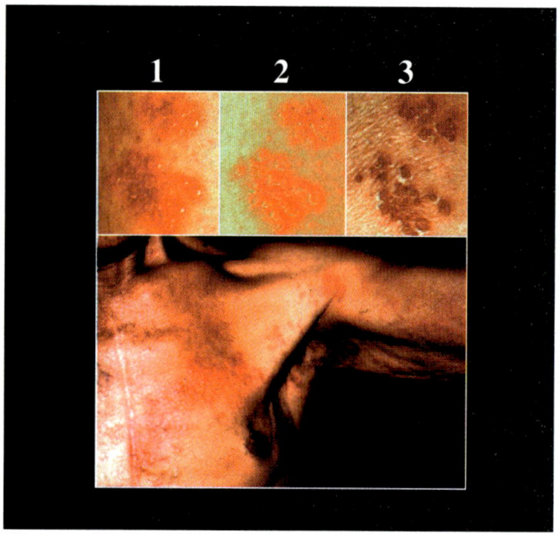

VISUAL PEARL

What is your diagnosis based on the appearance of this rash? The rash evolved as per the listed sequence. The patient complained of burning pain in the areas of the lesions over the left hemithorax and left upper extremity for several days prior to the appearance of the rash.

ANSWER

Varicella-zoster with thoracic neuralgia presents with multiple, small, erythematous, grouped vesicles which evolve into crusted ulcerations. Impaired immunity, elderly age, debilitation or malnourishment may all contribute to activation of the virus. Diagnosis of neuralgia can be difficult if vesicles are not evident, but the patient has pain within a dermatome (zoster sine herpete). Acute thoracic radiculopathy may precede the rash by many days. Treatment may include systemic steroids (some studies show a decrease incidence of postherpetic neuralgia if given early) and oral (or intravenous) acyclovir.

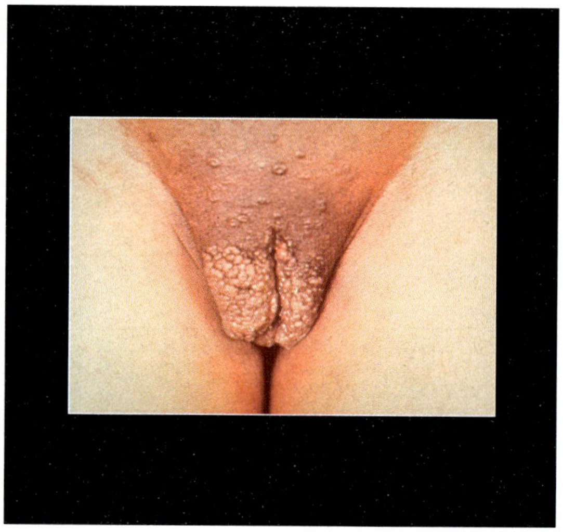

VISUAL PEARL

This female patient presents with a progressive area of granulation tissue which is elevated, red and painless. She has had the problem for "several months." The lesions began as a papule which ulcerated. What is the most likely diagnosis?

ANSWER

Granuloma inguinale (Donovanosis) is a mildly contagious, chronic, progressive, autoinocuable, ulcerative disease. It involves skin and lymphatics of perianal and genital areas. It is sexually transmitted and associated with the presence of an intracellular microorganism (the Donovan body) in affected tissues. Lesions appear within 30 days after sexual exposure. Lesions in women progress anteriorly over the genitalia in a V shape along the vulva. Extragenital lesions may occur. Erythromycin or trimethoprim-sulfamethoxazole are effective antimicrobial therapy.

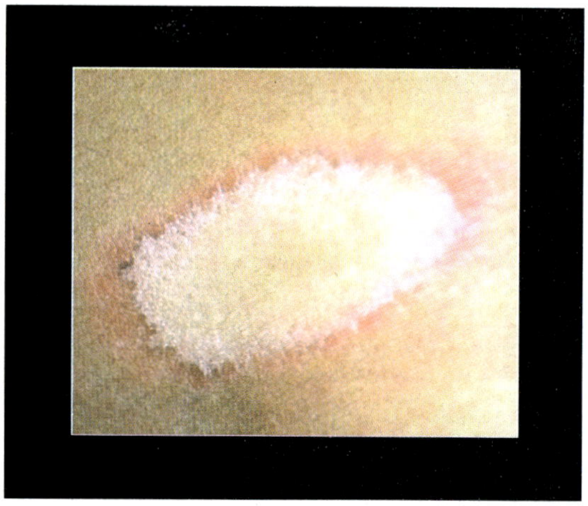

VISUAL PEARL

This adult patient complained of a mild viral syndrome with a subsequent rash which began as a single lesion on the posterior thorax. Subsequently, multiple small patches of skin became covered with a dry epidermis and then desquamated to form a collarette of scale at their periphery. What is the most likely diagnosis and management? What else should the physician consider?

ANSWER

The first lesion of pityriasis rosea is a solitary erythematous or salmon-colored herald plaque. It is most often seen on the trunk and extremities, followed by the development of smaller maculopapular lesions similiar to the initial lesion. These latter lesions erupt over time in groupings and often appear in the pattern of a christmas tree following the lines of skin tension on the posterior thorax. Other regions of the skin may be affected. This is probably a viral condition and may last 3-8 weeks. Care is only symptomatic. Lesions heal without sequelae. In general, a diagnosis of secondary syphilis should be ruled out.

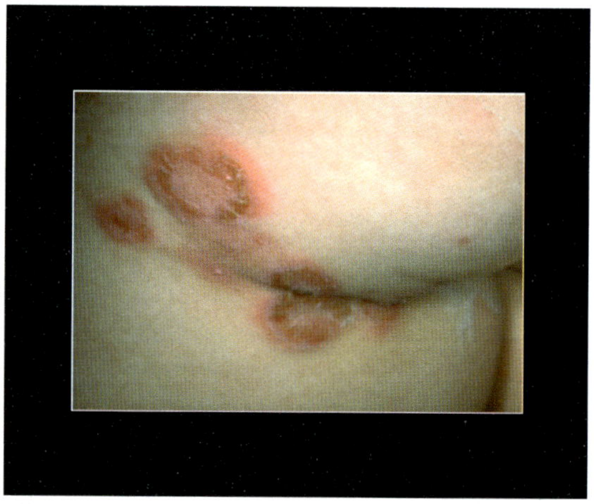

VISUAL PEARL

This 7-year-old male child presented with multiple lesions of the left buttock and upper thigh. There is no history of injury to the area. The original lesion appeared as a red papule. This progressed over several days to multiple lesions with erythema, a rim of adherent golden crust, and central clearing. The child is not acutely ill. What is the diagnosis and the treatment?

ANSWER

The diagnosis is impetigo contagiosa. The causative organism is Group A ß-hemolytic streptococcus, but it may occasionally be due to staphylococcus. Effective therapy includes one of these: parenteral PCN, erythromycin, cephalexin, dicloxacillin, or mupurocin topically. Glomerulonephritis is associated with nephritogenic strains of streptococcus and is not prevented by antibiotic therapy.

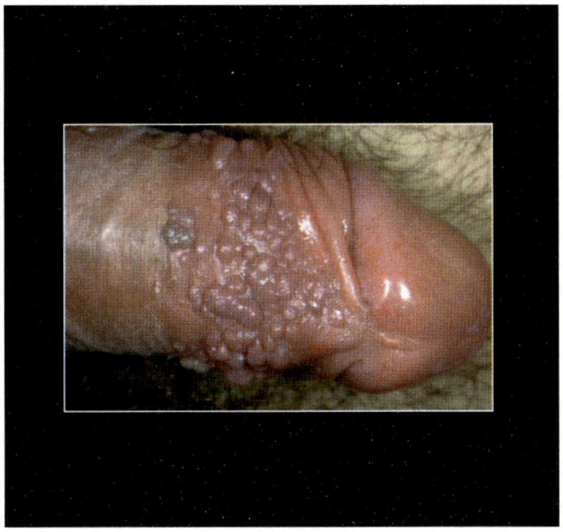

VISUAL PEARL

This adult patient complained of painless "bumps" on his penis. He admits to a history of homosexual behavior. What is your diagnosis based on this clinical appearance?

ANSWER

This photograph demonstrates genital warts. The incidence is significantly increasing even exceeding that for genital herpes. There is a strong correlation between genital warts due to human papilloma virus, HPV (several types), and genital cancer. Warts may spread rapidly and may extend into the urethra, rectum, or, in the female, into the vagina. Visualization is enhanced after application of dilute acetic acid. Treatment includes podophyllum resin and may result in significant pain with local inflammation.

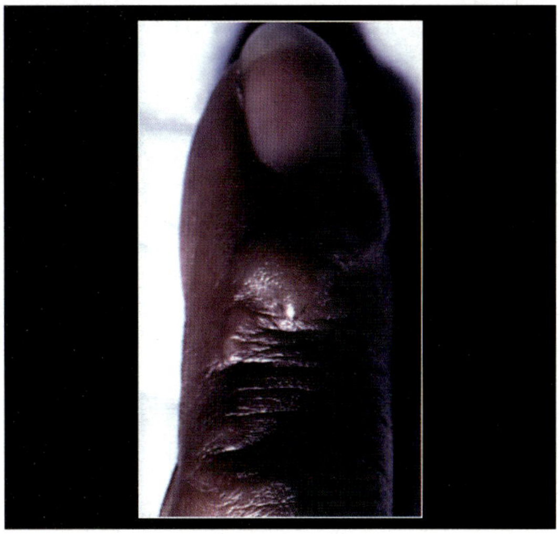

VISUAL PEARL

This adult female complained of pruritis and a migratory rash with tracks that changed position and shape on her skin. She had episodes of abdominal pain and diarrhea containing some mucus and blood. Her blood demonstrated eosinophilia. What is the diagnosis and treatment?

ANSWER

Creeping eruption (cutaneous larva migrans) is an infestation of migrating hookworm larva (most common is *Ancyclostoma braziliense*) after they penetrate the skin. The patient has usually been walking barefoot on soil. Moderate itching and eosinophilia occur. Loffler's syndrome is a transitory, patchy pulmonary infiltrate in patients with a severe cutaneous infestation. Parasites may be found in the sputum. Treatment includes topical thiabendazole or ivermectin. Oral antibiotics and topical steroids are used for secondary bacterial infection or eczematous inflammation. Oral thiabendazole induces nausea, vomiting and dizziness in a significant number of patients but may be indicated.

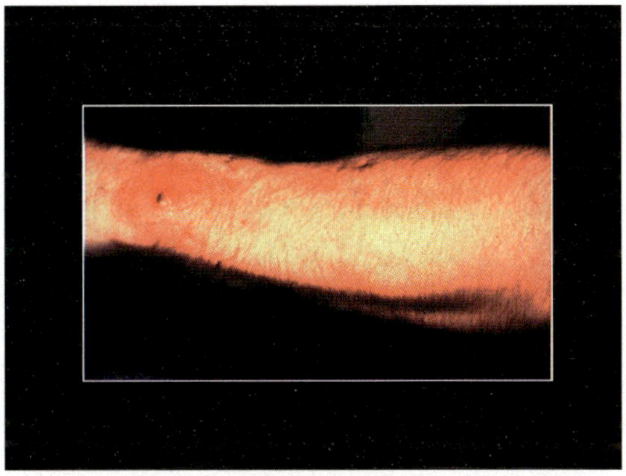

VISUAL PEARL

This adult male awoke in the morning with this problem on his left dorsal wrist. He had been drinking heavily and fell asleep in his barn. His temperature is 100.2°F. He complains of chills, nausea, and muscle aches. What is your diagnosis based upon this appearance and clinical information?

ANSWER

The initial bite of a brown recluse spider usually produces a minor burning or sudden sharp pain. Severe bites may demonstrate necrosis of the bite area within 4 hours and severe pain. Within 12 hours after the bite the victim may demonstrate systemic toxicity. The toxin may induce thrombocytopenia, generalized hemolysis, DIC, renal failure, or even death (severe reactions are more likely in children). Primary treatment includes bedrest, elevation, tetanus toxoid, antibiotics, dapsone, and pain management. Immediate surgical excision is avoided.

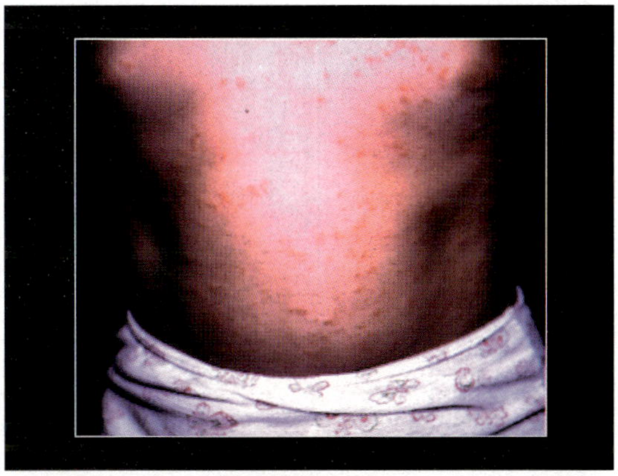

VISUAL PEARL

This child had been on vacation in Florida and developed a sudden pruritic dermatitis after swimming in the ocean. She had been wearing a bathing suit that covered her abdomen. This is the appearance of the rash after 3 days. She had associated headache and conjunctivitis. The dermatitis resolved after 10 days. She had no sequelae. What is the diagnosis?

ANSWER

Seabather's eruption is a pruritic dermatitis that primarily involves skin surfaces previously covered by a bathing suit after exposure to the larval form of the thimble jellyfish, *Linuche unguiculata*. Systemic complaints may occasionally occur and include general malaise, headache, conjunctivitis, and urethritis. Treatment is symptomatic. Swimmer's itch (due to parasitic flatworm schistosomes in fresh water–usually in the Great Lakes region of the United States) occurs on any exposed areas and may be associated with secondary infection. Treatment for this infestation may include cool compresses, calamine lotion, and antihistamines. Topical steroids are occasionally indicated.

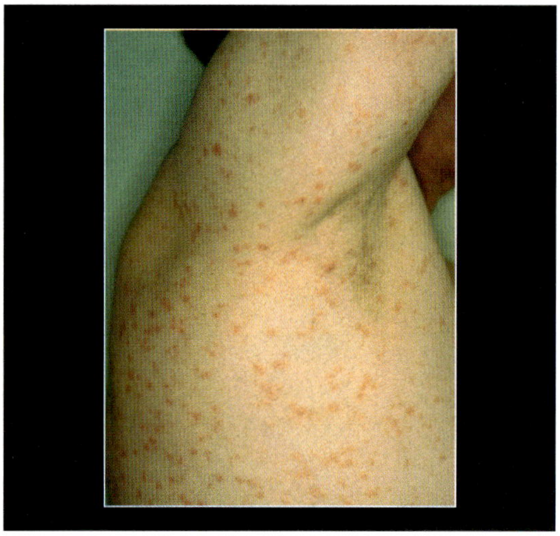

VISUAL PEARL

This adult male complained of rash, low grade fever, swollen glands and general malaise. He had no known tick exposure. His GU exam is normal. Bilateral nontender inguinal lymphadenopathy is present. Small ulcerations are visible in the mouth. The musculoskeletal examination is normal. What is the most likely diagnosis?

ANSWER

This patient presents with a maculopapular rash with intraoral lesions all consistent with secondary syphillis. The rash may be maculopapular, papular, macular, annular, psoriasiform, or follicular. The intraoral lesions are hightly contagious as are the lesions of condylomata lata. The patient requires antibiotic therapy with parenteral benzathine penicillin G. A falling RPR after measurement of a baseline serum titer indicates successful therapy. Alternate antibiotics for PCN sensitive patients include tetracycline and doxycycline; spectinomycin is not effective.

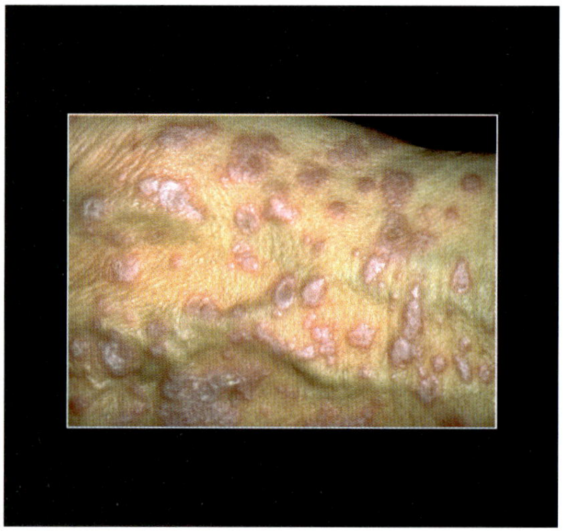

VISUAL PEARL

This adult male presents with a chronic pruritic rash with flat topped closely spaced pink-purple papules. Fine white scale is visible on the surface of the lesions. Some of the papules have angular margins. He is otherwise well and afebrile. There is no known exposure to medication or toxins. What is your diagnosis?

ANSWER

Lichen planus is an inflammatory cutaneous reaction of unknown etiology. It may affect the mucous membranes. Drugs and toxins have been implicated; there is no known viral or bacterial etiology associated. 10% of patients have a positive family history primarily as adults. The lesions are pruritic, planar, polyangular, purple papules (*the five P's*). The fine lacy scale or lines on the surface are called Wickham's stria (areas of epidermal thickening). Treatment includes topical steroids for localized disease, intralesional steroids, and sometimes systemic steroids. Antihistamines effectively relieve itching.

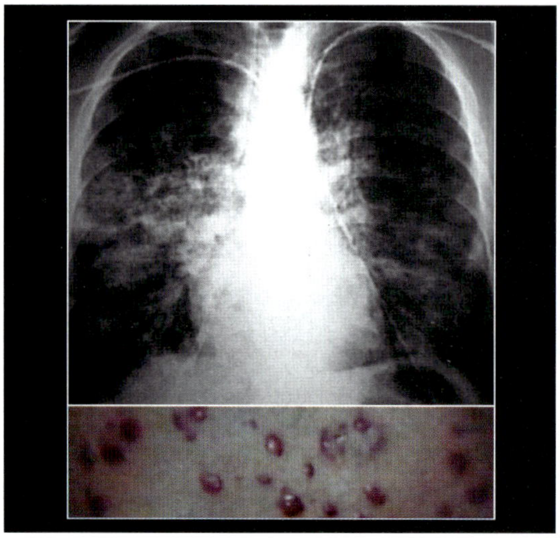

VISUAL PEARL

This patient was confused and has a history of intravenous drug abuse. He is severely dyspneic with a rectal temperature of 104.2°F and a nonproductive cough. His posterior thorax also demonstrates skin lesions with this appearance (lower portion of image). What is the likely diagnosis? What do the skin lesions represent?

ANSWER

Bilateral alveolar and interstitial infiltrates on chest film in this patient were due to pneumocystis carinii pneumonia (PCP). This is a classic appearance, although the initial chest film may be falsely normal in some symptomatic patients. The skin lesions are Kaposi's sarcoma (KS). This patient had previously contracted the HIV virus. PCP is the most common opportunistic infection (manifestation) of AIDs; KS is the second most common manifestation.

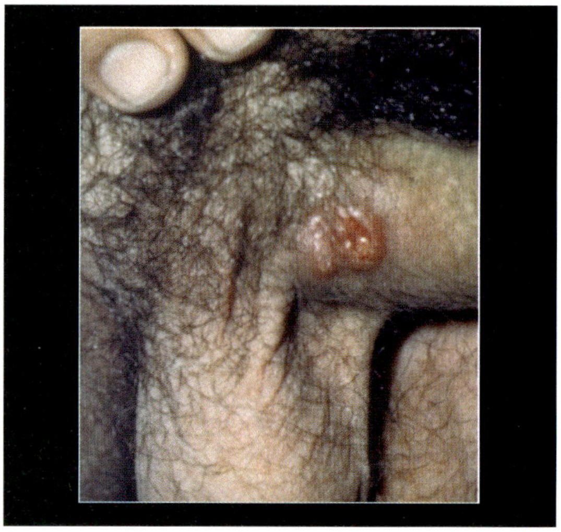

VISUAL PEARL

This adult male presents with a painless lesion on his proximal penis. What is the likely diagnosis?

ANSWER

3 serotypes of *Chlamydia trachomatis* cause lymphogranuloma venereum. A small papule or herpetiform vesicle appears on the genitalia after an incubation period of 5-21 days. Rapid evolution leads to painless ulcer formation and healing occurs without scarring. Primary lesions are rare in women and the initial lesion may go unnoticed. Unilateral or bilateral inguinal lymphadenopathy develops 1-4 weeks after healing of the ulcer. This is accompanied by headache, fever, arthralgia, and migratory polymyalgia. Rupture of lymph nodes (buboes) and lymphatic obstruction with genital edema (the latter in females) are chronic sequelae. Diagnosis is made using microimmunofluorescent techniques or culture. Treatment is with tetracycline.

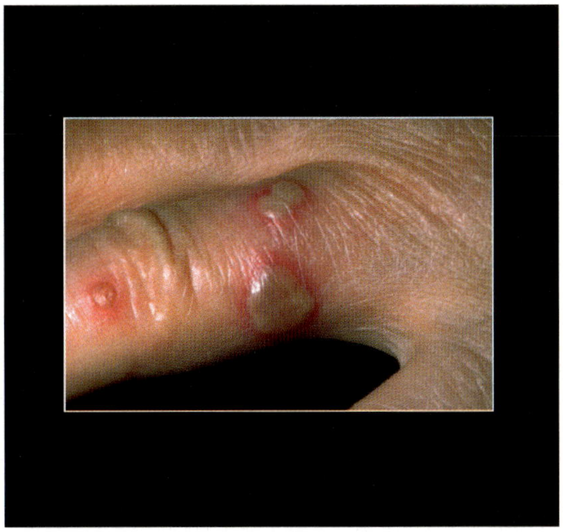

VISUAL PEARL

This adult male complained of blisters with this appearance on the hand. There is no history of burn or injury. On presentation, he was afebrile and appeared well. There are no other lesions on the skin surfaces. There is no regional lymphadenopathy. What is your diagnosis based on this appearance?

ANSWER

Bullous impetigo is caused by an epidermolytic toxin which causes separation of the skin at the granular layer. The lesions usually are not contaminated by streptococci. Respiratory colonization predates colonization of normal skin (opposite sequence occurs in vesicular, i.e., streptococcal impetigo) by more than 10 days. The condition is most common in infants and children, especially on the face, and lesions may persist for months. Regional lymphadenitis is uncommon. Rarely, serious secondary infections (e.g., septic arthritis, pneumonia) develop.

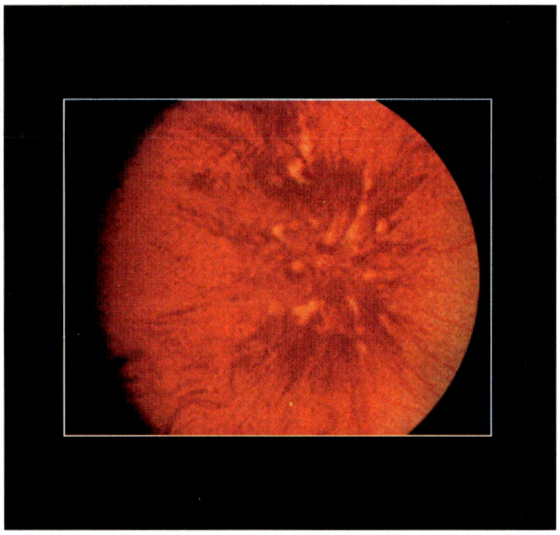

VISUAL PEARL

This adult patient complained of a relatively sudden uniocular complete loss of vision? He denied any pain. He has a history of hypertension. What is the most likely diagnosis?

ANSWER

The diagnosis in this case is central retinal vein occlusion. Pressure from the retinal artery has collapsed the retinal vein preventing the egress of blood out of the eye. The retina appears chaotic with blood-streaked areas. There is no immediate therapy the emergency physician can provide that will ameliorate the problem. The patient requires immediate ophthalmologic consultation.

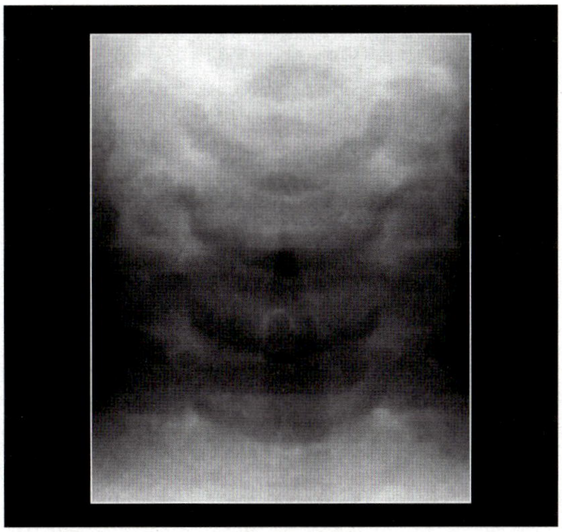

VISUAL PEARL

This 3-year-old child presented with a temperature of 101.5 °F, a mild sore throat and a brassy cough. The parents became concerned when they heard a "noise" on inspiration. There was no drooling, and the child was taking po liquids without difficulty. He appeared moderately ill, but was not in obvious distress. What is your diagnosis based on this AP film?

ANSWER

"Steeple sign" seen in croup (laryngotracheal bronchitis). The noise was stridor (it typically begins abruptly at night). Croup mainly affects children less than 4 years old and is usually caused by viruses (especially the parainfluenza group). Other etiologies include influenza virus, respiratory syncytial virus, and measles. Primary treatment includes oxygen and humidification. Corticosteriods are generally not utilized. Antibiotics are only indicated in the uncommon situation of secondary bacterial infection.

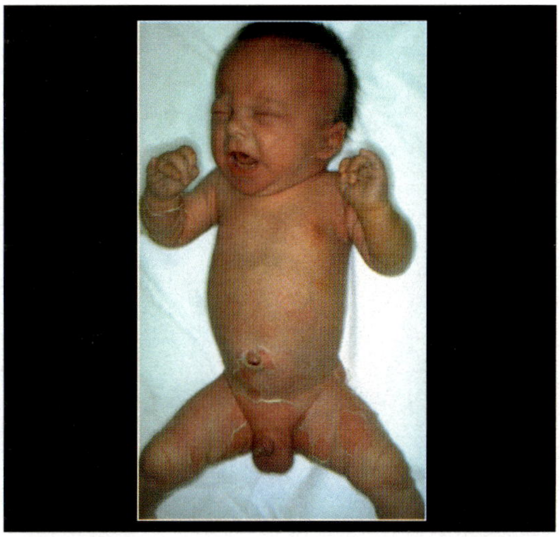

VISUAL PEARL

This baby had an initial umbilical infection. Moderate dehydration was managed with intravenous fluids. The illness also required intravenous methicillin, but corticosteroids were specifically withheld. Healing occurred without scar formation. Cultures from intact bullae were negative. What is your diagnosis based on this information and clinical appearance?

ANSWER

Staphylococcal scalded skin syndrome (*Ritter's disease)* is a staphylococcal epidermolytic toxin-mediated syndrome that begins with a localized *S. aureus* infection. A diffuse erythema with tenderness evolves with bullae formation, wrinkling of the skin and subsequent desquamation in large sheets. Minor pressure will induce skin separation (Nikolsky's sign). Nikolsky's sign is *not* specific for SSSS.

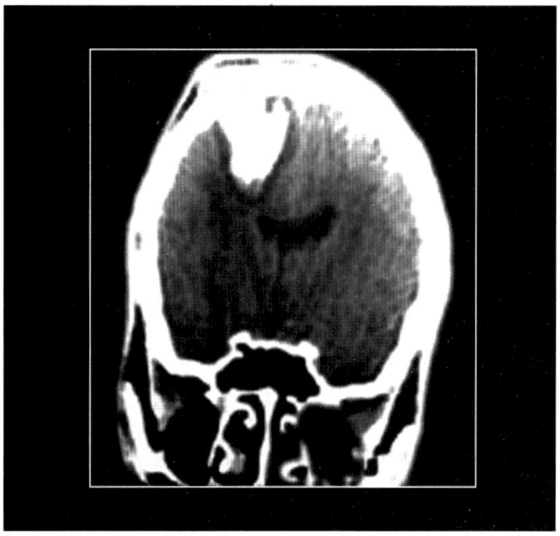

VISUAL PEARL

This patient was found unconscious after a "gang fight." What is the most likely diagnosis?

ANSWER

This is a coronal reformatted cranial CT. The finding is a penetrating injury to the skull with an irregularly shaped intracranial hematoma of high density (acute hemorrhage) and subcutaneous hematoma. Note the low density border surrounding the hematoma; this is representative of cerebral edema. There is some shift of the midline structures to the left. When an intracranial hematoma is irregular in shape, think of a traumatic injury. Spontaneous intracranial hemorrhage is more typically round in appearance.

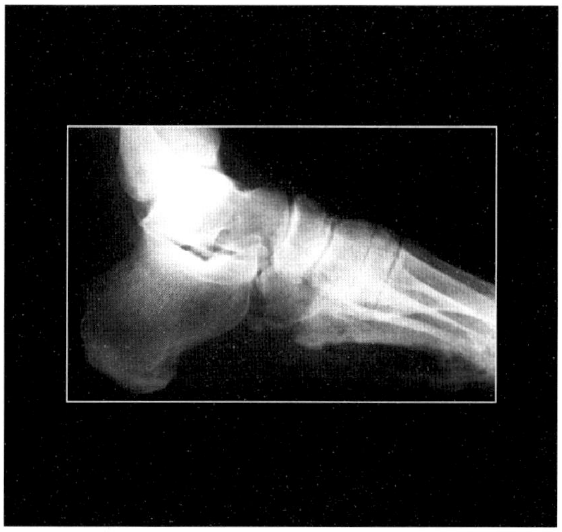

VISUAL PEARL

This diabetic was febrile with severe erythema, swelling and a dusky appearance to the foot after minor trauma to the soft tissues of the volar surface several days ago. There is also blister formation on the dorsal skin. A lateral radiograph was obtained. What is your concern? What is the most likely diagnosis?

ANSWER

There is a large amount of subcutanenous gas visible within the plantar and distal posterior soft tissues. This implies a gas-forming infection. The primary concern is gas gangrene due to *Clostridium perfringens* although other organsisms (synergistic infections) may produce this radiographic appearance. The patient requires tetanus prophylaxis, immediate surgical consultation, and broad spectrum, parenteral antibiotics. Hyperbaric oxygen therapy might also be employed.

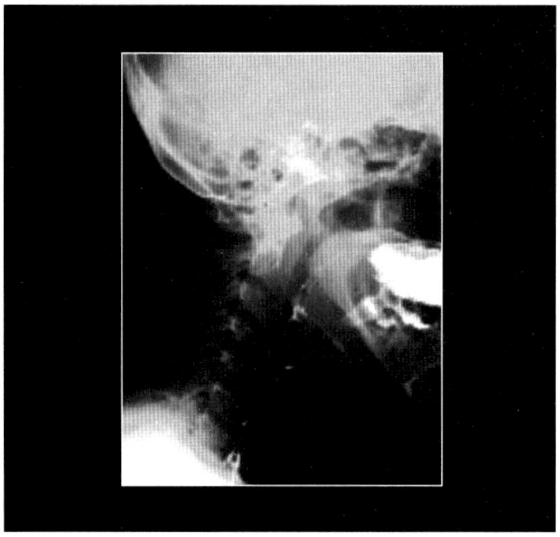

VISUAL PEARL

This patient complained of a sudden choking spell. What is your diagnosis?

ANSWER

This film highlights a radiolucent foreign body in the esophagus anterior to the vertebral bodies of C^{6-7} after water soluble contrast ingestion.

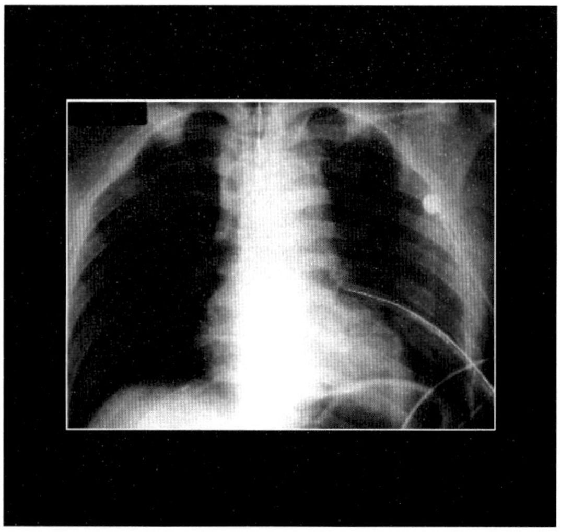

VISUAL PEARL

This adult male was intoxicated, but complained of left chest pain after a motor vehicle accident. A chest tube was placed and immediately drained 250 mL of blood. The patient's vital signs improved after 1500 mL of isotonic crystalloid were administered. What are the key findings and primary diagnostic concern?

ANSWER

There is obvious widening of the upper mediastinum with bilateral apical capping. Widening of the superior mediastinum is significant if it is more than 8 cm on an upright PA CXR. Although this is a portable AP film, the findings strongly suggest traumatic rupture of the aorta (TRA), or mediastinal venous bleeding which is significant enough to warrant suspicion for TRA. The patient requires angiography to establish the nature of the injury and the need for urgent surgical repair.

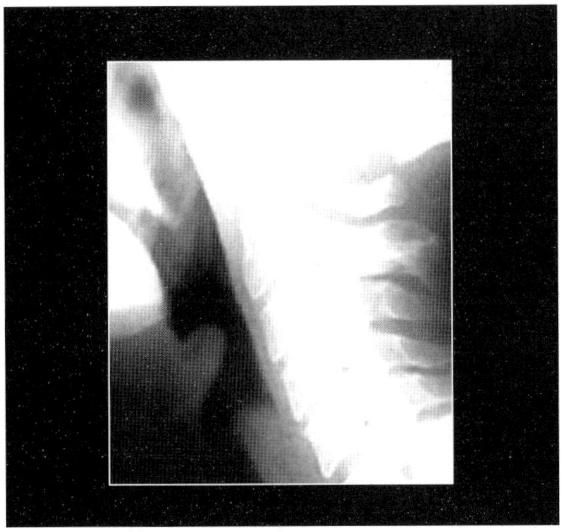

VISUAL PEARL

This adult patient complained of a severe sore throat and dysphagia of several hours duration. He was febrile and appeared acutely ill, but was not initially in respiratory distress. What is your diagnosis based on this lateral neck film?

ANSWER

This film demonstrates a markedly swollen epiglottis with a dilated proximal airway, i.e., acute epiglottitis in an adult. The primary age for this infection is 2 to 7 years old, but it may occur at any age. It is most commonly due to *H. influenzae* type B, but may also be caused by *Streptococcus* or *Staphylococcus* species. After protection of the airway, the primary therapy includes the parenteral administration of a third generation cephalosporin. Adults with epiglottitis may be managed in an intensive care setting without intubation.

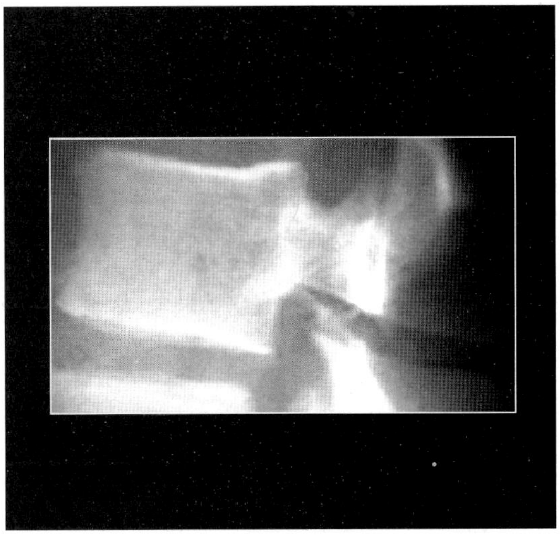

VISUAL PEARL

This ambulatory 12-year-old female complained of back pain after a motor vehicle accident. She was a rear-seat passenger and her vehicle was struck from the rear. She was restrained by a lap belt without a shoulder harness. What is your diagnosis?

ANSWER

There is a large horizontal-oblique fracture extending from the spinous process of L1 anteriorly through the laminae and pedicles, to the posterior border of the vertebral body–a Chance fracture. This injury is seen with hyperflexion of the thoracolumbar (TL) region. Distraction of the posterior and middle column occurs with simultaneous impaction of the anterior column of the TL spine. This bony injury may be associated with a neurologic deficit. Up to 50% have an associated intraperitoneal injury, involving primarily the intestine.

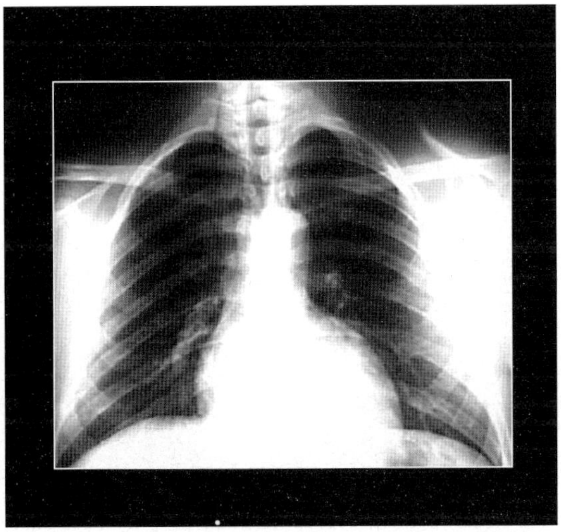

VISUAL PEARL

This 17-year-old male complained of a sore throat two days after playing football. He stated, "I had the wind knocked out of me during the game." On presentation, he was afebrile and appeared well. There were no findings on the initial physical examination. What is your diagnosis based on this chest film?

ANSWER

This film demonstrates a vertical linear lucency in the right paramediastinal region which travels cephalad into the neck. The diagnosis is pneumomediastinum (not a ruptured esophagus). The patient had an uneventful recovery.

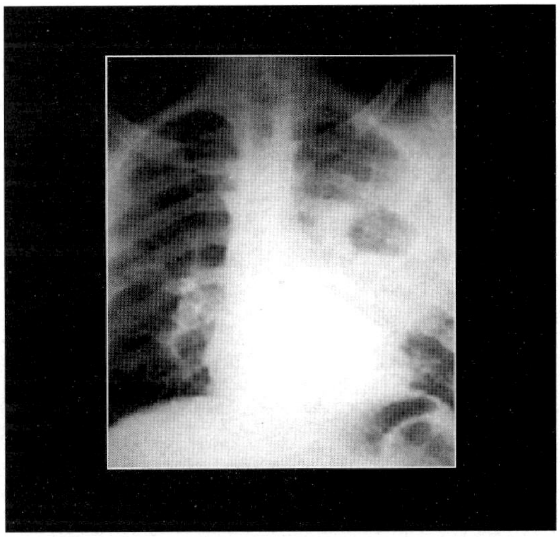

VISUAL PEARL

This known alcoholic adult patient was confused, severely dyspneic with a rectal temperature of 104°F and a productive cough. There is a foul odor to the breath. What are the primary findings on this chest film? What is the likely diagnosis?

ANSWER

There is a large, diffuse infiltrate in the left hemithorax with elevation of the left hemidiaphragm. There is a central lucency with a meniscus within the infiltrate. The most likely diagnosis is anaerobic lung abscess after an episode of emesis with aspiration. Anaerobic lung abscess is more common in patients with dental caries.

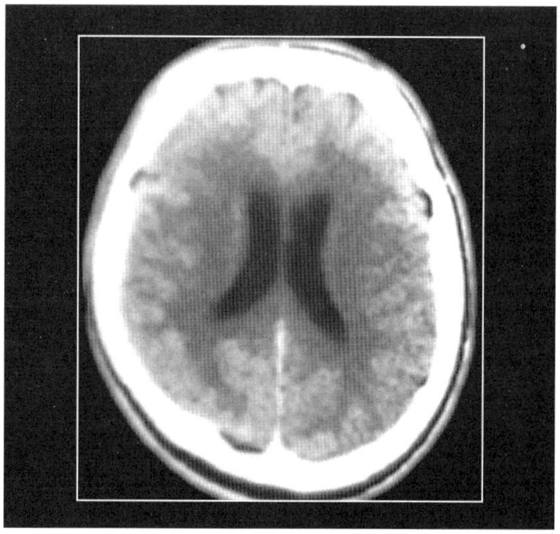

VISUAL PEARL

This adult patient complained of a severe generalized headache and subsequently became severely obtunded. What is your diagnosis based on the general appearance of this axial cranial CT? This study was obtained without radiographic contrast enhancement, i.e., it is a C "–" CT.

ANSWER

This particular cut demonstrates a diffuse subarachnoid hemorrhage (note the increased fuzzy density along the sulci and gyri) and bilateral ventricular enlargement. Blood in the subarachnoid space is causing a convexity (outflow) obstruction, i.e., it is preventing the normal flow of cerebrospinal fluid from the arachnoid granulations into the venous sinuses. Expansion of the body of both lateral ventricles is strong evidence for the presence of a convexity block in this circumstance.

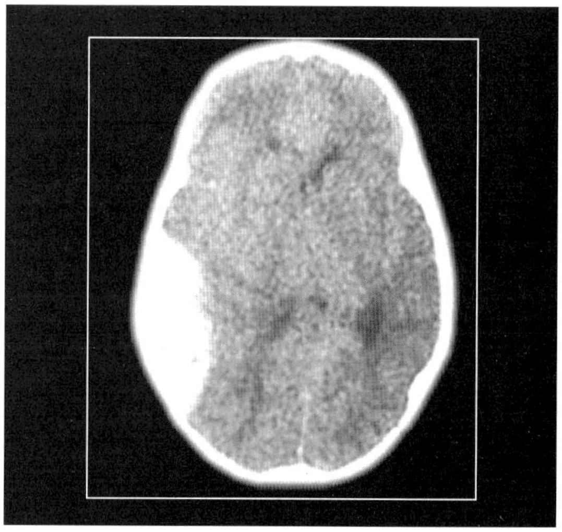

VISUAL PEARL

This adult patient was intoxicated with ethanol. She suddenly became unresponsive in the emergency department. She was immediately intubated and managed with controlled hyperventilation, a loop diuretic, fluid restriction and elevation of her head. What is your diagnosis based on the appearance of her axial cranial C – CT?

ANSWER

There is a large epidural (lenticular shape) hematoma of the right parieto-occipital region with a shift of the intracranial structures to the left. The anterior horn of the right lateral ventricle is compressed. This is usually a high pressure hemorrhage from an arterial vessel injury. Occasionally, epidural hemorrhage is venous in origin since the location of the dural venous sinuses is between the periosteal (lateral) and meningeal (medial) layers of the dura. Dural venous sinus injury will therefore produce a lens shaped collection of blood on a CT image.

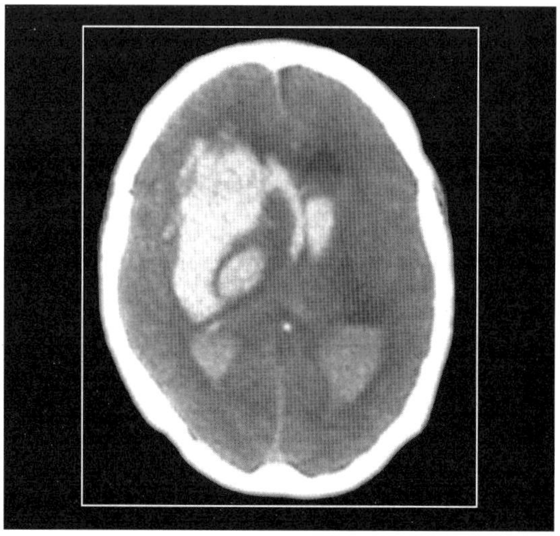

VISUAL PEARL

This adult patient complained of a severe headache which began on the right after an episode of syncope. He had vomited at the time of arrival to the hospital and then displayed decorticate posturing. What is your interpretation of this axial cranial CT obtained without radiographic contrast enhancement (C – CT)?

ANSWER

There is a large, irregular very hyperintense right intracerebral hemorrhage (acute) associated with moderately increased intensity in the posterior horns of the lateral ventricles bilaterally. In the left posterior horn there is a meniscus which is seen as an interface between a collection of posterior horn blood (higher intensity) and the CSF (lower intensity). The interface has been identified with three dotted markers.

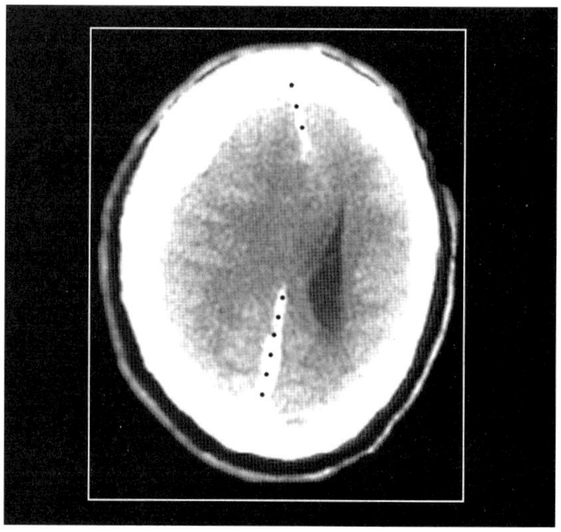

VISUAL PEARL

This adult male patient complained of a severe generalized headache and subsequently had a rapid decline in his mental status. He was then markedly obtunded. What is your diagnosis based on the appearance of his axial cranial CT obtained without radiographic contrast enhancement (C – CT)?

ANSWER

There is a large subdural (crescent shaped) hematoma compressing the entire right hemispheric region. The right lateral ventricle is not visible because it is completely compressed. This hemorrhage also extends along the falx cerebri (dotted markers) and is causing a shift of the intracranial structures to the left.

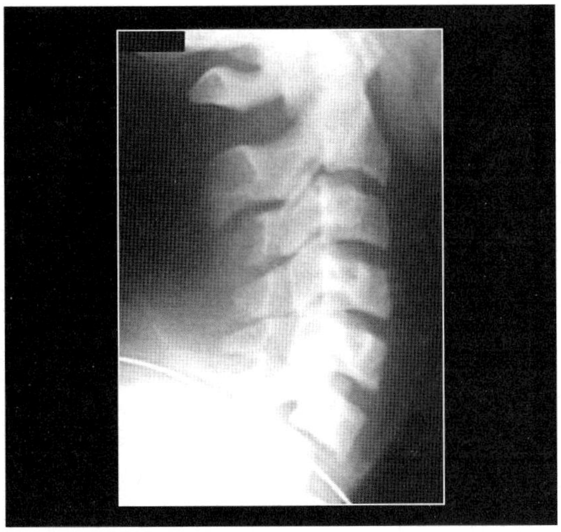

VISUAL PEARL

This 22-year-old male complained of midline low neck pain after being kicked in the back of the head with a boot. He was ambulatory and had an odor of ketones on his breath. There was no obvious neurologic deficit. What is your diagnosis based on this clinical information and the film?

ANSWER

This patient presents with bilateral interfacetal dislocation of C^6 on C^7. Fifty percent or more override of one vertebral body anteriorly over the subjacent body implies this injury. The mechanism is hyperflexion without rotation. This is an unstable injury and would likely present with, or develop, an acute neurologic deficit. The patient requires immediate C-spine immobilization, further diagnostic evaluation and orthopedic and/or neurosurgical consultation.

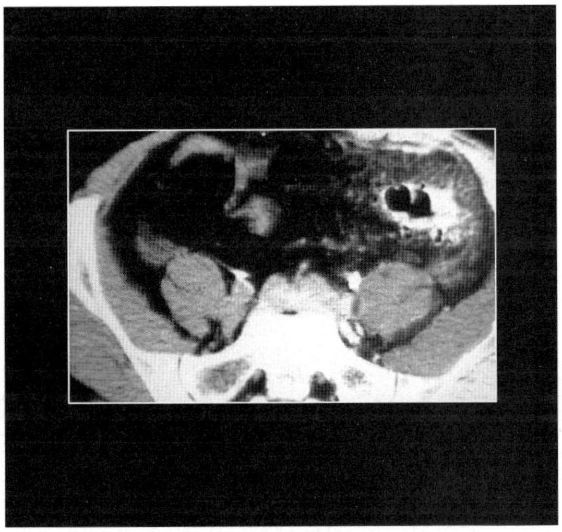

VISUAL PEARL

This 37-year-old physician complained of severe pain in the left inguinal region. He presented with a chief complaint of left inguinal hernia. On physical examination no hernia was detectable. He had direct tenderness in the left lower abdomen with some tenderness on rectal examination. Genitourinary examination was normal. What is your diagnosis?

ANSWER

This patient has a diverticular abscess (phlegmon). Multiple tiny dark gas-filled pockets surround a hyperintense (white) thickened bowel wall on the patient's left side of the study. A fever would be expected although its absence does not rule out the diagnosis. The patient was treated with broad spectrum intravenous antibiotics and did not require surgery.

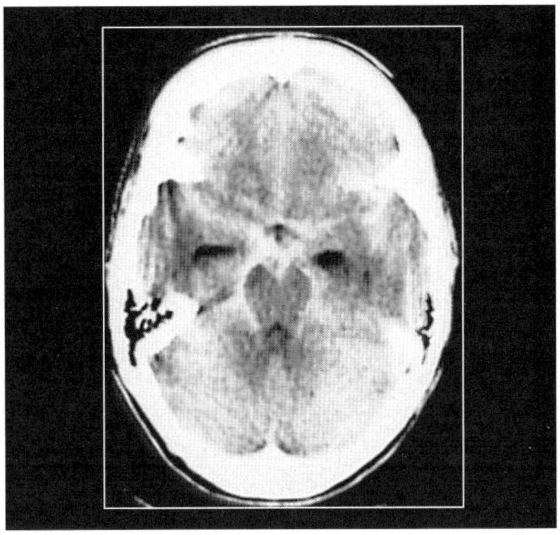

VISUAL PEARL

This male patient presented with acute loss of consciousness after complaining of a severe headache. Decerebrate posturing, hyperreflexia and a positive Babinski reflex were present. His breathing pattern was irregular and rapid with pauses. He died shortly after this study was obtained. What is your diagnosis?

ANSWER

TThe diagnosis is acute subarachnoid hemorrhage seen as a hyperintense outlining of the brainstem in the center of the image. This is an axial cranial CT without contrast (C - CT). New hemorrhage greatly attenuates the x-ray fan beam on CT, and therefore, appears white. The findings in this patient indicated a moribund presentation with increased intracranial pressure.

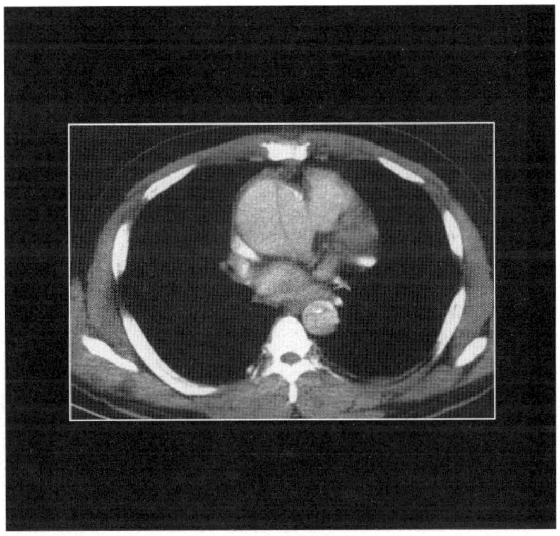

VISUAL PEARL

This 65-year-old male fell from a ladder. He complained of sudden, severe, anterior chest pain and became profoundly hypotensive and anuric shortly after his arrival in the ED. A systolic murmur was heard over the posterior thorax. The initial CXR was normal. The following study was obtained just prior to the episode of hypotension. What is your diagnosis?

ANSWER

This CT demonstrates acute traumatic rupture of the ascending aorta with extension into the descending aorta. A portion of the calcified aortic wall is seen centrally in the descending aorta. Both true and false lumen are visible in the ascending and descending aorta. This is a surgical emergency. Untreated, the condition is lethal. Preoperative aortography is performed, when possible, to define anatomy and delineate the extent of injury. Pulse deficits and asymmetric bilateral blood pressure measurements may be present. Sudden anuria indicates obstruction of blood flow to the kidneys or severe hypotension with renal hypoperfusion.

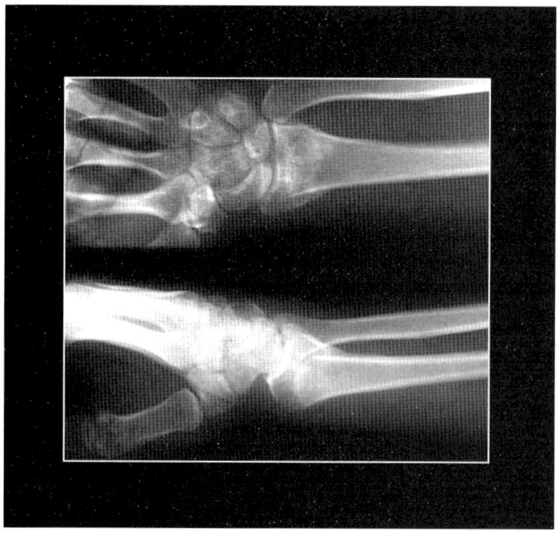

VISUAL PEARL

Describe the injury and its typical mechanism. What is the treatment? What associated bony injury may be found? Which nerve is most likely to be injured in association with this type of fracture?

ANSWER

This pair of films demonstrates a classic Colles' fracture. This is a distal radius fracture involving the metaphysis. The distal fragment is dorsally displaced and angulated. The mechanism for a Colles' fracture is typically a fall on the patient's outstretched hand. An ulnar styloid fracture may be associated with a Colles' fracture. Closed reduction is usually possible after a local hematoma block. The patient is then treated with immobilization in a cast. Median nerve injury is only one of several potential complications.

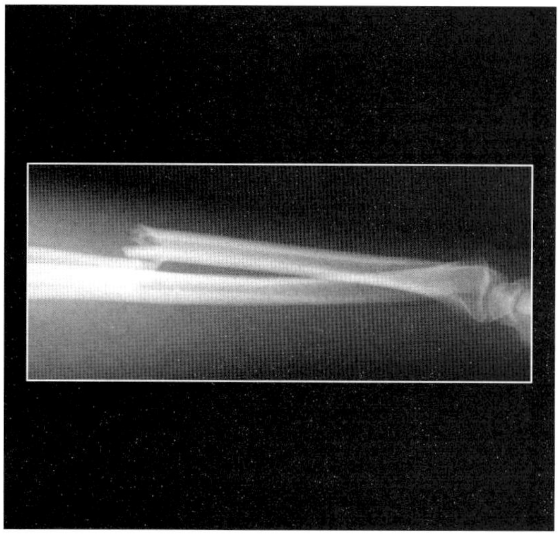

VISUAL PEARL

Describe the injury, its typical mechanism and the appropriate management in this case. What is an associated injury to consider? What would you suspect if the mechanism for a similar fracture in a child was described as a fall on the outstretched hand?

ANSWER

This is a *nightstick* fracture of the ulna. It is due to a direct blow. In this patient there is significant displacement of the fragments at the site of the fracture. This requires open reduction and internal fixation. Look for an associated radius fracture or dislocation. Fracture of the shaft of the ulna with dislocation of the radial head is referred to as a *Monteggia fracture-dislocation*. Suspect abuse if the mechanism was described as a fall on the outstretched hand in a child.

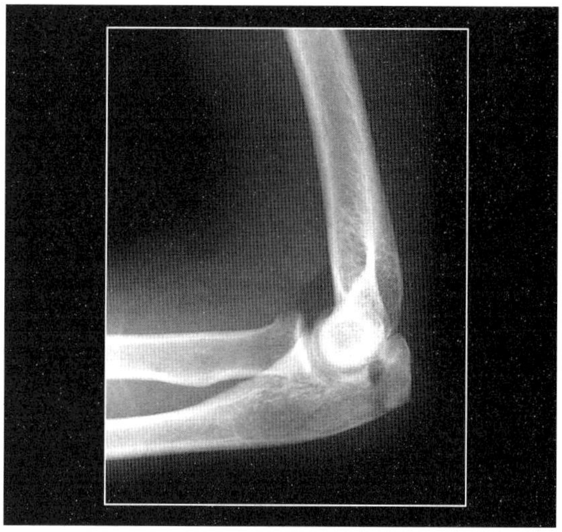

VISUAL PEARL

Describe the injury and its mechanism. The neurovascular examination of the upper extremity was normal. What other finding is present and what does it signify? Is a posterior fat pad sign visible? What initial treatment is indicated

ANSWER

This is a displaced olecranon fracture. This injury was the result of a direct blow to the posterior elbow. The anterior fat pad is visible and indicates an intraarticular fracture. The posterior fat pad is not seen on this film. The posterior fat pad is normally never visible on a plain film unless an adjacent fracture is present. Hematoma may then displace the posterior fat pad out of the olecranon fossa. This injury requires a long arm plaster splint and orthopedic consultation. Don't forget to address the patient's acute pain management.

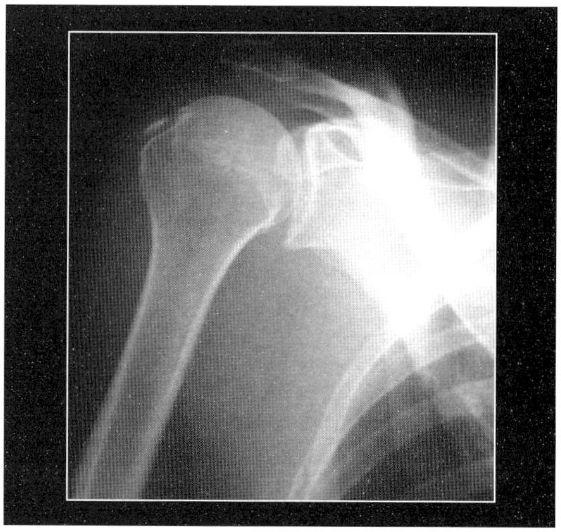

VISUAL PEARL

Describe the key finding you see on this shoulder film. What prior mechanism or condition does it signify? What is the related injury that may occur to the glenoid rim as a result of the same mechanism?

ANSWER

There is a compression fracture of the head of the humerus. This is often referred to as a *Hill-Sachs lesion*. It implies a *prior* anterior dislocation of the humerus. At the time of the dislocation, the humeral head was compressed as it impacted against the inferior rim of the glenoid. The shoulder dislocation has been reduced. The associated glenoid fracture that may also occur is called a *Bankart lesion*. It is a fracture of the inferior rim of the glenoid and may eventually appear as a rim defect (the inferior glenoid would appear irregular and incomplete).

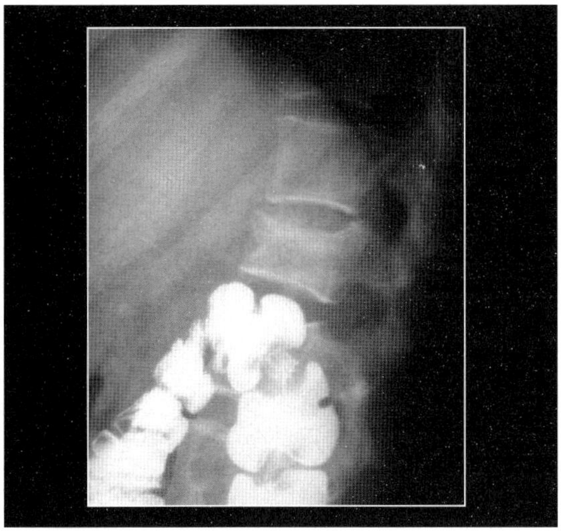

VISUAL PEARL

This 57-year-old male complained of persistent back pain five days after a syncopal episode. A lumbar spine film on his original date of injury was reported to be uremarkable. A contrast study had been requested one day ago as part of his ongoing evaluation. What finding did the radiologist now report?

ANSWER

This lateral film demonstrates a compression fracture of the eleventh thoracic vertebra. This finding was originally missed. The constrast study is a barium enema and it is normal. However, it is not possible to come to that conclusion from this single, partial view. The patient had no neurologic deficit. His back pain resolved without sequelae after several months.

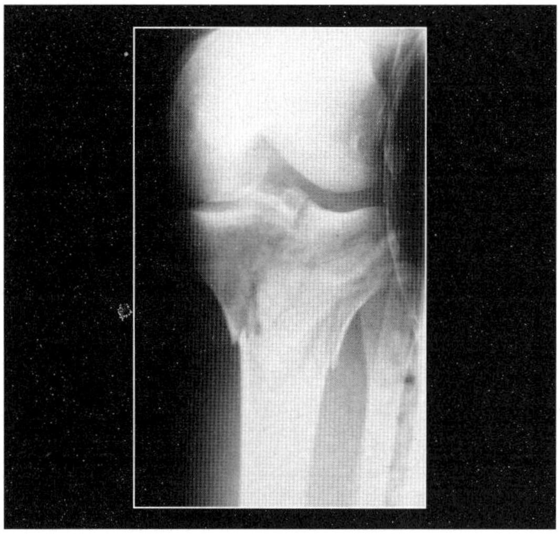

VISUAL PEARL

This patient sustained this injury late at night after being struck by the bumper of a car when he was attempting to walk across a street. Describe all of the elements of this injury. What are the associated local injuries to consider? What is the appropriate management?

ANSWER

This patient has sustained a comminuted tibial plateau fracture onvolving both medial and lateral tibial plateaus. There is a large oblique fracture line passing through the proximal tibia from the lateral plateau down to the medial proximal tibia. There is some local central depression of the lateral plateau. Multiple smaller fracture lines of comminution are visible in the proximal tibia. A proximal fibular fracture and injury to the knee ligaments and menisci would be commonly associated. The most frequent serious complications include nonunion (or malunion) and posttraumatic arthritis. This complex injury requires surgery.

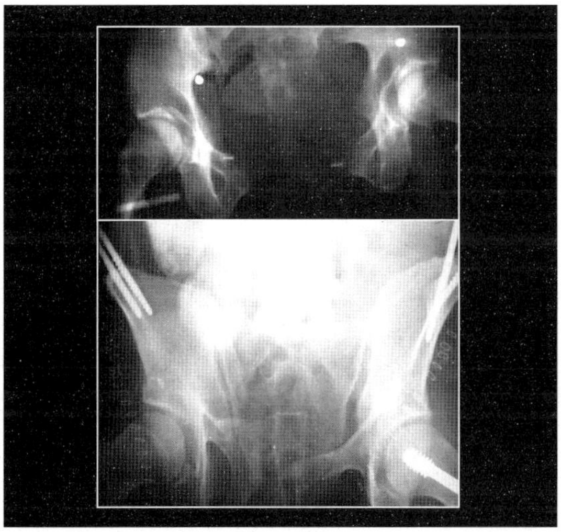

VISUAL PEARL

This trauma victim was involved in a high-speed motor vehicle accident. Describe all of the findings which best represent the pelvic abnormalities depicted in these two films. What other local injuries are commonly associated with this form of pelvic trauma?

ANSWER

This unstable pelvic injury is frequently referred to as an *open book* pelvic dislocation or a bilateral sprung pelvis. There is complete and wide disruption of the pubic symphysis in the upper film. There is significant diastasis in the left sacroiliac joint best visualized here in the lower film. However, there is also minimal widening of the right sacroiliac joint. The lower film was obtained after partial pelvic stabilization was achieved. Severe bleeding from disruption of pelvic blood vessels and genitourinary injury (urethral and/or urinary bladder rupture) are commonly associated injuries.

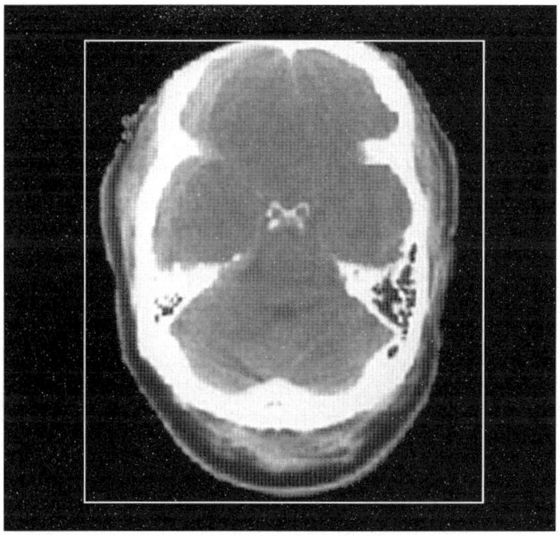

VISUAL PEARL

This adult male trauma patient became increasingly obtunded after repair of an occipital scalp laceration. A head CT was performed. What is your diagnosis based on this appearance? What is the most common form of intracranial hemorrhage after trauma? What is the least common type of hemorrhage in this circumstance? (Hint: it is much less common than subdural hemorrhage after trauma.)

ANSWER

There is moderately intense crescentic hematoma of the right frontal and parietal areas. This is consistent with a subdural hematoma. This is representative of a *contrecoup* injury since the patient struck his occiput. A large posterior (occipital) scalp hematoma is visible. A small subarachnoid hemorrhage is the most common intracranial hemorrhage after trauma; epidural hematoma is the least common intracranial hemorrhage after trauma.

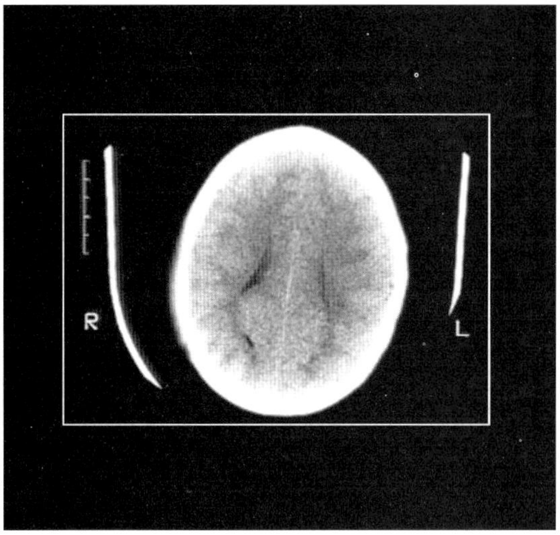

VISUAL PEARL

This two-year old male toddler fell backward striking his head against a marble fireplace when he attempted to pop a balloon with his foot. His neurologic examination is normal. There was no loss of consciousness. What is your diagnosis based on his axial cranial CT without contrast (C - CT)?

ANSWER

Given the normal neurologic examination, it is questionable that this child required an initial CT of the head. The brain structures are rotated, but are normal. Rotation of the head in the axial and coronal planes is causing the asymmetric appearance of the lateral ventricles. The falx is normal (looks like a pencil line). There is a faintly visible right parietal skull fracture at the posterior margin of a small right scalp hematoma. The patient was discharged after a brief period of observation. He had a normal examination at a subsequent follow-up appointment with his pediatrician.

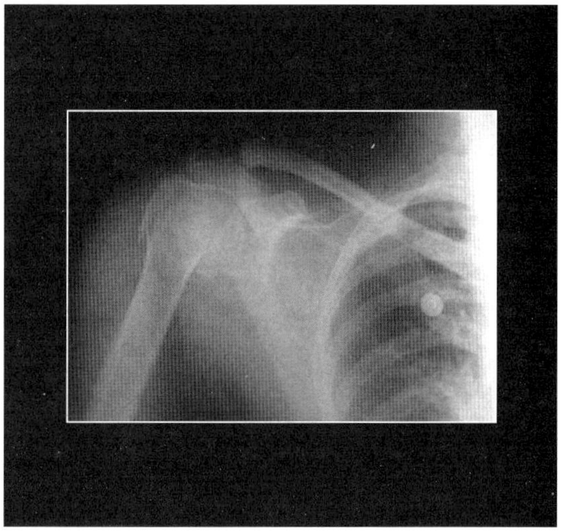

VISUAL PEARL

This 52-year-old male complained of right shoulder pain after falling on his right shoulder. His shoulder is ecchymotic, swollen and tender. Describe the injury. What is the usual mechanism for this type of injury? What is the importance of a displaced fracture of the greater tuberosity?

ANSWER

This is at least a three-part comminuted humeral head fracture. There are two large fracture lines, one passing through the surgical neck, and one passing through the medial border of the greater tuberosity, separating it from the humeral head. It is difficult to make out the lesser tuberosity. If it is a separate fragment, that would then make this a four-part fracture. This type of injury is due either to a direct blow *or* to a fall on the outstretched upper extremity (especially in the elderly). Although the greater tuberosity fragment is not markedly displaced in this case, one that is may imply a rotator cuff tear which will require surgical repair.

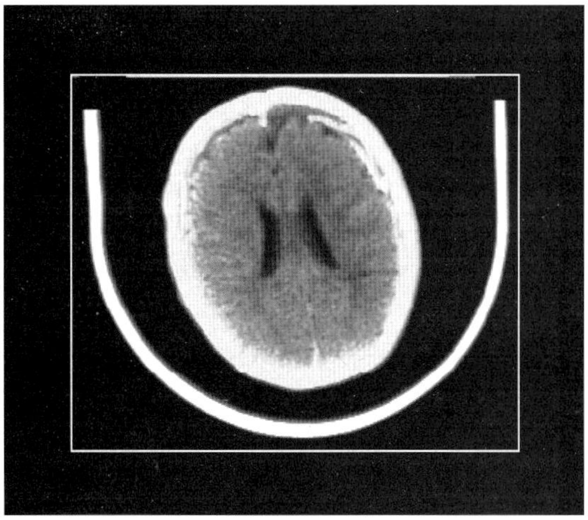

VISUAL PEARL

This baby was lethargic, febrile and feeding poorly. The parents also reported that the baby had one episode of vomiting today. Initially the physician suspected meningitis or sepsis. What are the key findings on this axial cranial CT scan performed without radiographic contrast? What is your diagnosis? What is the only physical finding you may detect in an infant to suspect this diagnosis?

ANSWER

The is *shaken-impact* (shaken-baby) *syndrome*. There is a bifrontal and bitemporal collection of new (hyperintense) subdural hemorrhage (much more prominent on the left). There is old bifrontal subdural hemorrhage represented by the gray areas adjacent to atrophied left frontal brain. There is a hypointense linear parenchymal laceration of the brain just posterior to the left lateral ventricle. The ventricles are dilated indicating some obstruction of CSF flow. Multiple areas of injury of differing ages implies multiple episodes of trauma. This is classic for shaken-baby syndrome. On physical examination you might find retinal hemorrhages; rarely, an upper extremity bruise (grip mark) might be found.

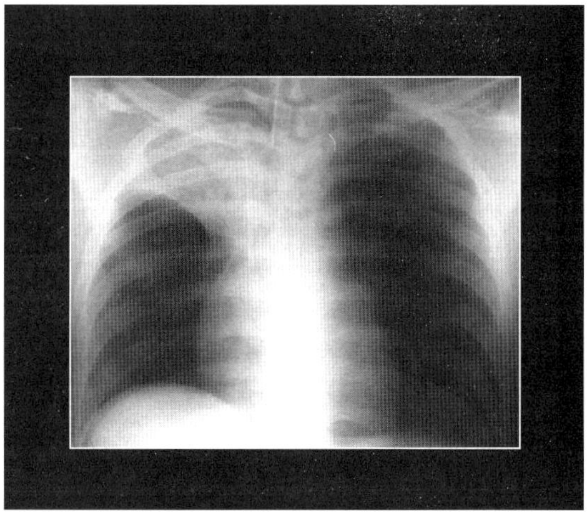

VISUAL PEARL

This adult male patient developed a fever after he was intubated for emergency abdominal surgery. What *tubes* are in place on his chest film? The patient recovered from this problem in a relatively short period of time after specific management. What is your diagnosis based on this information and his chest film?

ANSWER

This patient has a right subclavian line and an endotracheal tube in place. There is loss of volume in the right upper lobe with upward displacement of the minor fissure. The increased density in the right upper lobe in this case is most consistent with simple atelectasis of the right upper lobe. Pulmonary toilet with suctioning of the ET tube and proper ventilation resulted in complete resolution of the problem. One should always consider the possibility of an iatrogenic complication when a patient has had a procedure such as placement of a central catheter or endotracheal intubation.

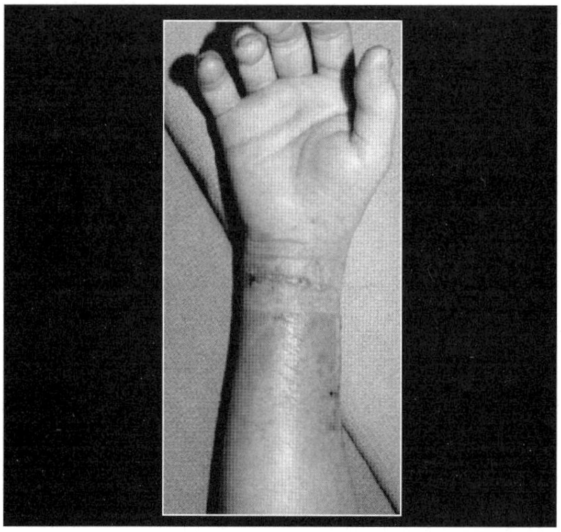

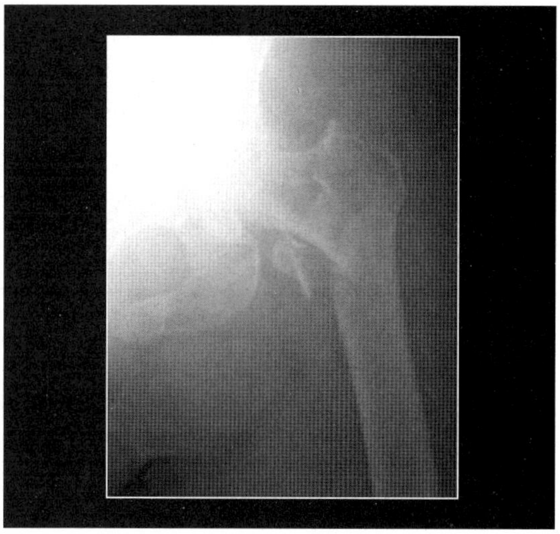

VISUAL PEARL

This child was bitten by a neighbor's dog when she attempted to play with it. The patient complained of forearm pain with passive stretching of the fingers and her active flexor function appeared to be markedly limited because of pain. Erythema and swelling is noted along the forearm. Radiographs did not reveal any foreign body, gas, or fracture. What is your diagnosis? What treatment is indicated?

ANSWER

This child has developed an infection involving the flexor tendon sheaths with suppurative tenosynovitis. She requires intravenous antibiotics, tetanus prophylaxis (depending on her immunization status) and orthopedic consultation for surgical management including debridement and drainage. Infection from a dog bite is typically due to *S. aureus*, Streptococcal species, and/or *Pasteurella multocida*. Gram negatives may also be involved in an infected a dog bite. An inquiry should be made regardings the dog's prior vaccination for rabies.

VISUAL PEARL

An adult male patient presented with this injury after sustaining a fall. Describe the anatomic location of the injury. Is it likely to interrupt the blood supply to the femoral head? How does this compare to an intracapsular fracture of the proximal femur? In the latter circumstance, what is the likely complication?

ANSWER

This film demonstrates a comminuted intertrochanteric fracture of the proximal femur. Intertrochanteric fractures are extracapsular injuries which do not typically disrupt the blood supply to the femoral head, i.e., the circumflex femoral arteries, which are located subcapsularly around the femoral neck. Thus, compared to intracapsular fractures of the proximal femur, they are less likely to cause osteonecrosis of the femoral head. Intracapsular fractures are four basic types and occur at subcapital (the most common), capital (uncommon), basicervical (uncommon) and midcervical (rare) locations.

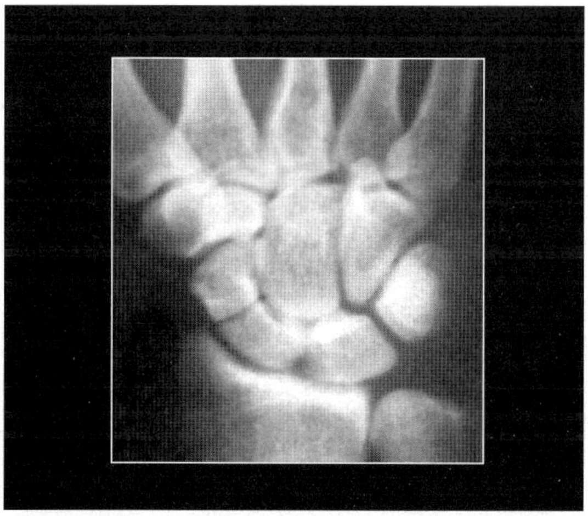

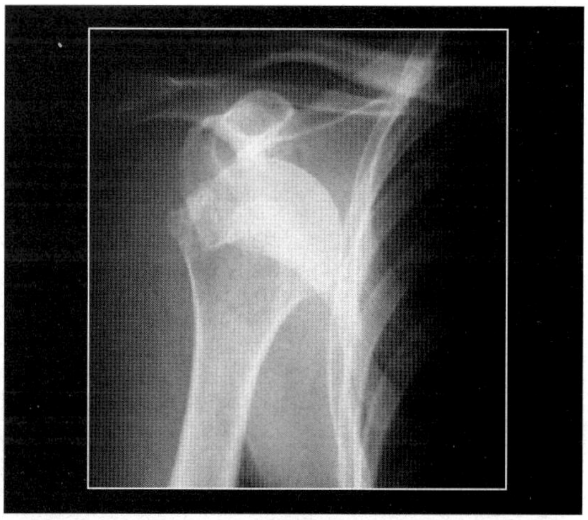

VISUAL PEARL

This 35-year-old female complained of persistent right wrist pain and swelling after falling on her right hand six weeks previously. Describe the finding. How common is this injury? What are the potential posttraumatic complications and their treatment?

ANSWER

This is a dorsovolar view of the wrist with an obvious scaphoid fracture without callus formation. Scaphoid fractures represent slightly more than half of all fractures and dislocations in the wrist. This makes them the most common fracture of the carpus. The two most common complications are nonunion and osteonecrosis. Osteonecrosis is visible on plain film as increased density of the affected fracture fragment. Posttraumatic arthritis may also occur. Nonunion is treated with bone grafting. If this is not successful, the scaphoid may have to be excised and replaced with a prothesis.

VISUAL PEARL

This known alcoholic adult patient was complaining of right shoulder pain after falling off of a bar stool. Witnesses stated that the patient did not lose consciousness or display any obvious seizure activity. What is the diagnosis? What nerve injury may be associated and therefore should be assessed? What clinical finding and films are important in evaluating a patient for a posterior dislocation of the shoulder?

ANSWER

This patient has sustained an *anterior* dislocation of the right glenohumeral joint. You should test the function of *both* the axillary and musculocutaneous nerves. A closed reduction is indicated. *Posterior shouder dislocation* may occur in alcoholic patients with seizures (and in any patient with seizures or severe muscle contractions). In general, a posterior shoulder dislocation is uncommon. It is suspected when there is flattening of the normal anterior shoulder contour. An AP projection may reveal overlap of the huneral head (which is displaced medially and posteriorly) with the glenoid. A compression fracture line may be noted in the humeral head. An axillary projection will usually display a posterior dislocation and any associated humeral head fracture.

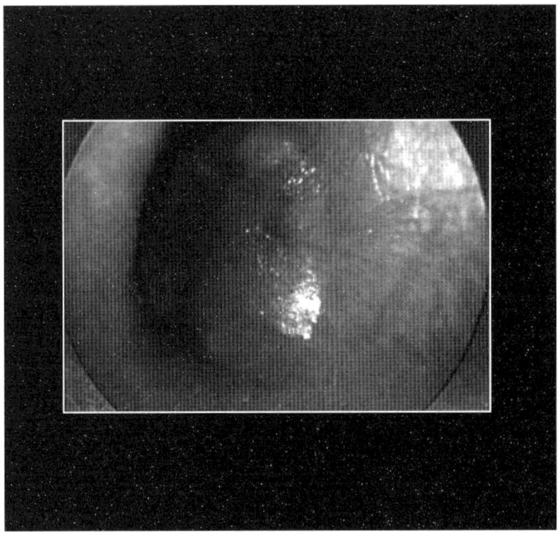

VISUAL PEARL

This 14 month-old male presented with fussiness, apparent otalgia and a temperature of 101.2°F. There is limited movement of the left TM on pneumatic otoscopy; it is grossly injected. This toddler is consolable, alert and taking fluids by mouth in the ED. What is the diagnosis? What are the most common causative organisms?

ANSWER

The diagnosis in this case is just acute otitis media (AOM). The peak incidence is in the 2nd half of the first year of life. *Streptococcus pneumoniae* is the most common bacterial cause of AOM at any age. Other important pathogens include *Hemophilus influenzae* and *Branhamella catarrhalis*. Gram-negative enterics, *Staphylococcus aureus* and Group B Streptococcus are primary pathogens in AOM during the first two weeks of life. *Mycoplasma pneumoniae* is the most common cause of bullous myringitis. Group A strep infections of the middle ear are infrequent.

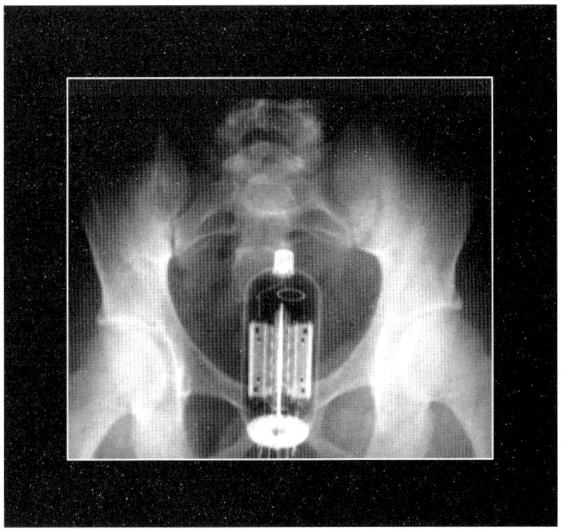

VISUAL PEARL

This adult male was brought to the hospital in a very intoxicated state from ethanol ingestion. He was subsequently admitted because of a persistently altered mental state, hypothemia and concern that he might be septic. An abdominal film was obtained two days after his hospitalization when his condition deteriorated. What happened?

ANSWER

A rectal foreign body has the potential to cause bowel perforation with leakage of bowel contents into the peritoneal cavity and subsequent sepsis. Bowel obstruction is another potential risk. In this case, the initial evaluation did not include a rectal examination; therefore, a foreign body was not suspected. Despite an aggressive fluid resuscitation and appropriate parenteral antibiotics on the second hospital day, the patient expired before any surgical management could be attempted. The point of this film is to remind you that all *sick* patients need a complete physical examination.

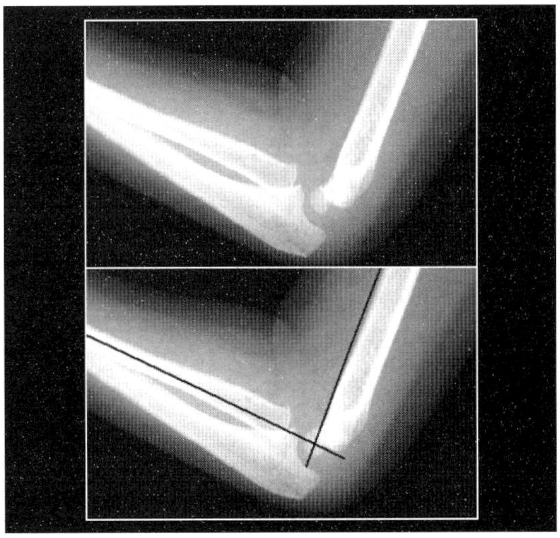

VISUAL PEARL

This four-year-old child complained of elbow pain after falling on her right upper extremity. What can you conclude from this film? The anterior humeral line and long radial axis have been drawn for your examination on a duplicate image below. Do you suspect a supracondylar fracture of the elbow?

ANSWER

This film depicts the normal relationship of the anterior humerus, capitellum, and radius on a lateral view of the elbow. No fracture is evident. The anterior humeral line should bisect the capitellum into two equal parts as it does in this patient. In a supracondylar fracture the capitellum will be displaced posterior to this line. Likewise, a line which defines the long axis of the radius should bisect the capitellum into two equally sized superior and inferior parts. The resulting appearance at the intersection of these two lines which yields 4 equal *capitellar quandrants* is normal.

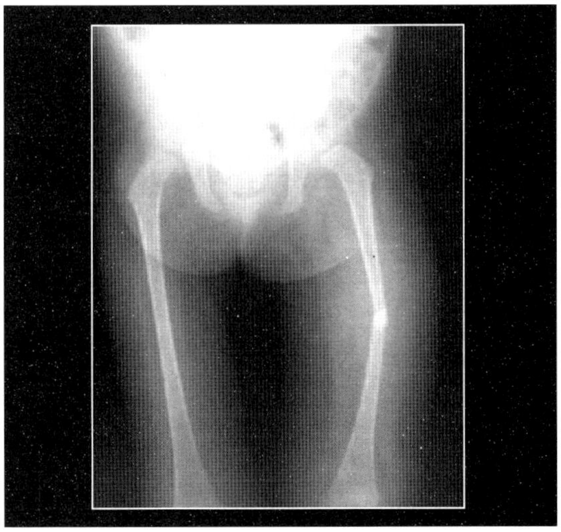

VISUAL PEARL

This toddler was brought to the hospital because he was unable to stand. He was crying persistently. The parents reported that he was falling down at home while learning to walk. They denied that he had fallen from a height or that he had sustained any other injury. What do you see? What do you suspect?

ANSWER

This child has a left femur fracture. The history that his parents provided does not substantiate a mechanism for this particular injury. You should suspect child abuse. The child should be admitted to the hospital for protection as well as for management of his injury. He should receive a complete evaluation looking for other evidence of injury or neglect. No other injuries were found in this child during his hospitalization. However, his body weight was noted to be significantly low for his age (15th percentile) and relative to his birth weight (60th percentile).

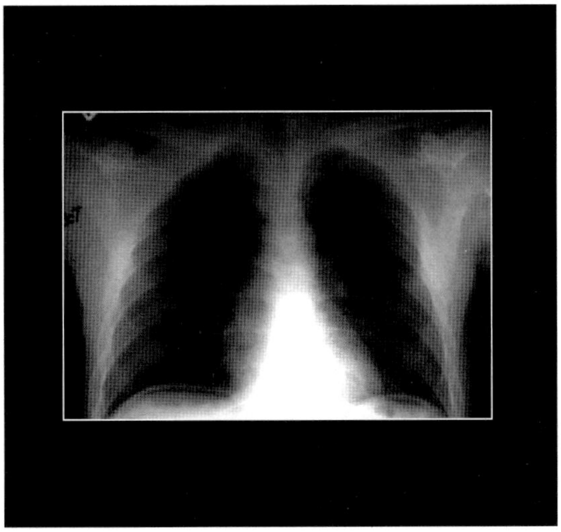

VISUAL PEARL

This 34 year-old male presented with nausea, bilious vomiting and upper abdominal pain. His temperature was 101.4°F on arrival in the ED and he was moderately hypotensive. He also complained of some shortness of breath, but denied chest pain. He admitted to recent heavy alcohol use. A 12-lead ECG revealed sinus tachycardia. What do you suspect?

ANSWER

The possibility of a ruptured esophagus should be considered when any patient presents in distress after an episode of vomiting. However, this chest film reveals free air *under* both leaves of the diaphragm. Thus, this patient must have a ruptured or perforated abdominal viscus. In this case, he had a perforated, benign anterior gastric ulcer and had developed peritoneal signs. The patient had no antecedent history of ulcer disease, but later admitted to frequent use of over-the-counter antacids. He required acute surgical intervention after a fluid resuscitation and intravenous antibiotic administration.

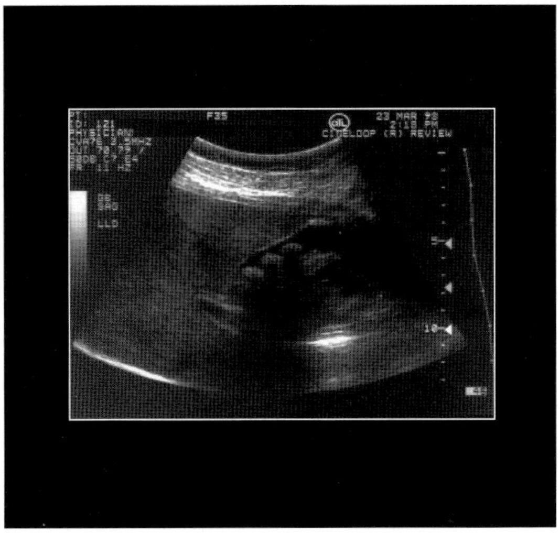

VISUAL PEARL

This obese 36 year-old female was awakened at night with severe RUQ abdominal pain. She was diaphoretic and believed she was having a heart attack. On arrival in the ED she was afebrile, pale and slightly diaphoretic. Her symptoms resolved spontaneously over a few hours. Her cardiac evaluation was unremarkable. This study was performed in the morning. What does it demonstrate?

ANSWER

This patient presented with an acute episode of biliary colic (symptomatic cholelithiasis). Her ultrasound of the gallbladder displays multiple gallstones which were freely floating within the gallbladder. The wall of the gallbladder was normal and no dilated ducts were visualized. Additional laboratory studies were normal except for a mild elevation of her alkaline phosphatase. A serum pregnancy test was negative. The patient had an uneventful recovery after a subsequent endoscopic cholecystectomy.

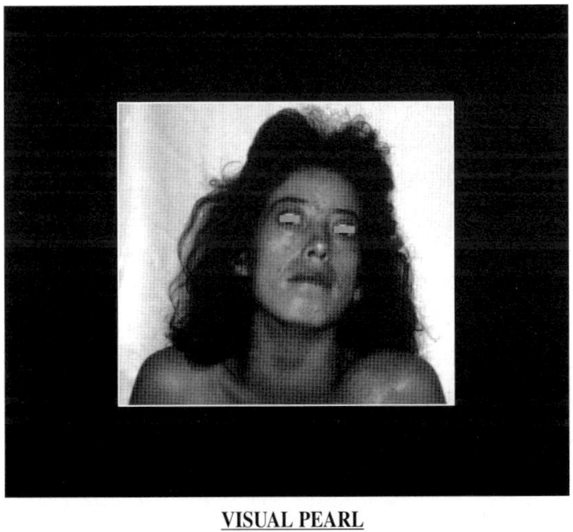

VISUAL PEARL

This woman presents with this appearance to her face. She is unable to speak or close her eyes. She appeared to have involuntary muscle spasms of her neck and was not able to change her posture. A friend reported that the patient might have just taken a "tranquilizer" pill. What is the diagnosis and the initial treatment? Discuss one serious idiosyncratic reaction that has been associated with the use of this type of medication.

ANSWER

This woman is experiencing an acute dystonic reaction. Most likely, she has taken a phenothiazine, e.g., chlorpromazine, or a neuroleptic, e.g., haloperidol. Initial treatment should involve parenteral administration of either 2 mg benztropine or 50 mg diphenhydramine. This problem will likely reoccur even if the patient does not take any more of the "tranquilizer." She should receive oral benztropine for the next several days. A rare but serious form of acute dystonia is laryngeal spasm. This can lead to acute compromise of both the airway and the adequacy of respiration.

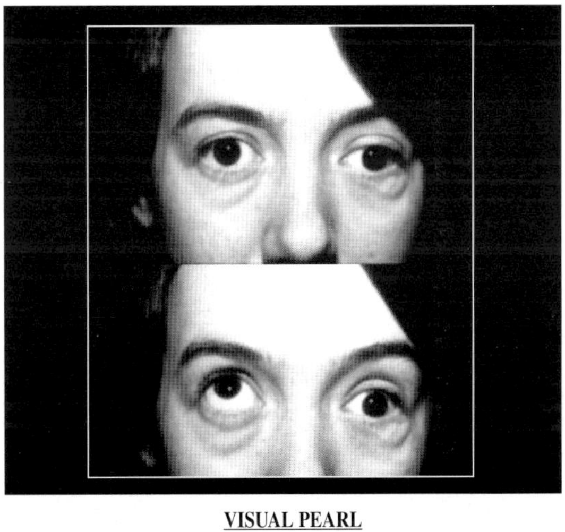

VISUAL PEARL

This woman had previously presented to the ED after being struck in the face with a blunt object. She had a black eye on the left side at that time as well as some facial contusions. There was no apparent injury to the globe. A Waters' (occipitomental) view was suspicious for an injury so she was referred to a specialist for further evaluation. She is complaining of frequent double vision. Based on these two photographs and the historical information, what do you suspect the physician saw on the initial film?

ANSWER

The initial film most likely displayed partial or complete opacification of the left maxillary sinus with or without apparent fracture of the orbital floor. In the upper photo with the patient looking directly foward, the gaze is disconjugate. The location of the corneal light reflex is different in each eye. Some enophthalmos is evident on the left and the left globe appears to be lower than the right. She is unable to elevate her left globe (lower photo) because of entrapment of soft tissues (including the inferior rectus muscle) with herniation into her left maxillary sinus. The patient requires surgical correction of her condition.